EMERGENCY MEDICINE

PEARLS OF WISDOM

Fourth Edition

Scott H. Plantz

Jonathan Adler

Dwight Collman

Copyright © 1997 by Boston Medical Publishing, Incorporated, Boston, MA.

Printed by Mount Auburn Press/IKON Office Solutions, Watertown, MA.

Graphic elements by Dwight Collman. The editors would like to extend thanks to Thomas Habif, M.D. and to to A. Colton, M.D. who each contibuted dermatologic photographs. Figures by Jonathan Adler.

This book was produced using Monaco, New Century Schoolbook, Times, Symbols and Zapf Dingbats fonts and computer based graphics with Macintosh® computers.

ISBN: 1-890369-00-4

9   8   7   6   5   4   3   2   1

In memory of my father, Alan Huntly Plantz, whose love, support and brilliance will always be my guiding light.

Scott

For my Pal, Scott Huntly Plantz, who has more from his father than his name, without whom this book, and other wonderful things in my life, would not be possible.

Jonathan

AUTHORS AND EDITORS, 4TH EDITION

Scott H. Plantz, M.D., FAAEM
Assistant Professor of Emergency Medicine
Chicago Medical School
Associate Chair, Emergency Medical Services
Mt. Sinai Medical Center
Chicago, IL

Jonathan Adler, M.D., FAAEM, FACEP
Associate Program Director
Harvard Affiliated Emergency Medicine
Residency (Massachusetts General Hospital)
Instructor in Medicine,
Harvard Medical School
Boston, MA

Dwight Collman, M.D.
President, The Collman Institute
Boca Raton, FL

CONTRIBUTING AUTHORS AND EDITORS, 4TH EDITION

Bobby Abrams, M.D., FAAEM
Attending Physician
Department of Emergency Medicine
Macomb Hospital

David F.M. Brown, M.D.
Assistant in Emergency Medicine
Massachusetts General Hospital
Instructor in Medicine
Harvard Medical School
Boston, MA

Eduardo Castro, M.D.
Assistant in Emergency Medicine
Massachusetts General Hospital
Instructor in Medicine
Harvard Medical School
Boston, MA

C. James Corrall, M.D., M.P.H.
Adjunct Associate Professor of Pharmacology
Clinical Assistant Professor of Emergency Medicine
Clinical Associate Professor of Pediatrics
University of Illinois College of Medicine
Peoria, IL

Leslie S. Carroll, M.D.
Assistant Professor of Emergency Medicine
Chicago Medical School
Toxicology Director
Mt. Sinai Medical Center
Chicago, IL

Craig Feied, MD, FACEP, FAAEM
Director, National Center for
Emergency Medicine Informatics
Director of Emergency Medicine Informatics,
Washington Hospital Center
Clinical Associate Professor of Emergency Medicine,
George Washington University

Bill Gossman, M.D., FAAEM
Assistant Professor of Emergency Medicine
Chicago Medical School
Mt. Sinai Medical Center
Chicago, IL

James F. Holmes, M.D.
Chief Resident
Division of Emergency Medicine
University of California, Davis
School of Medicine
Sacramento, California

Eddie Hooker, M.D., FAAEM
Assistant Professor
Department of Emergency Medicine
University of Louisville
Louisville, KY

Lance W. Kreplick, M.D., FAAEM
Assistant Professor
University of Illinois
Research Director
Department of Emergency Medicine
EHS Christ Hospital and Medical Center
Oak Lawn, IL

Bernard Lopez, M.D., FAAEM, FACEP
Assistant Professor of Surgery
Thomas Jefferson Medical College
Attending Physician
Department of Emergency Medicine
Thomas Jefferson University Hospital
Philadelphia, PA

Mary Nan S. Mallory, M.D., FAAEM
Instructor
Department of Emergency Medicine
University of Louisville
Louisville, KY

David Morgan, M.D., FAAEM, FACEP
Division of Emergency Medicine
University of Texas Southwestern Medical Center
Parkland Memorial Hospital
Dallas, TX

Edward A. Panacek, M.D., FAAEM
Program Director
Emergency Medicine Residency
Division of Emergency Medicine
Associate Professor of Medicine
University of California, Davis
School of Medicine
Sacramento, CA

Karen Rhodes, M.D.
Department of Emergency Medicine
University of Chicago Medical Center
Chicago, IL

Carlo Rosen, M.D.
Assistant Program Director
Harvard Affiliated Emergency Medicine
Residency (Massachusetts General Hospital)
Instructor in Medicine
Harvard Medical School
Boston, MA

Dana Stearns, M.D.
Assistant in Emergency Medicine
Massachusetts General Hospital
Instructor in Medicine
Harvard Medical School
Boston, MA

Jack "Lester" Stump, M.D., FAAEM
Attending Physician
Department of Emergency Medicine
Rogue Valley Medical Center
Medford, OR

Joan Surdukowski, M.D.
Assistant Professor of Emergency Medicine
Chicago Medical School
Mt. Sinai Medical Center
Chicago, IL

Loice Swischer, M.D., FAAEM
Assistant Professor of Emergency Medicine
Allegheny University of the Health Sciences
Philadelphia, PA

James Unger, M.D., FAAEM
Co-director
Center for Emergency Medicine
Redding Medical Center
Redding, CA

Table of Contents

Introduction

Congratulations! Emergency Medicine *Pearls of Wisdom*, Fourth Edition, will help you learn some emergency medicine. Originally designed as a study aid to improve performance on the EM Written Boards/Recertification or EM Inservice exam, "Pearls" is full of useful information. First intended for EM specialists, we have learned that "Pearls" unique format has also been found to be useful by house officers and medical students rotating in the ED. A few words are appropriate discussing intent, format, limitations and use.

"Pearls" is intended to serve as a study aid to improve performance on the EM Written Boards/Recertification or EM Inservice Exam. To achieve this goal the text is written in rapid-fire question/answer format. Questions receive immediate gratification with a correct answer. Misleading or confusing "foils" are <u>not</u> provided. This eliminates the risk of erroneously assimilating an incorrect piece of information that made a big impression. Questions themselves often contain a pearl intended to be reinforced in association with the question/answer. Additional "hooks" are often attached to the answer in various forms including mnemonics, evoked visual imagery, repetition and humor. Additional information not requested in the question may be included in the answer. Emphasis has been placed on distilling true trivia and key facts that are easily overlooked, are quickly forgotten and that somehow seem to be needed on Board exams.

Many questions have answers without explanations. This enhances ease of reading and rate of learning. Explanations often occur in a later question/answer. Upon reading an answer the reader may think - "Hmm, why is <u>that</u>?!" or, "Are you sure...?!." If this happens to you, GO CHECK! Truly assimilating these disparate facts into a framework of knowledge <u>absolutely requires</u> further reading of the surrounding concepts. Information learned in response to seeking an answer to a particular question is retained much better than that passively observed. Take advantage of this! Use "Pearls" with your preferred source texts handy and open!

The short question/answer format of the First Edition has been retained. The first half of the text is presented in descending order of relative importance on the EM board exam. Information presented is mostly limited to straightforward and more basic facts. The second section of the book consists of random pearls - questions grouped into small clusters by topic presented in no particular order. This section repeats some of the factual information previously covered and builds on this foundation with emphasis on linking information and filling in gaps from the topical chapters.

A significant change in the fourth edition has been the incorporation of questions produced by several new Contributing Editors and Authors. We extend heartfelt thanks on behalf of ourselves and the readers for the contributions of these individuals. The Fourth Edition contains several hundred additional improvements to questions and now contains 2850 questions! The photographs, x-rays and ECGs added by Dr. Dwight Collman further enhance the Fourth Edition.

"Pearls" has limitations. We have found many conflicts between sources of information. Variations between half-life of paralyzing agents and of naloxone, or between rankings of stability of cervical spine fractures, provided in Tintinalli vs. Rosen are concerning. We have tried to verify in other references the most accurate information. Some texts have internal discrepancies further confounding clarification of information.

"Pearls" risks accuracy by aggressively pruning complex concepts down to the simplest kernel - the dynamic knowledge base and clinical practice of emergency medicine is not like that! For the most part, the information taken as "correct" is that indicated in the texts, The Clinical Practice of Emergency Medicine, Second Edition, edited by Harwood-Nuss, Linden, Luten, Shepherd, and Wolfson, and Emergency Medicine A Comprehensive Study Guide, Fourth Edition, edited by Tintinalli, Krome and Ruiz.

Further, new research and practice occasionally deviates from that which likely represents the "right" answer for test purposes. The Fourth Edition updates much information; we hope that the test is similarly keeping up with advancements in knowledge and practice. This text is designed to maximize your score on a test. Refer to your most current sources of information and mentors for direction for practice.

"Pearls" is designed to be used, not just read. It is an *interactive* text. Use a 3x5 card and cover the answers; attempt all questions. A study method we recommend is oral, group study, preferably over an extended meal or pitchers. The mechanics of this method are simple and no one ever appears stupid.

One person holds "Pearls", with answers covered, and reads the question. Each person, including the reader, says "Check!" when he or she has an answer in mind. After everyone has "checked" in, someone states their answer. If this answer is correct, on to the next one, if not, another person says their answer or the answer can be read. Usually the person who "checks" in first gets the first shot at stating the answer. If this person is being a smarty-pants answer-hog, then others can take turns. Try it, its almost fun!

"Pearls" is also designed to be re-used several times to allow, dare we use the word, memorization. Two check boxes are provided for any scheme of keeping track of questions answered correctly or incorrectly.

We welcome your comments, suggestions and criticism. Great effort has been made to verify these questions and answers. Some answers may not be answer you would prefer. Most often this is attributable to variance between original sources (previously discussed). Please make us aware of any errata you find. Thank you to those who have done so; the Fourth Edition is more accurate because of your contributions. We hope to make continuous improvements and would greatly appreciate any input with regard to format, organization, content, presentation, or about specific questions. Leave a message with our managing editor at Boston Medical, Dr. Schlegel, at (Toll Free) 1-888- MBOARDS. We look forward to hearing from you.

Study hard and good luck!

S.H.P. & J.N.A.

CARDIOVASCULAR PEARLS

"Extreme remedies are very appropriate for severe diseases."

Hippocrates

❑❑ What is the most common symptom of aortic dissection?

Interscapular back pain.

❑❑ What is the most common side effect of esmolol, labetalol, and bretylium?

Hypotension.

❑❑ What side effect is expected with too rapid an infusion of procainamide?

Hypotension. Other side effects include: QRS/QT prolongation, V-fib, and torsade de pointe.

❑❑ Adverse drug effects of lidocaine?

Drowsiness, nausea, vertigo, confusion, ataxia, tinnitus, muscle twitching, respiratory depression, and psychosis.

❑❑ What are the three stages of CXR findings in CHF?

1st - PAWP 12-18 mmHg. Blood flow increases in upper lung fields (cephalization of pulmonary vessels).
2nd - PAWP 18 -25 mmHg. Interstitial edema with blurred edges of blood vessels and Kerley B lines.
3rd - PAWP > 25. Fluid exudes into alveoli with generation of the classic butterfly pattern of perihilar infiltrates.

❑❑ Do nitrates affect predominantly preload or afterload?

Mostly preload.

❑❑ Does hydralazine affect preload or afterload?

Afterload.

❑❑ Do prazosin, captopril, and nifedipine affect predominantly preload or afterload?

Afterload.

❑❑ When is dobutamine used in CHF?

Potent inotrope with some vasodilation activity, used when heart failure is not accompanied by severe hypotension.

❑❑ When is dopamine selected in CHF?

Vasoconstrictor and positive inotrope, used if shock is present.

❑❑ Causes of MAT?

COPD is a common cause. CHF, sepsis, and methylxanthine toxicity are other causes, particularly among the elderly. Treat the underlying disorder. Magnesium, verapamil, and ß-adrenergic agents are thought to be helpful.

❏❏ **How is atrial flutter treated?**

Initiate A-V nodal blockade with ß-adrenergic or calcium channel blockers or with digoxin. If necessary, in a stable patient, attempt chemical cardioversion with a class IA agent such as procainamide or quinidine after digitalization. If such treatment fails, or if patient is unstable and requires immediate electrocardioversion, do so with 25-50 J.

❏❏ **What are the causes of atrial fibrillation?**

Hypertension, rheumatic heart disease, pneumonia, thyrotoxicosis and ischemic heart disease are common causes. Pericarditis, EtOH intoxication, PE, CHF and COPD are other causes.

❏❏ **How is atrial fibrillation treated?**

Control rate with ß-blockade or verapamil then convert with procainamide, quinidine, or verapamil. Digoxin may be considered, though its effect will be delayed. Synchronized cardioversion at 100 to 200 J in an unstable patient requiring cardioversion. In a stable patient with a-fib of unclear duration, anticoagulation for 2-3 wk should be considered prior to chemical or electrical cardioversion. Watch for hypotension with administration of negative inotropes.

❏❏ **Causes of SVT?**

Ectopic SVT may be due to digitalis toxicity (25% of digitalis induced arrhythmias), pericarditis, MI, COPD, preexcitation syndromes, mitral valve prolapse, rheumatic heart disease, pneumonia, and EtOH.

▮❏ **How is SVT caused by digitalis toxicity treated?**

Stop digitalis, treat hypokalemia. Give Mg or phenytoin. Provide digoxin specific antibodies in the unstable patient. Avoid cardioversion. *and Calcium*

❏❏ **Treatment of stable SVT not caused by dig toxicity or by WPW syndrome?**

Adenosine, vagal maneuvers, verapamil, ß-blockers, Mg.

❏❏ **Describe the key features of Mobitz I (Wenckebach) 2° AV block.**

Progressive prolongation of the PR interval until atrial impulse is not conducted. If symptomatic, atropine and transcutaneous/transvenous pacing.

❏❏ **Describe the features and treatment of Mobitz II 2° AV block.**

Constant PR interval. One or more beats fail to conduct. Treat with atropine and transcutaneous/transvenous pacing.

❏❏ **What artery is most commonly associated with embolism in mesenteric ischemia?**

Superior mesenteric artery.

❏❏ **Name 5 causes of mesenteric ischemia.**

Arterial thrombosis at sites of atherosclerotic plaques, emboli from left atrium in patients with a-fib or rheumatic heart disease who are not anticoagulated, arterial embolism most commonly to the superior mesenteric artery, insufficient arterial flow, and venous thrombosis.

❑❑ **What is the most common source for acute mesenteric ischemia?**

Arterial embolism 40-50%. Source is usually the heart, most often from a mural thrombus. Most common point of obstruction is the superior mesenteric artery.

❑❑ **What lab abnormalities are expected in a patient with mesenteric ischemia?**

Leukocytosis >15,000, metabolic acidosis, hemoconcentration, and elevation of phosphate and amylase.

❑❑ **For how long do ST and T changes persist after an episode of pain in unstable angina?**

Up to several hours.

❑❑ **What is the cause of Prinzmetal's variant angina?**

Spasm of epicardial coronary arteries.

❑❑ **Contraindications to ß-blockers?**

CHF, variant angina, AV block, COPD, asthma (relative), bradycardia, hypotension and IDDM.

❑❑ **What percentage of LV myocardium must be damaged to cause cardiogenic shock?**

40%. 25% results in heart failure.

❑❑ **What percentage of MI's are clinically unrecognized?**

About 5 - 10%.

❑❑ **What may a new systolic murmur indicate in a patient with an AMI?**

Ventriculoseptal rupture or mitral regurgitation as a result of papillary muscle rupture or dysfunction.

❑❑ **A non-Q-wave infarction is associated with:**

Non-Q-wave infarctions are more commonly associated with subsequent angina or recurrent infarction. They also have a lower in-hospital mortality than Q-wave MIs.

❑❑ **Why do T waves invert in an AMI?**

Infarction or ischemia causes a reversal of the sequence of repolarization (endocardial-to-epicardial as opposed to normal epicardial-to-endocardial).

❑❑ **What ECG changes are seen in a true posterior infarction?**

Large R-wave and ST depression in V1 and V2.

❑❑ **What conduction defects are commonly seen in an AWMI?**

The dangerous kind. Damage to the conducting system results in a Mobitz II 2° or in a 3° AVB.

❑❑ **What conduction defects are commonly seen in an IWMI?**

IWMI affects the autonomic fibers in the atrial septum which increases vagal tone and impairs AV nodal conduction; 1° AV block and Mobitz type I 2° (Wenckebach) AV block are common.

❑❑ **How should PSVT be treated during an AMI?**

Vagal maneuvers, adenosine, or cardioversion. Stable patients may be able to tolerate verapamil or even ß-adrenergic blockers which are negative inotropes.

❑❑ **A patient presents 1 day after discharge for an AMI with a new harsh systolic murmur along the left sternal border and pulmonary edema. Diagnosis?**

Ventricular septal rupture. Diagnosis is confirmed with Swan-Ganz catheterization or echo. Treatment includes nitroprusside for afterload reduction and possible intra-aortic balloon pump followed by surgical repair.

❑❑ **In a patient who has suffered an AMI, when would cardiac rupture be expected?**

50% in the 1st 5 d and 90% within the 1st 14 d post MI.

❑❑ **What type of infarct commonly leads to papillary muscle dysfunction?**

IWMI. Signs and symptoms include a mild transient systolic murmur and pulmonary edema.

❑❑ **A patient presents 2 wk post AMI with chest pain, fever, and pleuropericarditis. A pleural effusion is seen on CXR. Diagnosis?**

Dressler's (postmyocardial infarction) syndrome which is caused by an immunologic reaction to myocardial antigens.

❑❑ **Can patients be retreated with streptokinase or APSAC?**

Antibodies persist for 6 mo. Retreatment is not recommended.

❑❑ **What type of thrombolytic agent is fibrin specific?**

Tissue plasminogen activator. It is a human protein with no antigenic properties.

❑❑ **What maneuvers will increase hypertrophic cardiomyopathy murmurs?**

Valsalva, standing, and amyl nitrate.

❑❑ **What maneuvers will decrease hypertrophic cardiomyopathic murmurs?**

Handgrip, squatting and leg elevation in the supine patient.

❑❑ **What is the most common symptom of acute pericarditis?**

Sharp or stabbing retrosternal or precordial chest pain. Pain increases when supine and decreases when sitting-up and leaning forward. Pain may be increased with movement and deep breaths. Other symptoms include fever, dyspnea described as pain with inspiration, and dysphagia.

❑❑ **What physical findings are associated with acute pericarditis?**

Pericardial friction rub is the most common. Rub is best heard at the left sternal border or apex in a sitting leaning forward position. Other findings include fever and tachycardia.

❑❑ **What ECG changes are seen in acute pericarditis?**

ST segment elevation in the precordial leads, especially V5 and V6 and in lead I. PR depression is seen in leads II, aVF, V4-V6.

❑❑ **What percentage patients with angiogram proven pulmonary embolism have an initial ventilation-perfusion scan reported as low probability?**

12%!

❑❑ **What are the most common symptoms and signs of PE?**

CP (88%).
Tachypnea (92%).
Dyspnea (84%).
Anxiety (59%).
Fever (43%).
Tachycardia (44%).
DVT (32%).
Hypotension (25%).
Syncope (13%).

❏❏ **Can a patient with a PE have a PaO$_2$ greater than 90 mmHg?**

About 5% have a PaO$_2$ > 90 mmHg.

❏❏ **What is the most common CXR finding in PE?**

Elevated dome of one hemidiaphragm as a result of decreased lung volume observed in 50% of PEs. Other common findings include pleural effusions, atelectasis, and pulmonary infiltrates.

❏❏ **What are two relatively specific findings in PE on CXR?**

Hampton's Hump - Area of lung consolidation with a rounded border facing the hilus.
Westermark's sign - Dilated pulmonary outflow tract ipsilateral to the emboli with decreased perfusion distal to the lesion.

❏❏ **What does a normal perfusion scan rule out?**

Rules out a PE. An abnormal scan can be caused by PE, asthma, emphysema, bronchitis, pneumonia, pleural effusion, carcinoma, CHF, and atelectasis.

❏❏ **What does normal ventilation with decreased perfusion suggest?**

PE.

■❏ **What are some of the indications for pulmonary angiography in a patient thought to have a PE?**

1. Patients at high risk for bleeding complications with anticoagulation.
2. Negative test for DVT and low or medium probability lung scans.
3. Unstable patients for whom fibrinolytic therapy is being considered.

❏❏ **What is the most common cause of mitral stenosis?**

Rheumatic heart disease. The most common initial symptom is dyspnea.

❏❏ **What is the earliest chest x-ray finding seen with mitral stenosis?**

Straightening of the left heart border as a result of left atrial enlargement.

❏❏ **What physical findings may be found with mitral stenosis?**

Prominent a-wave, early-systolic left parasternal lift, 1st heart sound is loud and snapping, and early-diastolic opening snap with a low-pitched, mid-diastolic rumble that crescendos into S1.

❏❏ **What are the most common causes of acute mitral regurgitation?**

Rupture of the chordae tendineae, rupture of the papillary muscles, or perforation of the valve leaflets. Common causes include AMI and infectious endocarditis.

❏❏ **What are the two <u>most</u> <u>common</u> causes of valvular aortic stenosis?**

Rheumatic heart disease or congenital bicuspid valve.

❑❑ **What triad of symptoms is characteristic of aortic stenosis?**

Syncope, angina, and left heart failure. As the disease progresses, systolic BP decreases and pulse pressure narrows.

❑❑ **What are the signs and symptoms of <u>acute</u> aortic regurgitation?**

Dyspnea, tachycardia, tachypnea, and chest pain. Causes include: infectious endocarditis, acute rheumatic fever, trauma, spontaneous rupture of valve leaflets, or aortic dissection.

❑❑ **What physical findings are characteristic of <u>chronic</u> aortic regurgitation?**

Bobbing of the head with systole, bounding carotid pulse (water-hammer), pistol shot sound, the to-and-fro murmur of Duroziez's sign over the femoral arteries, and capillary pulsation of the nailbeds (Quincke's sign).

❑❑ **What is the most common cause of tricuspid stenosis?**

Rheumatic heart disease.

❑❑ **A patient presents to the ED one month after placement of a mechanical prosthetic valve with fever, chills, and a leukocytosis. Endocarditis is suspected. What type of bacterium is most common?**

Staph aureus or Staph epidermidis.

❑❑ **Define a hypertensive emergency.**

Increased BP with associated end-organ dysfunction or damage. A controlled drop in BP over one h should be attempted.

❑❑ **Define a hypertensive urgency.**

BP elevated to dangerous level, typically a diastolic greater than 115 mmHg. Gradually reduce BP over 24 to 48 h.

❑❑ **Define uncomplicated hypertension.**

Diastolic BP less than 115 mmHg with no symptoms of end-organ damage. Does not require acute treatment.

❑❑ **What lab findings would suggest a hypertensive emergency?**

UA - RBCs, red cell casts, and proteinuria.
BUN and CR - elevated.
X-ray - Aortic dissection, pulmonary edema, or coarctation of the aorta.
ECG - LVH and cardiac ischemia.

❑❑ **What are the signs and symptoms of hypertensive encephalopathy?**

Nausea, vomiting, headache, lethargy, coma, blindness, nerve palsies, hemiparesis, aphasia, retinal hemorrhage, cotton wool spots, exudates, sausage linking, and papilledema. Treat with labetalol or sodium nitroprusside, lower the mean arterial pressure to approximately 120 mmHg.

❑❑ **In general, how quickly should severe elevations in BP (>210/130) be treated?**

Initial diastolic decrease of 20 - 30% over 30 to 60 min.

❑❑ **At what point does magnesium sulfate become toxic?**

Loss of reflexes occurs at levels >8 mEq/l and respiratory arrest at levels >12 mEq/l.

❑❑ **Can eclampsia occur post-partum?**

YES. Up to 2 weeks.

❑❑ **What two drugs are used to treat eclampsia?**

Magnesium sulfate 4 to 6 g bolus IV followed by a 2 g/h infusion as well as hydralazine 10 to 20 mg IV.
Labetalol may also be used.

❑❑ **What drugs should be used to lower BP in a patient with thoracic aortic dissection?**

Sodium nitroprusside, propranolol, or labetalol.

❑❑ **A patient presents with a history of episodic elevations in BP. She complains of headache, diarrhea, and skin flushing. Diagnosis.**

Pheochromocytoma.

❑❑ **A patient with a psychiatric history taking a MAO inhibitor, has ingested a 12 pack of beer with a meal of pickled herring and a nice aged cheese. He complains of severe headache. On exam, BP is elevated. A diagnosis of acute hypertension is made secondary to hyperstimulation of the adrenergic receptors. Treatment?**

An α- and ß-adrenergic antagonist such as labetalol.

❑❑ **What drug can be used for all hypertensive emergencies?**

Sodium nitroprusside (not DOC for eclampsia). Sodium nitroprusside works through production of cGMP which relaxes smooth muscle. This results in decreased preload and afterload, decreased oxygen demand, slight increased heart rate with no change in myocardial blood flow, cardiac output, or renal blood flow. Duration of action is 1 to 2 min. Sometimes, ß-blockade is required to treat rebound tachycardia.

❑❑ **What is the most common complication of nitroprusside?**

Hypotension. Thiocyanate toxicity with blurred vision, tinnitus, change in mental status, muscle weakness, and seizures is seen more often in patients with renal failure and after prolonged infusions. Cyanide toxicity is uncommon, it may occur with hepatic dysfunction, after prolonged infusions, and in rates greater than 10 µg/kg per minute.

❑❑ **A patient presents with sudden onset chest pain and back pain. Further work-up reveals an ischemic right leg. Diagnosis?**

Suspect an acute aortic dissection when chest or back pain is associated with ischemic or neurologic defects.

❑❑ **What physical findings are suspicious for acute aortic dissection?**

BP differences between arms, cardiac tamponade, and aortic insufficiency murmur.
An abnormal ECG may also be present.

❑❑ **What CXR findings occur with a thoracic aortic aneurysm?**

Change in appearance of aorta, mediastinal widening, hump in the aortic arch, pleural effusion (most common on the left), and extension of the aortic shadow.

❑❑ **How are Stanford type A and B aortic dissections defined and treated?**

Type A - Ascending, proximal to left subclavian (DeBakey I & II) - surgery.
Type B - Descending, distal to left subclavian (DeBakey III) - usually medical treatment.

❑❑ A 74 y old male presents with acute onset testicular pain. Ecchymosis is present in the groin and scrotal sac. Diagnosis?

Ruptured aortic or iliac artery aneurysm.

❑❑ In a patient with an abdominal mass and a suspected ruptured AAA, what x-ray study should be ordered?

None. They should go to the OR ASAP. About 60% of AAA's will have calcification and appear on lateral abdominal x-ray.

❑❑ What percentage of patients beyond the age of 80 experience CP with a AMI?

50% experience CP. 20% experience diaphoresis, stroke, syncope, and/or acute confusion.

❑❑ In a patient with substantial aortic stenosis, what murmur would be expected?

Prolonged, harsh, loud (IV, V, or VI) systolic murmur.

❑❑ What historical findings suggest an embolus vs. a thrombosis in a lower extremity?

Embolus - arrhythmia, valvular disease, MI, no skin changes of chronic arterial insufficiency, and no symptoms in the opposite extremity.
Thrombosis - opposite extremity shows evidence of chronic arterial occlusive disease with history of rest pain claudication, etc.

❑❑ How is thrombus vs. embolus distinguished on arteriogram?

Thrombus - tapering lumen. Embolus - sharp cutoff.

❑❑ What is the risk of PE in a patient with an axillary or subclavian vein thrombus?

The risk of PE is about 15%.

❑❑ Rheumatic heart disease is the <u>most common</u> cause of stenosis of what 3 heart valves?

Mitral, aortic (along with congenital bicuspid valve) and tricuspid.

TRAUMA PEARLS

"The only missing clotting factor is silk."

Donald Trunkey, M.D.

❏❏ **How long does it take to prepare fully crossmatched blood?**

30-60 minutes.

❏❏ **Can tetanus occur after surgical procedures?**

Yes. While most cases of tetanus in the US occur after minor trauma, there have been numerous reports of tetanus following general surgical procedures, especially those involving the GI tract.

❏❏ **How long should an area of abraded skin or a laceration be kept out of the sun?**

For at least 6 months. Abraded skin will develop permanent hyperpigmentation after exposure to the sun.

❏❏ **What is the most sensitive indicator of shock in children?**

Tachycardia.

❏❏ **What is the initial fluid bolus that should be given to children in shock?**

20 ml/ kg.

❏❏ **Do posttraumatic seizures occur more frequently in children or adults?**

Children.

❏❏ **Is the incidence of epidural hematomas and subdural hematomas higher or lower in elderly patients?**

Epidural hematomas are less common and subdural hematomas are more common.

❏❏ **By what time does a subdural hematoma become isodense?**

Between 1-3 wk after the bleed. At that time it may not show up on a CT unless you use contrast.

❏❏ **What spinal level innervates the diaphragm?**

C4.

❏❏ **What percentage of C-spine fractures will be identified on the lateral x-ray?**

90%.

❏❏ **What is the initial treatment of tension pneumothorax?**

Large bore IV catheter placed in the 2nd intercostal space (not a chest tube).

❏❏ **What is the most common source of intrathoracic bleeding?**

Lungs.

❏❏ **What is the most important cause of hypoxia in a patient with flail chest?**

The underlying lung contusion.

❏❏ **What is Hamman's sign?**

Also called Hamman's crunch. Crunching sound over the heart during systole secondary to pneumomediastinum.

❏❏ **What is the most common complaint in a patient with traumatic aortic injury?**

Retrosternal or intrascapular pain.

❏❏ **A radial pulse on exam indicates a BP of at least _____.**

80 mmHg.

❏❏ **A femoral pulse on exam indicates a BP of at least_____.**

70 mm Hg.

❏❏ **A carotid pulse indicates a BP of at least_____.**

60 mm Hg.

❏❏ **What is the most common long bone fractured?**

The tibia.

❏❏ **A trauma patient presents with decreasing level of consciousness and an enlarging right pupil. Diagnosis?**

Probable uncal herniation with oculomotor nerve compression.

❏❏ **The corneal reflex tests?**

Ophthalmic branch (V_1) of the trigeminal (5th) nerve afferent and the facial (7th) nerve efferent.

❏❏ **Name five clinical signs of basilar skull fracture.**

Periorbital ecchymosis (raccoon's eyes), retroauricular ecchymosis (Battle's sign), otorrhea or rhinorrhea, hemotympanum or bloody ear discharge, and 1st, 2nd, 7th, and 8th CN deficits.

❏❏ **A trauma patient presents with anisocoria, neurological deterioration, and/or lateralizing motor findings. Treatment?**

Mannitol 1 g/kg infused rapidly. (Avoid if hypovolemic). Elevate head of bed 30°. Some authors recommend dexamethasone 1 mg/kg, and phenytoin 18 mg/kg at 20 mg/min.

❏❏ **How is posterior column function tested and why is it significant?**

Position and vibration sensation are carried in the posterior columns and are usually spared in anterior cord syndrome. Light touch sensation may also be spared.

Pain and temperature sensation cross near the level of entry and are carried in the more posterior spinothalamic tract.

❏❏ **At what point of airway obstruction will inspiratory stridor become evident?**

70% occlusion.

❏❏ **What is the most common cause of shock in patients with blunt chest trauma?**

Pelvic or extremity fractures.

❏❏ **What nerve should be avoided during pericardiotomy?**

Open the pericardium vertically, anterior (medial) to the phrenic nerve. The nerve runs along the superolateral aspect of the pericardium.

❏❏ **Differential diagnosis of distended neck veins in a trauma patient?**

Tension pneumothorax, pericardial tamponade, air embolism, and cardiac failure. Neck vein distention may not be present until hypovolemia has been treated.

❏❏ **A trauma patient presents with a "rocking-horse" type of ventilation. Diagnosis?**

Probable high spinal cord injury with intercostal muscle paralysis.

❏❏ **What should be checked prior to inserting a chest tube in an intubated patient with respiratory distress and decreased breath sounds on one side?**

Position of the ET tube.

❏❏ **Should a chest tube be placed into a bullet hole apparent in the 4th lateral interspace?**

No. The tube might follow the bullet track into the diaphragm or lung.

❏❏ **A trauma patient presents with subcutaneous emphysema. Diagnosis?**

Pneumothorax or pneumomediastinum; if emphysema is severe, consider a major bronchial injury.

❏❏ **A pneumothorax is suspected but does not show up on PA and Lat CXR. What other x-rays should be considered?**

Expiratory films. A pneumothorax is usually best seen on expiratory films.

❏❏ **What rib fracture has the worst prognosis?**

First rib. First and second rib fractures are associated with bronchial tears, vascular injury, and myocardial contusions.

❏❏ **What cardiovascular injury is commonly associated with sternal fractures?**

Myocardial contusions (blunt myocardial injury).

❏❏ **How much fluid needs to collect in the chest to be seen on decubitus or upright chest x-rays?**

200 to 300 ml; if supine, greater than 1 liter may be necessary to be seen on AP CXR.

■❏ Describe Beck's triad.

Muffled heart tones, hypotension, and distended neck veins. Causes include: myocardial contusion, AMI, pericardial tamponade, and tension pneumothorax. Tamponade may also cause pulsus paradoxus and distention of neck veins during inspiration. Total electrical alternans is highly specific for pericardial tamponade.

❏❏ Which valve is most commonly injured with blunt trauma?

Aortic valve.

❏❏ What is the most likely cause of a new systolic murmur and ECG infarct pattern observed in a patient with chest trauma?

Ventricular septal defect.

❏❏ With a myocardial contusion (blunt myocardial injury), when should the CPK-MB peak?

About 18 to 24 h.

■❏ What is the most accurate plain film x-ray finding indicating traumatic rupture of the aorta?

Deviation of the esophagus > 2 cm right of the spinous process of T4.

Great quotes series:

"Caution: Cape does not enable user to fly."

Batman costume warning label.

❏❏ What is the basic disorder contributing to the pathophysiology of compartment syndrome?

Increased pressure within closed tissue spaces compromising blood flow to muscle & nerve tissue. There are three prerequisites to the development of compartment syndrome:

1) Limiting space.
2) Increased tissue pressure.
3) Decreased tissue perfusion.

❏❏ What are the two basic mechanisms for elevated compartment pressure?

1) External compression -- by burn eschar, circumferential casts, dressings, or pneumatic pressure garments.
2) Volume increase within the compartment -- hemorrhage into the compartment, IV infiltration, or edema due to post-ischemic swelling and that 2° to injury.

❏❏ Which two fractures are most commonly associated with compartment syndrome?

Tibia (resulting most often in anterior compartment involvement) and supracondylar humerus fractures.

❏❏ What are the early general signs & symptoms of compartment syndrome?

Early findings: 1. Tenderness and pain out of proportion to the injury, 2. Pain with active and passive motion, and 3. Hypesthesia (paresthesia) -- abnormal 2-point discrimination. Late findings: 1. Compartment tense, indurated, and erythematous, 2. Slow capillary refill, and 3. Pallor and pulselessness.

What are the four compartments of the leg?

Anterior, lateral, deep posterior, and superficial posterior compartments.

What signs & symptoms would be noted for a compartment syndrome involving the superficial posterior compartment of the leg?

Pain on active and passive foot dorsi-flexion and plantar-flexion and hypesthesia of the lateral aspect of the foot (sural nerve).

What signs & symptoms would be noted for a compartment syndrome involving the deep posterior compartment of the leg?

Pain on foot eversion or toe dorsiflexion and hypesthesia of plantar surface of foot.

What intracompartmental pressure raises concern?

Normal pressure is less than 10 mm Hg. It is generally agreed that > 30 mm Hg mandates emergent fasciotomy. The treatment for compartment pressures between 20 and 30 mm Hg is controversial and may require surgical consultation especially if the patient is unreliable (i. e. with altered level of consciousness).

What are the two major wounding mechanisms of ballistic injuries?

Tissue crush and tissue stretch. Crush creates a permanent cavity; the degree of crush is largely determined by the missile. Stretch is primarily determined by the tissue itself.

What bullet characteristics determine the degree of tissue crushing?

Yaw, deformation, & fragmentation (of missile and bone). These three factors determine the surface area of the missile(s) and subsequent tissue damage.

Why are civilian bullets usually more damaging than military bullets?

Military bullets are usually jacketed and are less prone to fragmentation/"mushrooming" than hollow/soft point civilian bullets.

Which tissues are more prone to significant wounding due to temporary cavitation?

Less elastic tissues such as brain, spleen & liver; fluid-filled organs such as bladder, bowel, and heart; and dense tissue such as bone.

Why do simple through-and-through wounds of the extremities fare well regardless of velocity of bullet?

The short path in the tissue results in:
1) little or no deformation of slower bullets,
2) less time for higher velocity bullet to yaw, thereby resulting in a lesser degree of tissue damage.

Is the heat of firing significant enough to sterilize a bullet and its wound?

No, contaminants from body surface & from viscera can be carried along the bullet's path.

What features of the brain/skull result in higher severity of head wounds?

The brain is highly sensitive to cavitation due to poor elasticity & cohesiveness, enclosure of calvarium contains the cavitation forces.
Also, the brain is really important in most people and causes a lot of problems when it is shot.

❏❏ **What anatomic locations of bullets/pellets are associated with lead intoxication?**

Within bursa, joints, or disc spaces.

❏❏ **Other than lead intoxication, why should intraarticular bullets be removed?**

Potential for lead synovitis leading to severe damage of articular cartilage.

❏❏ **What causes a boutonnière deformity?**

A disruption of the extensor hood at the PIP joint of the finger.

■❏ **Describe a Gamekeeper's thumb.**

Disruption of the ulnar collateral ligament of the MP joint of the thumb (stress testing showing > 20° opening indicates need for surgical repair).

❏❏ **For which condition does Finkelstein's test test?**

Tenosynovitis of the extensor pollicis brevis & abductor pollicis (DeQuervan's stenosing tenosynovitis). To perform the Finkelstein test, the patient places the flexed thumb in the palm of the hand and closes the fist around it. The wrist is then actively deviated to the ulnar side. If this produces pain along the flexor aspect of the thumb, the test is positive.

❏❏ **What is the treatment of a felon?**

10 - 12 with time-off for good behavior.
A felon is a subcutaneous infection of the pulp space of the fingertip, usually S. aureus; treat by incising the pulp space.

❏❏ **What is a paronychia?**

An infection of the lateral nail fold. Usually from S. aureus or Streptococcus. Treat with I&D followed by warm soaks.

❏❏ **Define increased intracranial pressure.**

ICP > than 15 mmHg.

❏❏ **What is the most common site of a basilar skull fracture?**

Petrous portion of the temporal bone.

❏❏ **What is the most common artery involved with an epidural hematoma?**

Meningeal artery, specifically the middle.

❏❏ **Where are epidural hematomas located?**

Between the dura and inner table of the skull.

■❏ **Where are subdural hematomas located?**

Beneath the dura and over the brain and arachnoid. Caused by tears of pial arteries or of bridging veins. Subdurals typically become symptomatic within 24 h to 2 wk after injury.

❑❑ **For a trauma victim, which test is most helpful for evaluating retroperitoneal organs?**

CT.

❑❑ **How should a DPL be performed for a trauma victim with a fractured pelvis?**

Supraumbilical incision to avoid pelvic hematoma.

❑❑ **Absolute contraindication to DPL?**

None.
Relative contraindications: clear indication for laparotomy, previous abdominal surgery and gravid uterus (use open technique).

■❑ **What findings represent a positive DPL in blunt trauma?**

RBC > 100,000 cells/mm^3, WBC > 500 cells/mm^3, bile, bacteria, or vegetable material.

❑❑ **What clues are evident with duodenal injury?**

Increased serum amylase and retroperitoneal free air.

❑❑ **What organ is most frequently injured with blunt trauma?**

Spleen.

❑❑ **What is Kehr's sign?**

Left shoulder pain with splenic rupture.

❑❑ **What type of injury most commonly damages the pancreas?**

Penetrating.

❑❑ **Inability to pass a nasogastric tube in a trauma victim suggests damage to what organ?**

Diaphragm, usually on the left.

❑❑ **What type of contrast medium should be used to evaluate the esophagus if traumatic injury is suspected?**

Gastrografin.

■❑ **Describe the 3 zones of the neck and their evaluation.**

I -   Below the cricoid cartilage - Arteriogram.

II-   Between the cricoid and the mandible - Surgery. "2 surgery!"

III -   Above the angle of the mandible - Arteriogram.

❑❑ **Name the function of, and spinal level innervating, the biceps, triceps, flexor digitorum, interossei, quadriceps, extensor hallucis, biceps femoris, soleus and gastrocnemius, and rectal sphincter.**

Muscle	Action	Spinal Level
Biceps	Forearm flexion	C 5,6
Triceps	Forearm extensors	C7

Flexor digitorum	Finger flexion	C8
Interossei	Finger Add/Abd	T1
Quadriceps	Knee extension	L3,4
Extensor hallucis	Great toe dorsiflexion	L5
Biceps femoris	Knee Flexion	S1
Soleus and gastrocnemius	Foot plantar flexion	S1,2
Rectal sphincter	Sphincter tone	S2-4

What is the dose of methylprednisolone used to treat acute spinal cord injury?

30 mg/kg load over 15 min in the 1st h followed by 5.4 mg/kg per h over the next 23 h.

Sensory innervation to the nipple, umbilicus, and perianal region?

Nipple   - T4
Umbilicus - T10.
Perianal   - S2-4.

What percent of fractures are seen on lateral, odontoid, AP films of the neck?

Lateral 90%
Odontoid 10%.
AP just a few.

On lateral Csp, how much soft tissue prevertebral swelling is normal from C1-4?

Up to 4 mm is normal; >5 mm suggests fracture.

How much anterior subluxation is normal on an adult lateral Csp?

3.5 mm.

How much angulation is normal in an adult lateral Csp, measured across a single interspace?

Up to 10°, greater is abnormal.

On lateral Csp, what does "fanning" of the spinous processes suggest?

Posterior ligamentous disruption.

What are the three most unstable cervical spine injuries?

1 - Transverse atlantal ligament rupture.
2 - Dens fracture.
3 - Burst fracture with posterior ligament disruption.

Describe a Jefferson fracture.

Burst of ring of C1, usually from vertical compression force. Best seen on odontoid view.

Describe a Hangman's fracture.

C2 bilateral pedicle fracture. Usually caused by hyperextension.

What is a clay-shoveler's fracture?

In order of frequency C7, C6, or T1 avulsion fracture of the spinous process. Flexion or direct blow.

❏❏ **Most common thoracolumbar wedge fracture in the elderly?**

L1. Wedge > 50% usually requires admit for pain control and observation for ileus.

❏❏ **Describe the key features of spinal shock.**

Sudden areflexia which is transient and distal which lasts hours to weeks. BP is usually 80 to 100 mmHg with paradoxical bradycardia.

❏❏ **A trauma patient has blood at the urinary meatus. What test should be ordered?**

Retrograde urethrogram. 10 ml of radiocontrast solution is injected into the urinary meatus.

❏❏ **What are the 2 most commonly injured genitourinary organs?**

1. - Kidney.
2. - Bladder (associated with pelvic fracture).

❏❏ **In blunt trauma, what is the most common renal pedicle injury?**

Renal artery thrombosis.

❏❏ **Describe the leg position in a patient with a femoral neck fracture.**

Shortened, abducted, and slightly externally rotated.

❏❏ **Describe the leg position in a patient with an anterior dislocation.**

Hip is abducted and externally rotated. 10% of hip dislocations. Mechanism is forced abduction. If anterior superior, hip is extended. If anterior inferior, hip is flexed.

❏❏ **Describe the leg position in a patient with a posterior hip dislocation.**

Shortened, adducted, and internally rotated. 90% of hip dislocations. Force applied to a flexed knee directed posteriorly. Associated with sciatic nerve injury (10%) and avascular necrosis of the femoral head.

❏❏ **A pneumatic tourniquet can be inflated on an extremity to more than a patient's systolic blood pressure for how long?**

2 h without damage to underlying vessels or nerves.

❏❏ **For how long can wound care be delayed before proliferation of bacteria that may result in infection?**

3 h.

❏❏ **What mechanisms of injury create wounds that are most susceptible to infection?**

Compression or tension injuries. They are 100 times more susceptible to infection.

❏❏ **What are the 3 anatomic subdivisions of the body created by composition of skin microflora?**

Moist areas: axilla & peritoneum - 10^4 to 10^6/cm^2.
Dry areas: trunk, upper arms & legs - 10^1 to 10^3/cm^2.
Exposed areas: head, face, hands, feet - 10^4 to 10^6/cm^2.

❏❏ **What is the dose of bacteria necessary to cause wound infection without a foreign body & with a foreign body?**

Without foreign body - > 10^6 bacteria/gm of tissue.
With foreign body - 100 bacteria.

❏❏ **What 2 factors determine the ultimate appearance of a scar?**

Static & dynamic skin tension on surrounding skin.

❏❏ **What has been proven to decrease the pain of local anesthetic administration?**

Buffering the solution with sodium bicarbonate, decreasing the speed of injection and use of a subdermal injection instead of superficial or intradermal injections.

❏❏ **Why is epinephrine added to local anesthesia?**

To increase the duration of the anesthesia. Epinephrine also causes vasoconstriction & decreased bleeding, which weakens tissue defenses and increases the incidence of wound infection.

❏❏ **Where does one inject local anesthesia for an ulnar nerve block?**

On the anterior wrist, proximal volar skin crease, between the ulnar artery & the flexor carpi ulnaris.

❏❏ **Where does one inject local anesthesia for a median nerve block?**

On the anterior wrist, proximal volar skin crease, between the tendon of the palmaris longus & the flexor carpi radialis.

❏❏ **What nerve block is used for anesthesia of the sole of the foot?**

Tibial nerve block. Tibial nerve block does not provide anesthesia to the lateral aspect of the heel and foot.

❏❏ **What is the preferred route for anesthesia for deep lacerations of the anterior tongue?**

Lingual nerve block.

❏❏ **What local anesthetic, ester or amide, is responsible for most allergic reactions?**

Esters - procaine.

❏❏ **How should hair be removed prior to wound repair?**

By clipping the hair around the wound, not by using razor preparation which increases infection rates.

❏❏ **What are the 4 C's in determining muscle viability?**

Color, Consistency, Contraction, and Circulation.

❏❏ **How long should one wait before delayed primary closure?**

4 d. This will decrease the infection rate and is used for severely contaminated wounds.

❏❏ **Bacterial endocarditis secondary to soft tissue infections may be caused by which two organisms?**

Staphylococcus aureus & Staphylococcus epidermidis.

❏❏ **What factors increase the likelihood of wound infection?**

Dirty or contaminated wounds, stellate or crushing wounds, wounds longer than 5 cm, wounds older than 6 h, and infection prone anatomic sites.

❑❑ **Gabrianna Lucelli, the famous mountain bike racer, presents to your "fast-track" after stepping on a nail that went right through her favorite, oldest pair of tennis shoes. What organism might infect her puncture wound?**

Pseudomonas aeruginosa.

❑❑ **What is the common bacteria seen in cat bite wounds which can also occur with dog bites?**

Pasteurella multocida.

❑❑ **Which has greater resistance to infection, sutures or staples?**

Staples.

❑❑ **What types of wounds result in the majority of tetanus cases?**

Lacerations, punctures, & crush injuries.

❑❑ **Characterize tetanus prone wounds.**

Age of wound:	> 6 h.
Configuration:	Stellate wound.
Depth:	> 1 cm.
Mechanism of injury:	Missile, crush, burn, frostbite.
Signs of infection:	Present.
Devitalized tissue:	Present.
Contaminants:	Present.
Denervated &/or ischemic tissue:	Present.

❑❑ **T/F: It is acceptable to clip or shave an eyebrow if needed to repair the skin.**

False. Eyebrows are valuable landmarks. 15% will not regrow.

❑❑ **When is a scar considered mature so that scar revision can be performed?**

6 - 12 mo.

❑❑ **What is the risk associated with not treating a septal hematoma of the nose?**

Aseptic necrosis, followed by absorption of the septal cartilage resulting in septal perforation.

❑❑ **What are the important structures to be considered when repairing lacerations of the cheek?**

Facial nerve, and parotid duct & gland.

❑❑ **What is the resultant deformity if an auricular hematoma is not properly treated?**

Cauliflower ear.

❑❑ **Describe Tinel's and Phalen's tests.**

Tinel's - Tapping the volar aspect of the wrist over the median nerve produces paresthesias that extend along the index & long finger.
Phalen's - Full flexion at the wrist for one minute leads to paresthesia along distribution of median nerve. Both test for carpal tunnel syndrome.

❑❑ **What are the three most common carpal fractures?**

The scaphoid, dorsal chip (triquetrum), and the lunate. All may be 2° falls on an outstretched hand. Radiographs may initially be normal. The scaphoid is the most common.

❑❑ **What is Kienbock's disease?**

Avascular necrosis of the lunate with collapse of the lunate secondary to fracture. As with a navicular (scaphoid) fracture, initial wrist x-rays may not demonstrate the fracture. Therefore, tenderness over the lunate warrants immobilization.

❑❑ **A stress fracture is suspected of the 2nd or 3rd metatarsal, but none is found on initial x-rays. How long before a 2nd set of x-rays will likely be positive?**

14-21 d.

❑❑ **The three steps of bone healing after a fracture are:**

Union - consolidation - remodeling.

❑❑ **How long after a fracture does callus start to form?**

5 - 7 d.

❑❑ **The most common Salter-Harris class fracture?**

Type II. A triangular fracture involving the metaphysis and an epiphyseal separation.

■❑ **What tarsal bone is most commonly fractured?**

Calcaneus (60%). Calcaneal fractures are commonly associated with lumbar compression injuries (10%).

❑❑ **The tarsal-metatarsal joint is also called:**

Lisfranc's joint.

❑❑ **The second metatarsal is the locking mechanism of the mid-part of the foot. A fracture at the base of the second metatarsal should raise suspicion of:**

A disrupted joint - treatment may require ORIF.

❑❑ **What is a ballet fracture?**

An avulsion fracture at the base of the 5th metatarsal usually secondary to plantar flexion and inversion. Also called a Jones fracture. It is the most common metatarsal fracture.

❑❑ **What is the 2nd most common tarsal fracture?**

Talus.

❑❑ **What is the most common metatarsal fracture?**

5th.

❑❑ **What is the most common foot fracture?**

Calcaneus.

■❑ **Which patellar fracture requires orthopedic consultation?**

Displaced transverse fracture, comminuted fractures, and open fractures.

❏❏ **What is the most common mechanism for fractures of the femoral condyles?**

Direct trauma, fall or blow to the distal femur.

❏❏ **Of tibial plateau fractures, where is the most common site?**

Lateral, more common in the older population, usually presenting with swollen painful knee and limited range of motion.

❏❏ **With complete rupture of medial or collateral ligaments, how much laxity is expected on exam?**

>1 cm without endpoint as compared to uninjured knee.

❏❏ **What is the most common ligamentous injury to the knee?**

Anterior cruciate ligament, usually from non-contact injury.

❏❏ **Why 'tap' a knee with an acute hemarthrosis?**

Relieve pressure and pain and see if fat globules are present indicating a fracture.

❏❏ **How would you 'un-lock' a 'locked' knee?**

Hang leg over table at 90 degree flexion, allow relaxation and apply longitudinal traction with internal and external rotation.

❏❏ **Where is the most common site of compartment syndrome?**

Anterior compartment of the leg - contains tibialis anterioris, extensor digitorum longus, extensor hallucis longus, and peroneus muscles, as well as anterior tibial artery and deep peroneal nerve.

❏❏ **Who gets Achilles' tendon rupture?**

Middle aged men most commonly on the left side.

❏❏ **Where is the most common site for a palpable defect of Achilles' tendon?**

2 - 6 cm proximal to its insertion.

❏❏ **What are the most common lower extremity injuries to bone in children?**

Tibial and fibular shaft fractures, usually secondary to twist forces.

❏❏ **What radiograph would one order with suspected patellar fracture in a child?**

Standard radiographs including patellar or "sunrise" views, plus comparison radiographs of uninvolved knee.

❏❏ **What are the differences between Osgood-Schlatter disease and avulsion of tibial tubercle?**

Both occur at tibial tubercle, avulsion presents with acute inability to walk, lateral view of the knee is most diagnostic, treatment is surgical.
Osgood-Schlatter's has vague history of intermittent pain, is bilateral in 25% of cases, has pain with range of motion but not with rest; treatment is symptomatic and not surgical.

❏❏ **What is a toddler fracture?**

Common cause of limp or refusal to walk in this age group is a spiral fracture of the tibia without fibular involvement.

❏❏ **What is the most common cause of a painful hip joint in infants?**

Septic arthritis. Staphylococcus is the most common cause in infancy. Hip usually abducted, flexed, and externally rotated.

❏❏ **Most common cause of painful hip in older children?**

Transient synovitis. It can be difficult to distinguish from septic arthritis.

■❏ **8 y old male presents with a limp. On exam, hip range of motion is decreased. What rare disease should be considered?**

Children 5 - 9 y may get idiopathic avascular necrosis of the femoral heal (Legg-Calvé-Perthes Disease).

■❏ **Describe a common patient with a slipped capital femoral epiphysis.**

Obese boy, age 10 to 16 y. Groin or knee discomfort increases with activity; may have a limp. Often bilateral. The slip is best seen on a lateral view.

❏❏ **What is the most important complication of a proximal tibial metaphyseal fracture?**

Arterial involvement, especially when there is a valgus deformity.

❏❏ **What is the most common ankle injury?**

75% of ankle injuries are sprains with 90% of these involving the lateral complex.
90% of lateral ligament injuries are anterior talofibular.

❏❏ **What is the most helpful physical exam test for anterior talofibular ligament injury?**

Anterior drawer test, >3 mm of excursion might be significant (compare sides), >1 cm is always significant.

❏❏ **How are sprains classified?**

1st° - stretching of ligament, normal x-ray.
2nd° - severe stretching with partial tear, marked tenderness, swelling, pain, normal x-ray (now stressed).
3rd° - complete ligament rupture, marked tenderness, swelling and obviously deformed joint. X-ray may show an abnormal joint.

❏❏ **What is unique about avulsion fractures at the base of the fifth metatarsal?**

It is one of the most commonly missed fractures, history is of ankle injury from plantar flexion and inversion.

❏❏ **A 21 y old female complains of pain and 'clicking' sound located at the posterior lateral malleolus. You sense a 'fullness' beneath the lateral malleolus. Dx?**

Peroneal tendon subluxation, with associated tenosynovitis.

❏❏ **What percentage of distal tibial (medial malleolus) fractures treated closed result in non-union?**

10 - 15%.

❏❏ **Traumatic arthritis occurs in what percentage of ankle fractures?**

20 - 40%.

❏❏ **Which bone is most commonly fractured at birth?**

The clavicle.

❑❑ **Most common shoulder dislocation?**

Anterior (95%).

❑❑ **A patient cannot actively abduct her shoulder. What injury does this suggest?**

Rotator cuff tear. The cuff is comprised of the supraspinatus, infraspinatus, subscapularis, and the teres minor muscles and tendons.

❑❑ **Why is the displaced supracondylar fracture (of distal humerus) in a child considered a true emergency?**

The injury often results in injury to brachial artery or median nerve. It can also cause compartment syndrome.

❑❑ **What is the significance of the fat pad sign with an elbow injury?**

Fat pad sign or radiolucency just anterior to the distal humerus is indicative of effusion or hemarthrosis of the elbow joint; this suggests an occult fracture of the radial head.

❑❑ **What signs and symptoms would be noted for a compartment syndrome involving the anterior compartment of the leg?**

Pain on active and passive dorsi-flexion and plantar-flexion of the foot and hypesthesia of the first web space of the foot.

❑❑ **How is a scaphoid fracture diagnosed?**

Frequently, the initial radiograph will appear normal. Therefore if the patient has tenderness in the anatomical snuff box, a scaphoid (navicular) fracture is presumed and the hand splinted. A follow-up radiograph 10-14 d following the injury may then reveal the fracture.

❑❑ **What is the common feared complication of a scaphoid fracture?**

Avascular necrosis. The more proximal the fracture, the more common is avascular necrosis.

❑❑ **What type of Salter (Salter-Harris) fracture have the worst prognosis?**

Type V--compression injury of the epiphyseal plate.

❑❑ **What metatarsal fracture is highly associated with a disrupted tarsal-metatarsal joint?**

Fracture to the base of the 2nd metatarsal. Treatment may require open reduction and internal fixation.

❑❑ **Which is the more sensitive test used to determine an anterior cruciate ligament tear in the knee: the anterior drawer test or the Lachman test?**

Lachman test. While the knee is held at 20 degrees flexion and the distal femur is stabilized, the lower leg is pulled forward. Greater than 5 mm anterior laxity compared to the other knee is evidence of an anterior cruciate ligament tear.

❑❑ **What fracture is frequently missed when the patient complains of an ankle injury?**

Fracture at the base of the fifth metatarsal. Caused by plantar flexion and inversion. Radiographs of the ankle may not include the fifth metatarsal.

❑❑ **What is the Young classification system for pelvic fractures?**

The Young system divides pelvic fractures into 4 categories depending on the type and direction of force.
    (1) Lateral Compression (LC)
    (2) Anterior-Posterior Compression (APC)
    (3) Vertical Sheer (VS)
    (4) Combination Mechanical-mixed (CM)

❑❑ **Describe a lateral compression pelvis fracture (LC).**

Most common (50%). Usually caused by a motor vehicle collision in which the car and patient are broadsided. The lateral force causes: (1) a sacral fracture, iliac wing fracture, or a sacral-iliac ligamentous injury and (2) a transverse fracture of the pubic rami. There is no ligamentous injury at the pubic symphysis.

❑❑ **Describe an anterior-posterior compression pelvic fracture (APC).**

About 20% of pelvic fractures. Usually caused by a head-on motor vehicle collision. These always have (1) a disruption of the pubis symphysis and (2) usually have a disruption (of different degrees) of the sacral-iliac joint.

❑❑ **Describe a vertical sheer pelvic fracture (VS).**

About 6% of pelvic fractures. Usually caused by a fall from a height. These have (1) an injury of the sacral-iliac ligaments and (2) either a disruption of the pubis symphysis or vertical fractures through the pubic rami. The iliac wing is vertically displaced.

❑❑ **What life-threatening injury is associated with pelvic fractures?**

Severe hemorrhage, usually retroperitoneal. Up to 6 liters of blood can be accommodated in this space.

■❑ **Which pelvic fracture is most likely to have severe hemorrhage?**

Vertical sheer fractures (75%).

■❑ **Which pelvic fracture is most likely to have bladder rupture?**

Lateral compression fractures, Type III (20%).

■❑ **Which pelvic fracture is most likely to have urethral injury?**

Anterior-posterior compression fracture, Type III (36%).

❑❑ **Describe the leg position in a patient with an intertrochanteric hip fracture.**

Shortened, markedly externally rotated, and abducted.

❑❑ **Which fracture is associated with avascular necrosis of the femoral head?**

Femoral neck fractures. Avascular necrosis occurs with 15% of non-displaced femoral neck fractures and with near 90% of displaced femoral neck fractures.

❑❑ **What is a stress fracture?**

A stress or "fatigue" fracture occurs from repetitive small forces usually involving the metatarsal shafts, the distal tibia, and the femoral neck. These fractures may not be seen on initial radiographs.

❏❏ **What is "nursemaid's elbow"?**

Subluxation of the radial head. During forceful retraction, some fibers of the annular ligament that encircle the radial neck become trapped between the radial head and the capitellum. On presentation, the arm is held in slight flexion and pronation.

❏❏ **Describe the leg position associated with an anterior inferior hip dislocation.**

Hip is flexed, externally rotated, and abducted.

EENT PEARLS

"I have never let my schooling interfere with my education."

Mark Twain

❏❏ **What is the most common cause of odontogenic pain?**

Carious tooth. The offending tooth when percussed with a tongue blade will produce a sharp pain. The pain may be felt in the ear, throat, eyes, temple and other side of the jaw.

❏❏ **A child presents after falling and knocking out his front tooth. How would the management differ if the child was 3 versus 13?**

With primary teeth no reimplantation should be attempted because of the risk of ankylosis or fusion to the bone. However, with permanent teeth reimplantation should occur as soon as possible. Remaining periodontal fibers are a key to success. Thus, the tooth should not be wiped dry as this may disrupt the periodontal ligament fibers still attached.

❏❏ **A 20 year old presents with both his upper central incisors in hand after an altercation. How can you tell which is the right tooth and which is left?**

When looking at the facial (anterior) surface of the tooth, the sharper angle faces midline. So when replacing the teeth, the two sharp angles should be midline.

❏❏ **What is the best transport medium for an avulsed tooth?**

Hank's solution, a pH balanced cell culture medium, which can even help restore cell viability if the tooth has been avulsed for more than 30 min. Milk is an alternative or the patient, if able to keep from aspiration, may place the tooth underneath their tongue.

❏❏ **A patient accidentally swallowed his crown while eating. He cannot afford another crown and wants to know if this one could be used again once it passes?**

Yes. It can be sterilized and replaced.

❏❏ **A patient complains of a tongue irritation from a slightly chipped tooth after a fall. No dentin is exposed. What treatment can be offered to this patient?**

Tooth fractures only involving the enamel are called Ellis Class I fracture. The sharp edges can be filed with an emery board for immediate relief and the patient can be referred to a dentist for cosmetic repair.

❏❏ **How can one differentiate a Ellis Class II and III fracture?**

Class II fractures involve the dentin and enamel. The exposed dentin will be pinkish.
Class III fractures involve enamel, dentin and the pulp. A drop of blood is frequently noted in the center of the pink dentin.

❏❏ **Why should topical analgesics not be used in Ellis Class III tooth fractures?**

Severe tissue irritation or sterile abscesses may occur with their use. Treatment includes application of tinfoil, analgesics and immediate dental referral.

❑❑ **A patient presents 3 d after tooth extraction with severe pain and a foul mouth odor and taste. Diagnosis and treatment?**

Alveolar osteitis (dry socket) results from loss of the blood clot and local osteomyelitis. Treat by irrigation of the socket and application of a medicated dental packing or iodoform gauze moistened with Campho-Phenique or eugenol.

❑❑ **A patient presents with gingival pain and a foul mouth odor and taste. On exam, fever and lymphadenopathy are present. The gingiva is bright red and the papillae are ulcerated and covered with a gray membrane. Diagnosis and treatment?**

Acute necrotizing ulcerative gingivitis. Antibiotics (tetracycline or penicillin) and topical anesthetic. A possible complication of this disease is destruction of alveolar bone.

❑❑ **What is the most common oral manifestation of AIDS?**

Oropharyngeal thrush. Some other AIDS-related oropharyngeal diseases are Kaposi's sarcoma, hairy leukoplakia, and non-Hodgkin's lymphoma.

❑❑ **A 47 year old female present to the ED with a complaint of excruciating waxing and waning "electric shock type" pain in the right cheek. Diagnosis and treatment?**

Tic douloureux. The most significant finding is that the pain follows the distribution of the trigeminal nerve. Often minor trigger zone stimulation can consistently reproduce the pain. Carbamazepine (100 mg bid starting dose and increasing to 1200 mg daily if needed). Referral to a neurologist and a dentist to rule out cerebellopontine angle tumors, MS, nasopharyngeal carcinoma, cluster headaches, polymyalgia rheumatica, temporal arteritis and oral pathology.

❑❑ **A three year old child presents with a unilateral purulent rhinorrhea. Most likely diagnosis?**

Nasal foreign body.

❑❑ **What potential complications of nasal fractures should always be considered on physical examination?**

Septal hematoma and cribriform plate fractures. A septal hematoma appears as a bluish mass on the nasal septum and if not drained aseptic necrosis of the septal cartilage and septal abnormalities may occur. A cribriform plate fracture should be considered in a patient who has a clear rhinorrhea after trauma.

❑❑ **What physical exam findings would make posterior epistaxis more likely than anterior epistaxis?**

a) Inability to see the site of bleeding. Anterior nosebleeds usually originate at Kiesselbach's plexus, an area easily visualized on the nasal septum.
b) Blood from both sides of the nose. In a posterior nosebleed the blood can more easily pass to the other side because of the proximity of the choanae.
c) Blood trickling down the oropharynx.
d) Inability to control bleeding by direct pressure.

❑❑ **What is the most common site of bleeding in posterior nosebleeds?**

The sphenopalatine artery's lateral nasal branch.

❑❑ **A patient returns to the emergency department with fever, nausea, vomiting and hypotension two d after having nasal packing was placed for an anterior nosebleed . What potential complication of nasal packing should be considered?**

Toxic shock syndrome.

❏❏ A child with a sinus infection presents with proptosis, a red swollen eyelid and a inferolaterally displaced globe. Diagnosis?

Orbital cellulitis and abscess associated with ethmoid sinusitis.

❏❏ A patient with a frontal sinusitis presents with a large forehead abscess. Diagnosis?

Pott's puffy tumor. This is a complication of frontal sinusitis where the anterior table of the skull is destroyed allowing the formation of the abscess.

❏❏ An ill-appearing patient presents with a fever of 103 °F, bilateral chemosis, 3rd nerve palsies, and untreated sinusitis. Diagnosis?

Cavernous sinus thrombosis. This life-threatening complication occurs from direct extension through the valveless veins. Complication of sinusitis may be local (osteomyelitis), orbital (cellulitis), or within the central nervous system (meningitis or brain abscess).

❏❏ Retropharyngeal abscess is most common in what age group? Why?

Six months to three years. This is because the retropharyngeal lymph nodes regress in size after the age of three.

❏❏ How do patients with retropharyngeal abscesses appear?

These children are often ill appearing, febrile, stridorous, drooling and in an opisthotonic position These children may complain of difficulty swallowing or may refuse to feed.

❏❏ What radiographic sign can be used to make the diagnosis of a retropharyngeal abscess?

A widening of the retropharyngeal space (normal 3-4 mm or less than half the width of the vertebral bodies). False widening may occur if the x-ray is not done during inspiration with the patient's neck extended. (Occasionally, an air fluid level may be noted in the retropharyngeal space.)

❏❏ What is the most common organism to cause a retropharyngeal abscess?

ß-hemolytic streptococcus.

❏❏ A 48 year old male presents with a high fever, trismus, dysphagia, and swelling inferior to the mandible in the lateral neck. Diagnosis?

Parapharyngeal abscess.

❏❏ Peritonsillar abscesses are <u>most common</u> in what age group?

Adolescents and young adults. Symptoms may include ear pain, trismus, drooling and alteration of the voice.

❏❏ What is the <u>most common</u> origin of Ludwig's angina?

Lower 2nd and 3rd molar. It is a swelling in the region of the submandibular, sublingual and submental spaces. This soft tissue swelling may cause displacement of the tongue upward and posteriorly. The most common organisms are hemolytic Streptococci, Staphylococcus, and mixed anaerobe and aerobes.

❏❏ Why is needle aspiration preferred over incision and drainage for a fluctuant acute cervical lymphadenitis?

Development of a fistula tract is possible if the patient has atypical mycobacterium or cat scratch fever rather than a bacterial lymphadenitis.

❑❑ **Can a patient lose more of the upper lip or the lower lip without cosmetic problems?**

Up to 1/3 of the lower lip can be avulsed or débrided and the patient still may have an acceptable cosmetic appearance. The upper lip is less forgiving due to the relationship with the columella, alar bases and philtrum.

▮❑ **What are the signs and symptoms of a mandibular fracture?**

Malocculsion, pain, opening deviation or abnormal movement, decreased range of motion, bony deformity, swelling, ecchymosis, and lower lip (mental nerve) anesthesia.

❑❑ **What is the most common type of mandible fracture?**

Alveolar. Most commonly the incisors.

❑❑ **Bilateral mental fractures may cause what acute complication?**

The tongue may cause acute airway obstruction because of loss of anterior support.

❑❑ **A patient was yawning and now is unable to close his mouth. He is having difficulty talking and swallowing. Diagnosis ?**

Bilateral dislocation of the mandibular condyles. This can occur when the mouth is opened excessively wide as in yawning, laughing, over stretching the mouth during general anesthesia and hysteria. X-rays can rule out bilateral condyle fractures which may have a similar clinical appearance.

❑❑ **A 42 year old female presents with dull right ear and jaw pain and a burning sensation in the roof of her mouth. The pain is worse in the evening. She also hears a "popping" sound when she opens and closes her mouth. Exam reveals tenderness of the joint capsule. Diagnosis and treatment?**

TMJ syndrome. Treat with physiotherapy, analgesia, soft diet, muscle relaxants and occlusive therapy. Apply warm moist compresses 4 to 5 times daily for 15 min for 7 to 10 d.

❑❑ **When there is internal derangement of the TMJ due to meniscal displacement, in which direction is the meniscus displaced?**

Anteromedially which may cause the joint to lock in a closed position. The jaw may deviate towards the affected side. The articular disc may become displaced due to tears, perforation or stretching of the posterior ligamentous attachments.

❑❑ **What is the best radiographic view to visualize a zygomatic arch fracture?**

Modified basal view of the skull (also known as jug-handle, submentaloccipital or submental-vertical views).

❑❑ **Signs and symptoms of fracture of the zygomaticomaxillary complex?**

Subcutaneous emphysema, edema, ecchymosis, facial flattening, subconjunctival hemorrhage, ecchymosis around the orbit, unilateral epistaxis, anesthesia of the cheek upper lip and gum from infraorbital nerve injury, step deformity, decreased mandibular movement and diplopia.

▮❑ **What are the two most common findings with an orbital floor fracture?**

Diplopia and globe lowering.

❑❑ **What radiographic finding might be seen with an orbital blowout fracture?**

a) fracture lines or bony fragments in the maxillary sinus.
b) subcutaneous or orbital emphysema.
c) air-fluid level in the maxillary sinus.
d) a "teardrop" sign where a soft tissue mass may protrude into the maxillary sinus.

❏❏ **Define a Le Fort I fracture.**

Fracture line runs from the nasal opening along the wall of the maxillary sinuses bilaterally, across the pterygomaxillary tissue to the lateral pterygoid plates (also called a horizontal maxillary fracture.) X-rays often miss this fracture. Mobility of the maxilla without movement at the nasal bridge or zygoma is noted on physical examination.

❏❏ **Describe a Le Fort II fracture.**

Fracture involves facial aspects of the maxillae extending to the nasal and ethmoid bones. The fracture also involves the maxillary sinuses and infraorbital rims bilaterally and cross the nasal bridge. This is also called a pyramidal fracture. Swelling of the nose, lips and midface may be noted. Subconjunctival hemorrhage may present with blood in the nares. Suspect cerebrospinal involvement and check for CSF rhinorrhea. Diagnosis can be made clinically by crepitation or movement at the nasal bridge when the maxilla is moved.

❏❏ **Describe a Le Fort III fracture.**

The fracture line runs through the frontozygomatic suture lines bilaterally extending through the orbits, the base of the nose and the ethmoid region. Movement of the zygoma and midface is suggestive. This is also called a "Dishface" fracture or complete craniofacial dysjunction.

❏❏ **In which Le Fort fracture is CSF rhinorrhea most common?**

III.

❏❏ **What plain radiographic views are most helpful in visualizing facial fractures?**

a) Water's view. This will show the frontozygomatic area, the infraorbital area and the lateral walls of the maxillary sinus and is particularly helpful in evaluating for zygomaticomaxillary complex, orbital blowout, and Le Fort type fractures.
b) Modified basal view of the skull. Useful for zygomatic arch fractures.
c) Panorex. This is the best view for mandibular fractures as the three view mandible series (PA and bilateral obliques) have superimposition of bone.

❏❏ **What three clinical signs would cause a physician to consider disruption of the medial canthal ligaments with nasal skeletal fracture?**

Widened nasal bridge, increased intercanthal distance (normal is approximately 35 mm) and almond-shaped palpebral fissures.

❏❏ **A 48 y old diabetic male presents with pain, itching and discharge from the right ear. The tympanic membrane is intact. Diagnosis?**

Otitis externa. Treat by suctioning ear and one week of antibiotic steroid otic solution. An ear wick may improve delivery of the antibiotic. Suspect malignant otitis externa in the diabetic patient.

■❏ **A patient presents with ear pain and fluid-filled blisters on the tympanic membrane. Diagnosis?**

Bullous myringitis, commonly caused by Mycoplasma or viruses. Treat with erythromycin.

❏❏ **A 16 y old boxer presents with right ear pain and swelling after receiving a blow to the ear. Treatment?**

The ear should be aseptically drained by incision or aspiration and a mastoid conforming dressing should be applied. ENT follow-up is mandatory. If the ear is not treated appropriately a cauliflower deformity may result.

A patient presents with a swollen, tender, red left auricle. Diagnosis?

Perichondritis caused by Pseudomonas.

What is the most frequent cause of hearing loss?

Cerumen impaction.

What would the physical finding be in unilateral sensory hearing loss?

The patient will lateralize, have air conduction greater than bone conduction (i.e. normal Rinne test) indicating no conductive loss. The Weber test will lateralize to the normal ear. The most common cause of this is viral neuronitis.

If a patient has bilateral sensory hearing loss what causes should be suspected?

Noise or ototoxins such as certain antibiotics, loop diuretics, antineoplastics as well as others.

What is the most common neuropathy associated with acoustic neuroma?

Due to trigeminal nucleus involvement the corneal reflex may be lost.

Name some causes of tympanic membrane perforation.

Blast injuries (water or air), foreign bodies in the ear (particularly Q-tips), lightning strikes, otitis media, associated temporal bone fractures.

A young male was involved in a bar room brawl complains of ear pain, significantly decreased hearing and vertigo. A tympanic membrane rupture is seen on exam. What is the concern?

Injury to the ossicles, temporal bone, or labyrinth. Emergent ENT consult is necessary.

On vacation a diver decided to go scuba diving despite his cold. On decent the patient had acute ear pain followed by vertiginous symptoms and vomiting. What happened?

Middle ear squeeze. This is the most common form of barotrauma in amateur scuba divers. With abnormal eustachian tube function due to the upper respiratory infection, the pressure from the middle ear could not equalize. The middle ear volume decreased until the tympanic membrane retracted to the point of rupture. The cold water which rushed in caused vestibular stimulation. Similar problems can occur on planes.

What is the most common organism which causes pediatric acute otitis media?

Strep. pneumoniae followed by Haemophilus influenzae and Moraxella catarrhalis.

Why are preschool children more susceptible to acute otitis media?

Eustachian tube dysfunction is most important factor contributing to acute otitis media. Children's shorter, more horizontal eustachian tubes may prevent adequate drainage and allow aspiration of nasopharyngeal bacteria into the middle ear particularly with URI's.

What is a Bezold abscess?

A complication of acute mastoiditis where infection spreads to the soft tissues below the ear and sternocleidomastoid muscle.

❑❑ **What is the most common cause of sialoadenitis?**

Mumps.

❑❑ **A patient presents with an erythematous, tender parotid gland; trismus; and fever. Pus is expressed from Stenson's duct. What conditions may predispose a person to bacterial parotitis?**

Any situation which decreases salivary flow. Irradiation, phenothiazines, antihistamines, parasympathetic inhibitors, dehydration or debilitation. Up to 30% of cases occur postoperatively.

❑❑ **In which salivary gland do stones most likely occur?**

Eighty percent are submandibular. The least likely is the sublingual gland.

❑❑ **What does grunting versus inspiratory stridor indicate?**

Stridor localizes respiratory obstruction to the level at or above the larynx. Grunting is specific for lower respiratory tract disease such as pneumonia, asthma, or bronchiolitis.

❑❑ **What is the most common cause of epiglottitis?**

Hemophilus influenzae.

❑❑ **What is the most common cause of laryngeal trauma?**

Blunt trauma secondary to motor vehicle accidents.

❑❑ **A patient presents with well demarcated swelling of the lips and tongue. She had been started on an antihypertensive agent three weeks ago. Which agent is most likely?**

Angiotensin converting enzyme inhibitor. Although, angioneurotic edema may occur anytime during therapy with an ACE inhibitor it is most likely in the first month of treatment.

❑❑ **A lower airway foreign body is suspected. What will plain films show?**

Plain films may show air trapping on the affected side. Inspiration and expiration views demonstrate mediastinal shift away from the affected side.

❑❑ **What two conditions are true ophthalmologic emergencies?**

Chemical burns requiring immediate irrigation and central retinal artery occlusion requiring re-establishment of blood flow within 90 min.

❑❑ **How is a Schiötz tonometer interpreted?**

Low scale readings suggest high pressure and high scale readings suggest low pressure. With a 5.5 gm weight a scale of 4 or greater is equal to 20 mm Hg or less (normal).

❑❑ **A patient presents with an itching, tearing, right eye. On exam huge cobblestone papillae are found under the upper lid. Diagnosis?**

Allergic conjunctivitis.

❑❑ **A patient is seen with herpetic lesions on the tip of the nose. Why is this a problem?**

The tip of the nose and the cornea are both supplied by the nasociliary nerve. Thus, the cornea may also be involved.

❑❑ **A patient presents with inflammation of the conjunctiva and lid margins. Slit lamp exam reveals a "greasy" appearance of the lid margins with scaling, especially around the base of the lashes. Diagnosis?**

Blepharitis. Often caused by staphylococcal infection of the oil glands and skin next to the lash follicles. Treatment consists of scrubbing with baby shampoo and, in consolation with an ophthalmologist, sulfacetamide drops and steroids.

❑❑ **A patient presents with a painful red eye. On slit lamp exam, a localized white flocculent infiltrate is seen in the anterior chamber. Diagnosis?**

Hypopyon is an accumulation of white inflammatory exudate in the anterior chamber.

❑❑ **A welder presents with severe eye pain. What would be the expected findings on slit-lamp exam?**

Diffuse punctate keratopathy or "welder's flash". Multiple pinpoint area of fluorescein uptake representing ruptured corneal epithelial cells.

❑❑ **A patient presents with a pustular vesicle at the lid margin. Diagnosis and treatment?**

Hordeolum (stye). Acute inflammation of the meibomian gland most commonly of the upper lid. Treat with topical antibiotics and warm compresses. Surgical drainage may be necessary.

❑❑ **A patient presents with a chronic non-tender uninflamed nodule of the upper lid. Diagnosis?**

Chalazion. Treat with surgical curettage.

❑❑ **A patient presents with the sensation of a foreign body in the eye. Slit-lamp reveals a dendritic figure which has a Christmas tree pattern. Treatment?**

Antiviral agents and cycloplegics are used to treat herpes simplex keratitis. Steroids spell disaster!

❑❑ **A patient presents with sudden vision loss in one eye which returns quickly. Diagnosis?**

Amaurosis fugax. Usually caused by central retinal artery emboli from extracranial atherosclerosis.

❑❑ **A patient presents with painless visual loss in one eye described as a wall slowly developing in the visual field. What finding would be expected on exam?**

Gray detached retina. Patient may also complain of flashing lights in the peripheral visual field or "spider webs" in the visual field. Inferior detachment is treated with the patient sitting up. Superior detachment is treated with the patient lying flat.

❑❑ **When and where do retinal detachments occur after a blunt traumatic injury?**

Frequently there is a delay between the incident and detachment. Half occur in the first eight months. Two years following the accident 80% will be noted. The detachment most commonly occurs in the inferotemporal quadrant.

❑❑ **A patient was hit in the eye during a fight last night while intoxicated. He present eight h after the incident with proptosis and visual loss? Examination reveals an intact globe and an afferent pupillary defect. What is the problem?**

Retro orbital hematoma with ischemia of the optic nerve or retina. The pressure of the blood in the orbit exceeds the profusion pressure causing lack of blood flow and loss of function. Treatment is to release the pressure by lateral canthotomy. A similar situation can occur with orbital emphysema.

❏❏ **What five lid lacerations should be referred to an ophthalmologist?**

a) Near the lacrimal canaliculi (between the medial canthus and the punctum).
b) Near the levator (transverse lacerations of the upper lid).
c) Near the orbital septum (upper lid deep wounds, between the tarsus and the superior orbital rim).
d) Canthal tendons (wounds penetrating the lateral and medial canthi).
e) Lid margins (wounds through the tarsal plate and lid margins).

❏❏ **What are complications of a hyphema?**

The 4 S's - 1) Secondary rebleeds which usually occur between the second and fifth d post injury since this is the time of clot retraction. Rebleeds tend to be worse than the initial bleed. 2) Significantly increased intraocular pressure which can lead to acute glaucoma, chronic late glaucoma, and optic atrophy. 3) Staining of the cornea due to hemosiderin deposits. 4) Synechiae which interfere with iris function.

❏❏ **Why do patients with sickle cell anemia and a hyphema require special consideration when presenting with ophthalmologic concerns?**

Increased intraocular pressure can occur if the cells sickle in the trabecular network preventing aqueous humor from leaving the anterior chamber. Medication, such as hyperosmotics and Diamox, which increase the likelihood of sickling must be avoided

❏❏ **A patient presents with a history of trauma to the orbit with dull ocular pain, decreased visual acuity, and photophobia. Exam reveals a constricted pupil and ciliary flush. What will be found on slit-lamp exam?**

Flare and cells in the anterior chamber are present with traumatic iritis.

Great quotes series:

"There is a great deal of human nature in people."

Mark Twain

❏❏ **What are causes of a subluxed or dislocated lens?**

Trauma, Marfan's syndrome, homocystinuria, Weill-Marchesani syndrome.

❏❏ **Physiologically, what causes flare?**

Flare is caused by inflammatory proteins resulting in the "dust in the movie projector lights" or "fog in the headlights" phenomena in slit-lamp examination.

❏❏ **Which is worse, acid or alkali burns of the cornea?**

Alkali because of deeper penetration than acid burns. A barrier is formed from precipitated proteins with acid burns. The exception is hydrofluoric acid and heavy metal containing acids which can penetrate the cornea.

❏❏ **When should an eye not be dilated?**

With known narrow angle glaucoma and with an iris-supported intraocular lens.

❑❑ **Why shouldn't topical ophthalmologic anesthetics be prescribed?**

The anesthetics inhibit healing and decrease the patient's ability to protect his eye due to the lack of sensation.

❑❑ **What is the most common organism in contact lens associated corneal ulcers?**

Pseudomonas.

❑❑ **How can Krazy-Glue (cyanoacrylate) be removed if a patient has stuck their eyelids together?**

Copious irrigation immediately and then mineral oil. Acetone and ethanol are unacceptable in the eyes. Surgical separation must be done with extreme care to prevent laceration of the lids or globe. Often the patient will have a corneal abrasion and is treated in the usual manner.

❑❑ **An anxious 24 y old female presents with a complaint of blurred vision made worse when looking at objects far away. On exam, the eyes converge, the pupils constrict, and accommodation is at a maximum. Diagnosis?**

Spasm of accommodation. Treat anxiety. A short-acting cycloplegic may stop the cycle.

❑❑ **A very anxious 16 y old male present stating that his vision is like "looking down a gun barrel". How should physiologic versus hysterical scotoma be differentiated?**

Physiologic-double the distance between the patient and tangent screen (visual screen test) results in doubling of the size of the central visual field.
Hysterical- visual field remains the same.

❑❑ **What test can a physician use to determine if blindness is of a hysterical origin?**

An optokinetic drum can be used. If nystagmus eye movements occur the patient is seeing the stripes. Prisms may also be used.

❑❑ **Three h ago, a patient experienced sudden, painless visual loss in her right eye. Central retinal artery occlusion is suspected. What would be the expected finding on eye examination? What is the prognosis?**

Afferent pupillary defect, pale gray retina and a small pink dot hear the fovea. This cherry red spot is the choroidal vasculature being seen at the macula where the retina is the thinnest. After two h the prognosis is extremely poor for visual recovery. Digital massage or anterior chamber paracentesis may dislodge the clot.

❑❑ **What conditions have been associated with central retinal vein occlusion?**

Hyperviscosity syndromes, diabetes and hypertension. Funduscopic exam shows a chaotically streaked retina with congested dilated veins. There are superficial and deep retinal hemorrhages, cotton wool spots and macular edema.

❑❑ **A patient presents with atraumatic pain behind the left eye, an left pupil afferent defect, central visual loss, and a left swollen disc? Diagnosis and potential causes?**

Optic neuritis. This may be idiopathic or may be associated with multiple sclerosis, Lyme's disease, neurosyphilis, lupus, sarcoid, alcoholism, toxins or drug abuse.

❑❑ **After entering a dark bar a patient developed eye pain, nausea, vomiting, blurred vision and sees "halos" around lights. Why would this patient be given mannitol, pilocarpine and acetazolamide?**

This patient has acute narrow angle glaucoma. The goal of treatment is to decrease intraocular pressure. This can be done by
a) decreasing the production of aqueous (carbonic anhydrase inhibitor),
b) decrease of intraocular volume by making the plasma hypertonic to the aqueous humor (as with glycerol or mannitol) and to
c) constrict the pupil (as with pilocarpine) allowing increased flow of the aqueous out through the previously blocked canals of Schlemm.

❏❏ **A patient presents with multiple vertical linear corneal abrasions. What should be suspected?**

A foreign body under the upper lid. This pattern is sometimes called an "ice rink" sign.

❏❏ **How can a physician estimate if the anterior chamber of the eye is narrow?**

Tangential light (as with a penlight) is shone perpendicular to the line of vision across the anterior chamber. If the entire iris is in the light then the chamber is most likely a normal depth. If part of the iris is in a shadow, the chamber is narrow. This can occur with narrow angle glaucoma and with perforating corneal injuries.

❏❏ **What is the difference between a sympathomimetic and a cycloplegic medication when dilating the eye?**

A sympathomimetic simulates the iris's dilator muscle. The cycloplegic inhibits the parasympathetic stimulation which constricts the iris and inhibits the ciliary muscle. Thus, cycloplegics will cause blurred near vision.

❏❏ **A patient felt something fly into his eye while moving the lawn. On examination, there a brown foreign body on the cornea and a tear drop iris pointing towards the foreign body. What is the diagnosis?**

Perforated cornea with extruded iris. A similar foreign body may appear black on the sclera with scleral perforation.

❏❏ **A patient's cornea fluoresces prior to instillation of fluorescein. What should be considered?**

Pseudomonal infection. Several species fluoresce on their own.

❏❏ **How can one determine if a pupil is dilated by pharmacologic agents?**

Pharmacologic dilation should be suspected if the pupil does not constrict to 0.125% pilocarpine instillation. The pupil can be further tested with 1% pilocarpine.

❏❏ **A patient presents with sudden, painless, loss of vision in one eye. What physical findings would be expected?**

Central retinal artery occlusion typically results in a pale retina and a small pink dot near the fovea. Digital massage and immediate ophthalmic consultation with anterior chamber paracentesis is the treatment of choice.

❏❏ **A patient presents with a physical finding of a chaotically blood-streaked retina with congested and dilated veins. Diagnosis?**

Central retinal vein occlusion. Patients often complain of painless decrease in vision in one eye.

❏❏ **A patient presents with sudden loss of vision is one eye which returned quickly. Diagnosis?**

Amaurosis fugax. Usually caused by central retinal artery emboli from extracranial atherosclerosis.

Great quote series:

Get the facts first. You can distort them later.

Mark Twain

❑❑ **A patient presents with the sensation of painless loss of vision in one eye described as a wall slowly developing in the visual field. Findings expected on exam?**

Gray detached retina. Patient may also complain of flashing lights in the peripheral visual field or "spider webs" in the visual field. Inferior detachment is treated with the patient sitting up. Superior detachment is treated with the patient lying flat.

❑❑ **Which anesthetic works the fastest and which lasts the longest: proparacaine or tetracaine?**

Proparacaine - Rapid onset, duration 20 min.
Tetracaine - Delayed onset, duration 1 h.

❑❑ **Place the following mydriatic-cycloplegic medications in order of duration of activity: tropicamide, homatropine, atropine, and cyclopentolate?**

Tropicamide - Onset 15-20 min, brief duration.
Cyclopentolate - Onset 30-60 min, duration < 24 h.
Homatropine - Long lasting, 2-3 d.
Atropine - Very long lasting, 2 wk.

❑❑ **In what age group is retropharyngeal abscess most common?**

Children less than four. Symptoms may include difficulty breathing, fever, enlarged cervical nodes, difficulty swallowing, and a stiff neck. Exam may reveal a mass or fullness in the posterior pharyngeal area.

❑❑ **In what age group are peritonsillar abscesses most common?**

Adolescents and young adults. Symptoms may include ear pain, trismus, drooling, and alteration of voice.

PULMONARY PEARLS

"We rarely gain a higher or larger view except when it is forced upon us through struggles which we would avoid if we could."

Charles Cooney

❑❑ **What is the most common community acquired gram (-) rod pneumonia?**

Klebsiella pneumonia.

❑❑ **What bacterial agent that frequently causes community acquired pneumonia is not covered by erythromycin?**

Haemophilus influenzae.

❑❑ **What 2 antimicrobial agents are broadly effective against organisms that cause both typical and atypical pneumonias**

Azithromycin and Clarithromycin.

❑❑ **Hantavirus occurs most commonly in what geographic location?**

Southwestern United States, especially in areas with deer mice.

❑❑ **Where is aspiration most often seen on chest x-ray?**

Lower lobe of the right lung.

❑❑ **What is empyema necessitans?**

An encapsulated empyema that dissects into the subcutaneous tissues or through the chest wall.

❑❑ **What pH of aspirated fluid has the worst prognosis?**

pH < 2.5.

❑❑ **What single antibiotic is best for the treatment of uncomplicated lung abscess?**

Clindamycin.

❑❑ **What percentage of tuberculosis is drug resistant?**

About 14% but this mainly depends on location.

❑❑ **What are the side effects of INH?**

Hepatitis, neuritis, and lupus like syndrome.

❑❑ **What therapy may increase the body's absorption of a pneumothorax or pneumomediastinum?**

A high inspired FiO_2.

❑❑ **Life threatening hemoptysis should be suspected by.**

1) Large volume of blood, 2) fungus ball in a pulmonary cavity on chest x-ray 3) hypoxemia.

❑❑ **What is the hallmark symptom of COPD ?**

Exertional dyspnea.

❑❑ **What pulmonary function test correlates best with d-to-d function, morbidity, and mortality in the COPD patient?**

FEV_1/FVC.

❑❑ **What is the risk of placing a patient with COPD on a high FiO_2?**

Suppression of the hypoxic ventilatory drive.

❑❑ **Recommended therapeutic serum theophylline levels are?**

10-15 mg/L.

❑❑ **What therapies for asthma should be avoided in the pregnant patient?**

Parenteral ß-adrenergic agonists and epinephrine.

❑❑ **What is the role of salmeterol in the asthmatic patient?**

It is used in the long term management of these patients and not in the acute setting. Because of its long half-life, it may be ideal for chronic use in nocturnal break-through exacerbations.

❑❑ **What is an average, normal Peak expiratory flow rate (PEFR) in an adult male and an adult female?**

Male = 550-600 L/min and female = 450-500 L/min. However, this varies somewhat with body size.

❑❑ **What is the most common cause of bacterial pneumonia?**

Pneumococcus.

❑❑ **What percentage of upper respiratory infectious agents are non-bacterial?**

Non-bacterial agents account for over 90% of pharyngitis, laryngitis, tracheal bronchitis, and bronchitis.

❑❑ **Name two anti-viral medications that are useful for viral pneumonia.**

Amantadine for influenza A and aerosolized Ribavirin for RSV.

❑❑ **If a patient has a patchy infiltrate on a chest x-ray and bullous myringitis, what antibiotic should be given?**

Erythromycin for Mycoplasma.

❑❑ **What kind of pneumonia occurs in alcoholics and other persons who develop aspiration pneumonia?**

Anaerobe and gram-negative pneumonia.

❏❏ **What secondary bacterial pneumonia often occurs following a viral pneumonia?**

Staph. aureus pneumonia.

❏❏ **What 3 findings should be present to consider a sputum sample adequate?**

There should be > 25 PMNs and <10 squamous epithelial cells per low powered field along with a predominant bacterial organism.

❏❏ **A 40 y old alcoholic presents with rigors and shortness of breath. Currant jelly sputum shows short, plump gram-negative bacilli. Chest x-ray shows a necrotizing lobar pneumonia in the right upper lobe. What is the etiologic agent?**

Klebsiella pneumonia.

❏❏ **Legionella pneumoniae occurs mostly in summer or winter?**

Predominantly in the summer.
Staph pneumonia also occurs more frequently in summer.

❏❏ **An older patient with GI symptoms, hyponatremia, and a relative bradycardia most likely has what type of pneumonia?**

Legionella.

❏❏ **What is the treatment for Legionella pneumonia?**

IV erythromycin.

❏❏ **Should steroids be used in aspiration pneumonia?**

No.

❏❏ **Are aspirated foreign bodies more likely to be found in the right or left bronchus?**

Right.

❏❏ **T/F - Flora of lung abscesses are usually polymicrobial.**

True.

❏❏ **What are some common organisms of empyema?**

Staph, gram negatives, and anaerobes.

❏❏ **Describe the classic chest x-ray of Mycoplasma pneumonia.**

Patchy diffuse densities involving the entire lung are most common. Pneumatoceles, cavities, abscesses and pleural effusions can occur, but are uncommon. Rx. Erythromycin.

❏❏ **Describe the classic chest x-ray findings in Legionella pneumonia.**

Dense consolidation and bulging fissures. Expect elevated liver enzymes and hypophosphatemia.

❏❏ **What are the classic signs and symptoms of TB?**

Night sweats, fever, weight loss, malaise, cough, and a green/yellow sputum most commonly seen in the mornings.

❏❏ **What are some common extrapulmonary TB sites?**

Lymph node, bone, GI tract, GU tract, meninges, liver and the pericardium.

❏❏ **Right upper lobe cavitation with parenchymal involvement is classic for:**

TB.
Lower lung infiltrates, hilar adenopathy, atelectasis, and pleural effusion are also common.

❏❏ **T/F - People under 35 y of age with positive TB skin tests should have at least six months of isoniazid chemoprophylaxis.**

True.

❏❏ **Is there a higher incidence of spontaneous pneumothorax among males or females?**

Males.

❏❏ **What accessory x-rays may be obtained to diagnose a pneumothorax?**

1) Expiratory film and 2) Lateral decubitus film on the affected side.

❏❏ **What kind of pneumonias are commonly associated with a pneumothorax?**

Staph, TB, Klebsiella, and PCP.

❏❏ **What diagnostic test is helpful in sub-clinical PCP infection?**

Exertional pulse oximetry is positive for PCP if after 3 minutes of exercise the O_2 saturation decreases by 3% or the A-a gradient increases by 10 mm Hg from rest.

❏❏ **What laboratory tests aid in the diagnosis of PCP?**

A rising LDH or LDH > 450 and an ESR > 50. A low albumin implies a worse prognosis.

❏❏ **The initial therapy for PCP includes what antibiotics?**

TMP-SMZ or pentamidine.

❏❏ **When are corticosteroids recommended for severe PCP?**

p02 < 70 mm Hg or an A-a gradient > 35 mm Hg.

❏❏ **List two drugs that can cause ARDS.**

Heroin and aspirin.

❏❏ **How long after an initial insult does ARDS usually occur?**

12 to 72 h.

❏❏ **Are sedatives beneficial in anxious asthmatic patients?**

Very helpful if you are trying to kill them.
Appropriate to use during RSI.

❏❏ **Speaking of RSI, discuss some agents that may be used to induce unconsciousness.**

Agent	aka	Class	Onset	Duration	Dose
Thiopental	Pentothal	Barbiturate	≈ 30 s	2 - 30 min. dep. on source	2.0-5.0 mg/kg @ 40 mg/min
Methohexital	Brevital	Barbiturate	Fast	Very short	5-12 ml of 1% solution @ 1 ml/5 sec
Fentanyl	Sublimaze	Opiate	2 min	≈ 20 min	20 - 150 µg/kg
Midazolam	Versed	Benzodiazepine	≈ 5 min	≈ 30 min	0.1 mg/kg
Etomidate	Amidate	Benzoderiv.	1 min	3-12 min	0.2-0.4 mg/kg

❑❑ **How is the A-a gradient calculated for a patient breathing room air?**

$$A - a = 150 - Pa_{O_2} - (Pa_{CO_2} \times 1.25)$$ or 4 + age/4 Normal ≈ 2-10.

❑❑ **The summit of Mt. Everest is at 8,848 m (29,029 ft). What is the PaO_2 for a climber at this altitude?**

PaO_2 = 26 - 33 mm Hg. Measured $PaCO_2$ = 9.5 - 13.8 mm Hg with a corresponding SaO_2 of 58%. Whoa!

❑❑ **T/F- Pulse oximetry provides a reliable means of estimating oxyhemoglobin saturation in a patient suffering CO poisoning.**

False. COHb has light absorbance that can lead to a falsely elevated pulse oximeter transduced saturation level. The <u>calculated</u> value from a standard ABG may also be falsely elevated. The oxygen saturation should be <u>measured</u> using a co-oximeter that <u>measures</u> the amounts of unsaturated O_2Hb, of COHb and of MetHb.

❑❑ **What is the half-life of COHb for a patient breathing room air, breathing 100% oxygen and breathing 100% oxygen @ 3 atm pressure?**

Source	FIO_2 = 0.21	FIO_2 = 1.0	FIO_2 = 1.0 @ 3 atm
Tintinalli, 4th. Ed., pg 918.	4 - 5.3 h	50 - 80 min	23 min
Harwood-Nuss, 2nd Ed., pg 1280.	4 - 5 h	40 - 80 min	20 min
Rosen, 3rd Ed., pg 2675	4 - 6 h	90 min	30 min

Using weighted averages and throwing out the outlying values it seems safe to try to remember these values as ≈ **6** h, **1.5** h and **0.5** h.

GI PEARLS

"It is a good thing for the uneducated man to read books of quotations."

Sir Winston Churchill

❏❏ **After a week, an ill-appearing patient says her sore throat got worse and she complains of spiking fevers and central chest burning. What is your concern?**

Retro- or parapharyngeal abscess with extension to superior mediastinitis.

❏❏ **A child presents with odynophagia and drooling. What should you expect on examination of the oropharynx?**

Trouble, if you look with a tongue blade! A patient with suspected epiglottitis is at high risk for upper airway compromise; intubation with direct visualization, typically in the OR, is best. This dogma may be evolving.

❏❏ **A patient says food gets stuck in his mid-chest, then is regurgitated as a putrid, undigested mess. A barium study shows a dilated esophagus with a distal "beak." Diagnosis?**

Achalasia.

❏❏ **A woman with telangiectasias, "tight knuckles," and "acid indigestion" might have what findings on an upper GI series?**

Aperistalsis, characteristic of scleroderma.

❏❏ **A 40 y old smoker describes acute, crescendo substernal chest tightness going to his back, unrelieved by antacids. An ECG shows ST changes, and his pain resolves 7-10 minutes after a nitroglycerin tablet. Is this angina?**

Maybe, though the delayed response to nitrates characterizes "esophageal colic" caused by segmental esophageal spasm, often triggered by reflux.

❏❏ **An elderly woman has progressive trouble swallowing first solids, then liquids. She presents with sudden drooling after dinner. Your concern?**

A peptic stricture or esophageal cancer complicated by bolus obstruction.

❏❏ **A patient with an "acid stomach" develops melena and vomits bright red blood. Is esophagitis a likely cause?**

No. Capillary bleeding rarely causes impressive acute blood loss. Arterial bleeding (from a complicated ulcer, foreign body, or Mallory-Weiss tear) or variceal bleeding are much more likely.

❏❏ **A cirrhotic patient vomits bright red blood. He has a systolic blood pressure of 90 mm Hg. After an aggressive fluid resuscitation, 4 units of PRBC, and gastric lavage, his pressure is 90 mm Hg. What next?**

Assume a coagulopathy and transfuse fresh frozen plasma; start a vasopressin or octreotide drip; and arrange for emergent endoscopic evaluation/intervention usually for sclerotherapy or banding.

❏❏ **Recurrent pneumonias, especially in the right middle lobe or the superior segments of the bilateral upper lobes, suggests what syndrome?**

Aspiration, associated with motor diseases and gastroesophageal reflux.

❏❏ **List 4 contraindications to introduction of a nasogastric tube.**

> 1.) Suspected esophageal laceration or perforation.
> 2.) Near obstruction due to stricture.
> 3.) Esophageal foreign body.
> 4.) Severe head trauma with rhinorrhea.

❏❏ **Repeated, violent bouts of vomiting can result in both Mallory-Weiss tears and Boerhaave's syndrome. Differentiate the two.**

> Mallory-Weiss tears involve the submucosa and mucosa, typically in the right posterolateral wall of the GE junction.
> Boerhaave's is a full-thickness tear, usually in the unsupported left posterolateral wall of the abdominal esophagus.

❏❏ **After a high-speed MVA, an unrestrained driver develops abdominal and chest pain radiating to the neck. An upper chest film shows left pleural fluid. What gastroesophageal catastrophe might have occurred?**

> Impact against a steering wheel, can result in Boerhaave's syndrome with esophageal perforation and mediastinitis.

❏❏ **You suspect a perforated esophagus; what's the next test to order?**

> A water-soluble contrast study. In the mean time, start broad-spectrum antibiotics and call the surgeons ASAP.

❏❏ **Pediatric foreign bodies lodge at what esophageal levels?**

> Typically at levels of the cricopharyngeus muscles (most usual), thoracic inlet, aortic arch, tracheal bifurcation, and lower esophageal sphincter.

❏❏ **When is removing a button battery lodged in the esophagus indicated?**

> Always. If this corrosive foreign body was swallowed <u>less than 2 hours</u> ago, and endoscopy is <u>not</u> available, consider attempting Foley balloon removal. More wisely, find a scope doc for immediate endoscopic removal.

❏❏ **X-rays are crucial in the search for a suspected swallowed foreign body. In kids, what physical findings can tip you off?**

> Besides a child's distress, you may also find a red or scratched oropharynx, dysphagia, a high fever, or peritoneal signs. Subcutaneous air suggests perforation.

❏❏ **Most objects, even sharp ones, pass thorough the GI tract without incident. What objects should be removed?**

> Any object that obstructs or perforates, that is > 5 cm long and >2 cm wide (won't make it past the GE junction), or is toxic (batteries) should be removed, either endoscopically or surgically. Sharp or pointed objects (sewing needles and razor blades) should be removed if they haven't passed the pylorus.

❏❏ **An obstructing meat bolus should be removed within 12 hours. What's the best approach?**

> Endoscopy, through a trial of IV glucagon (given as 1 mg push after a small test dose, then repeated as a 2 mg dose at 20 min if no relief), or sublingual nifedipine, 10 mg, may work. Both relax esophageal smooth muscle. Meat tenderizer is best avoided, since perforation has occurred.

❑❑ **Which test is mandatory after the food bolus is cleared?**

A barium study or endoscopy to both confirm the passage/removal of the foreign body and to look for underlying pathology (present in virtually all adults with obstructing food boluses).

❑❑ **Are there clinical findings that reliably distinguish duodenal ulcer from gastric ulcer?**

No. Some findings are suggestive: A typical DU causes pain 2 h after a meal that may radiate to the back, and wake a patient from sleep, while GU often causes immediate postprandial pain and is more often due to ethanol or NSAID use.

❑❑ **Name two endocrine problems that cause peptic ulcer.**

Zollinger-Ellison syndrome and hyperparathyroidism (hypercalcemia).

❑❑ **Postprandial midabdominal pain might suggest what ectopic syndrome?**

Peptic ulcer in a Meckel's diverticulum.

❑❑ **T/F - H_2--blockers decrease the risk of perforation and rebleeding in peptic ulcer disease.**

False. However, cimetidine has reduced the need for surgery, improved rates of ulcer healing, and reduced the mortality from the initial bleeding episode.

❑❑ **Any worries in giving cimetidine to a wheezing, anticoagulated patient with a seizure disorder?**

Maybe. By decreasing blood flow to the liver and competing with the drug-eliminating cytochrome p450 system, cimetidine can increase the levels of theophylline, warfarin, and phenytoin, not to mention diazepam, propranolol, and lidocaine.

❑❑ **A patient with "half a stomach" after surgery for a bleeding ulcer presents with weight loss, epigastric burning, and diarrhea. Potential reasons?**

An obstructed afferent loop (Billroth II), bile reflux gastritis, dumping syndrome, malabsorption (poor mixing, of gastric/pancreatic juices, bacterial overgrowth), or gastric remnant carcinoma. Anemia (from B_{12}, iron, and folate malabsorption) and osteoporosis (from vitamin D and calcium malabsorption) are common.

❑❑ **Is a person with massive upper GI bleeding likely to have a perforated ulcer?**

No.

❑❑ **After fluid and blood resuscitation for a bleeding ulcer, the most useful diagnostic test?**

Endoscopy, which can also be therapeutic, with cryo- or electrocautery of an arterial bleeder.

❑❑ **In a patient with early satiety and ulcer symptoms, what clinical finding essentially rules out a gastric outlet obstruction?**

Bilious vomitus.

❑❑ **T/F - Upright abdominal, left lateral decubitus, or upright chest films show free air in most perforations.**

True, but just barely. Some 49% of cases show no free air (typically they are walled off). Insufflate 300-500 cc of air through a nasogastric tube, then clamp it, and have the patient sit up for 10 min to up the yield.

❑❑ **Are "stress ulcers" a surgical problem?**

Not usually. The diffuse gastric bleeding that results from CNS tumors, head trauma, burns, sepsis, shock, steroids, aspirin, or alcohol is usually mucosal, can be life-threatening, and can most often be managed medically. Endoscopic diagnosis is key.

❏❏ **Burning epigastric pain shooting to the back, hypovolemic shock, and a high amylase suggests . . .**

Posterior perforation of a duodenal ulcer.

❏❏ **Can non-gallstone cholecystitis perforate?**

Yes. Up to 40% of gall bladder perforations are associated with acalculous cholecystitis.

❏❏ **Who gets acalculous cholecystitis?**

Dehydrated post-op, post-trauma, and burn patients, as well as those with transfusion related hemolysis or narcotic use (illicit or prescribed).

❏❏ **Enteric coated potassium tablets, typhoid, tuberculosis, tumors, and strangulated hernia may cause what rare process?**

Non-traumatic small-bowel perforation.

❏❏ **The most common cause of lower GI perforation?**

Diverticulitis, followed by tumor, colitis, foreign bodies, and instrumentation.

❏❏ **A pregnant woman with right upper quadrant pain should be assumed to have what intraabdominal pathology until proven otherwise?**

Acute appendicitis.

❏❏ **Rovsing's, psoas, and obturator signs can all indicate an inflamed posterior appendix. Please describe these signs.**

Rovsing's sign - right lower quadrant pain on left lower quadrant palpation.
Psoas sign - right lower quadrant pain on right thigh extension.
Obturator sign - right lower quadrant pain on internal rotation of the flexed right thigh.

❏❏ **What does ultrasound show in acute appendicitis?**

A fixed, tender, non-compressible mass, but only in 75 to 90% of cases.

❏❏ **What does abdominal CT scanning show in acute appendicitis?**

Not much in early appendicitis; the study is useful to distinguish the causes of a right lower quadrant mass (late appendicitis, perforation/abscess, carcinoma, and pseudomyxoma).

❏❏ **What does laparoscopy show in acute appendicitis?**

Appendicitis, if you're lucky. Unfortunately, just seeing an inflamed appendix does not prove appendicitis; finding another cause of abdominal pain does not rule out appendicitis.

❏❏ **What about blood tests?**

An elevated WBC or a left shift are seen in 95 to 99% of cases; this is a sensitive test (helps rule out appendicitis), but nonspecific (can't rule it in).

❏❏ **So what's the point of the last four questions?**

Don't rely on diagnostic studies to diagnose acute abdominal pain. Rely instead on an exam by an experienced clinician, hospital admission, serial exams, and surgical consultation.

❑❑ **The most common cause of small bowel obstruction?**

Adhesions are the most common causes of <u>extra</u>luminal obstruction, followed by incarcerated hernia, while gallstones and bezoars are the most common causes of <u>intra</u>luminal obstruction.

❑❑ **Recurrent small bowel obstruction in an elderly woman associated with unilateral pain into one thigh suggests what occult process?**

Obturator hernia incarceration. May often present with pain down medial thigh to knee.

❑❑ **The most common causes of colonic obstruction?**

Cancer, then diverticulitis followed by volvulus.

❑❑ **An elderly man presents with new constipation without tenesmus, abdominal pain, nausea or vomiting. He has hard stool in the vault on rectal exam. A KUB shows a colon "full of stool." Is an enema all he needs?**

No. Fecal impaction with "obstipation" is both common and benign, but it is usually associated with tenesmus. He needs a workup for a colorectal tumor.

❑❑ **A KUB is suspicious for a large bowel obstruction. The next step(s) in evaluation?**

Unprepped sigmoidoscopy to confirm obstruction, then a barium study to determine the cause. If you suspect pseudo-obstruction (typically due to medications), **don't** order a barium study (for fear of concretion and obstruction). Colonoscopy can be diagnostic and therapeutic.

❑❑ **List three classes of drugs that cause pseudo-obstruction.**

Anticholinergics, antiparkinsonian drugs, and tricyclic antidepressants.

❑❑ **While you're at it, list three types of <u>internal</u> hernias.**

Diaphragmatic hernia, lesser sac hernia (through the foramen of Winslow), and omental or mesenteric hernia.

❑❑ **Which is more dangerous, a small hernia or a large one?**

Incarceration is more likely with small hernias.

❑❑ **Is a hernia in Hesselbach's triangle (between the inguinal ligament, inferior epigastric vessels, and lateral border of the rectus abdominis) likely to incarcerate?**

Direct hernias rarely incarcerate.

❑❑ **What about a hernia that is lateral to the epigastric vessels?**

Indirect hernias are much more likely to incarcerate.

❑❑ **Which is the most common hernia in women, inguinal or femoral?**

Inguinal, <u>not</u> femoral. While it's true that femoral hernias are more common in women than in men, inguinal hernias remain the most common hernia in women.

❑❑ **Distinguish between a groin hernia, a hydrocele and a lymph node.**

Hydroceles transilluminate and are non-tender. Lymph nodes tend to be freely moving, firm, and multiple. Hernias don't transilluminate and may have bowel sounds.

❑❑ **A patient tells you that 2 d ago his groin bulged and he developed severe pain with progressive nausea and vomiting. He has a tender mass in his groin. What <u>shouldn't</u> you do?**

Don't try to reduce a long-standing, tender incarcerated hernia! The abdomen is no place for dead bowel.

❑❑ **How does the pathology of Crohn's disease differ from that of ulcerative colitis?**

Crohn's is a trans-mucosal, segmental, granulomatous process, while ulcerative colitis is a mucosal, juxtapositional, ulcerative process.

❑❑ **A young man with atraumatic chronic back pain, eye trouble, and painful red lumps on his shins develops <u>bloody</u> <u>diarrhea</u>. What is the point of this question?**

To remind you of extraintestinal manifestations of inflammatory bowel disease, such as ankylosing spondylitis, uveitis, and erythema nodosum, not to mention <u>kidney</u> <u>stones</u>.

❑❑ **At least a third of patients with Crohn's disease have kidney stones. Why?**

Dietary oxalate is usually bound to calcium and excreted. When terminal ileal disease leads to decreased bile salt absorption, the resulting fattier intestinal contents bind calcium by saponification. Free oxalate is "hyper-absorbed" in the colon, resulting in hyperoxaluria and calcium oxalate nephrolithiasis.

❑❑ **Complications of** Crohn's **include perirectal** abscesses, **anal** fissures, **rectovaginal** fistulas, **and rectal prolapse. How often is perirectal disease present?**

Approximately 90 percent of patients.

❑❑ **A patient with chronic, occasionally bloody diarrhea develops severe diarrhea and abdominal pain with marked distention. What "can't-miss" diagnosis does this suggest?**

Toxic megacolon, a life-threatening complication of ulcerative colitis.

❑❑ **What are the odds that a patient with severe ileal disease will be cured by surgery?**

Virtually zero. Crohn's almost invariably recurs in the remaining GI tract. In contrast, total proctocolectomy with ileostomy is curative in ulcerative colitis.

❑❑ **A patient with new diarrhea and abdominal pain tells you she took antibiotics for sinusitis two weeks ago. Sigmoidoscopy might reveal what?**

Yellowish superficial plaques suggestive of pseudomembranous colitis. Stool studies would show C. difficile toxin.

❑❑ **What's the treatment?**

<u>Oral</u> vancomycin, 125 mg qid or <u>oral</u> metronidazole, 500 mg qid. Either regimen should be given for 7 to 10 d. Cholestyramine, which binds the toxin, can help limit the diarrhea. Follow-up stool studies should confirm clearance of the toxin.

❑❑ **Is diverticulitis the likely diagnosis in a patient with low abdominal pain and bright red blood per rectum?**

No. Typically diverticul<u>osis</u> bleeds, while diverticul<u>itis</u> doesn't. Diverticular bleeding is typically painless.

❑❑ **Is sigmoidoscopy or contrast x-ray study indicated in acute diverticulitis?**

A controversial topic. The conventional wisdom says wait until the acute inflammation resolves.

❏❏ **Crampy abdominal pain with mucus in the stool suggests what syndrome?**

The irritable bowel one. Patients are afebrile, and often improve after passing flatus.

❏❏ **What barium findings distinguish colonic obstruction due to acute diverticulitis from that due to colon cancer?**

Diverticulitis is extraluminal, so the mucosa appears intact and involved bowel segments are longer. Adenocarcinoma distorts the mucosa, involves a short segment of bowel, and has overhanging edges.

❏❏ **Abdominal pain in a gray-haired patient should always suggest _____ _____, until proven otherwise.**

Mesenteric ischemia.

❏❏ **Prescribe an outpatient antibiotic regimen for uncomplicated diverticulitis.**

Ciprofloxacin plus metronidazole.

❏❏ **Which is more sensitive for locating the source of GI bleeding, a radioactive Tc-labeled red cell scan, or angiography?**

A bleeding scan can find a site bleeding at a rate as low as 0.12 ml/min, while angiography requires rapid bleeding (greater than 0.5 ml/min).

❏❏ **A patient known to have gallstones presents with acute, postprandial right upper quadrant pain. What's the KUB likely to show?**

Nothing specific. Only around 10% of gallstones are radiopaque. Complications of cholelithiasis - emphysematous cholecystitis, perforation, and pneumobilia - are uncommon but useful findings.

❏❏ **A child with sickle cell disease presents with fever, shaking chills, and jaundice. The likely diagnosis?**

Charcot's triad suggests ascending cholangitis. The precipitating cause is most likely pigment stones resulting from chronic hemolysis.

❏❏ **A post-surgical patient develops right upper quadrant pain, nausea, and low-grade fevers. According to his surgeon, the gallbladder was normal intraoperatively. What's a probable diagnosis?**

Acalculous cholecystitis.

❏❏ **Eight years after her cholecystectomy, a woman develops right upper quadrant pain and jaundice. What's the chance of developing recurrent biliary tract stones after cholecystectomy?**

At least 10%, due either to retained stones or *in-situ* formation by biliary epithelium.

❏❏ **List the ultrasound findings suggestive of acute cholecystitis.**

Presence of gall stones (or sludge, in acalculous cholecystitis), gall bladder wall thickening > 5 mm, and pericholecystic fluid. A dilated common bile duct (>10 mm) suggests common duct obstruction.

❏❏ **Name two findings in acute cholecystitis that mandate emergent laparotomy.**

Emphysematous cholecystitis and perforation. Otherwise, timing of surgery is somewhat institution- and surgeon-dependent.

❏❏ **What simple test can distinguish between conjugated and unconjugated hyperbilirubinemia?**

A dipstick test for urobilinogen, which reflects conjugated (water soluble) hyperbilirubinemia.

❏❏ **In addition to conjugated hyperbilirubinemia, what liver function abnormalities suggest biliary tract disease?**

Elevated alkaline phosphatase out of proportion to transaminases.

❏❏ **Which two LFT abnormalities reflect a poor prognosis in acute viral hepatitis?**

A total bilirubin > 20 mg/dl, and prolongation of the prothrombin time > 3 seconds. The extent of transaminase elevation is not a useful marker.

❏❏ **Match the following hepatitis serologies with the right clinical description:**

(1) HBsAg (-), antiHBs(+)   ___ongoing viral replication; highly infectious.
(2) IgM HBcAg (+), antiHBs(-)   ___remote infection; not infectious.
(3) IgG HBcAg (+), antiHBs(-)   ___recent or ongoing infection; a high titer means high
                                            infectivity, while a low titer suggests chronic, active infection.
(4) HBeAg (+)   ___ prior infection or vaccination; not infectious.

Answers: 4,3,2,1.

HBeAg (+): "e" = "eeeek! I'm infectious!", for e ANTIGEN, anti-HBe implies decreased infectivity.
IgG HBcAg (+):   "G" = Gone.
IgM HBcAg (+):   "M" = Might be contagious still.
ANTIHBs (+):   "s" = Stopped, Pt. has antibodies to surface antigen.

WARNING! YOU <u>MUST</u> SPECIFY WHETHER THE <u>ANTIGEN</u> OR THE <u>ANTIBODY</u> IS PRESENT WHEN LEARNING THESE LETTER CODES, OTHERWISE YOU WILL LEARN THESE THINGS THE WRONG WAY AROUND!! Go over it ten times or so in the text of your choice, then it will make sense and remembering the letters won't be necessary.

❏❏ **T/F - The "delta agent" can cause hepatitis D in a patient without active hepatitis B.**

False. The d-agent is an incomplete, "defective," RNA virus responsible for hepatitis D. It is an obligate covirus and requires hepatitis B for replication.

❏❏ **You stick yourself with a needle from a chronic hepatitis B carrier. You've been vaccinated, but never had your antibody status checked. What would be the appropriate post-exposure prophylaxis?**

Have your anti-HBs titer measured. If it's adequate (>10 mIU), you need no treatment. If it's inadequate, you need a single dose of HBIG as soon as possible and a vaccine booster.

❏❏ **Match the following hepatotoxic drugs with the correct toxic syndrome:**

(1) Halothane, methyldopa, isoniazid.   ___chronic active hepatitis and cirrhosis.
(2) Anabolic steroids, oral contraceptives,   ___massive hepatic necrosis.
oral hypoglycemics, erythromycin
estolate.
(3) Carbon tetrachloride, phosphorus,   ___acute hepatitis.
acetaminophen, *Amanita* mushrooms.
(4) Vinyl chloride, arsenic.   ___steatosis, hepatocellular necrosis.
(5) Ethanol.   ___cholestatic jaundice.

(Answer: 4, 3, 1, 5, 2)

❏❏ **A high fever and leukocytosis accompanying acute alcoholic hepatitis is worrisome. Why?**

Alcohol is marrow toxic, so leukocytosis often reflects serious associated infection. Get a chest x-ray, and obtain blood cultures, a urinalysis, and ascitic fluid for cell count and culture.

❑❑ **A cirrhotic presents with weakness and edema. What electrolyte imbalances might be present?**

Hyponatremia (dilutional or diuretic-induced), hypokalemia (from GI losses, secondary hyperaldosteronism, or diuretics), and hypomagnesemia.

❑❑ **The best diuretic choice for most cirrhotics with ascites?**

Potassium-sparing agents (treat the hyperaldosterone state specifically).

❑❑ **A confused cirrhotic presents to the ED. She is afebrile and has asterixis. What should your exam consist of as you look for the precipitant of hepatic encephalopathy?**

Give thiamine and folate. Assess her mental status and search for localizing neurologic signs (occult head injury); look for dry mucous membranes and a low jugular venous pressure (hypovolemia and azotemia); check a stool guaiac (GI bleeding). Focused lab testing can pinpoint other causes (diuretic overuse and hypokalemia, hypoglycemia, anemia, hypoxia, and infection).

❑❑ **Aside from fixing the above, what therapy is useful?**

Lactulose, which produces an acidic diarrhea that traps nitrogenous wastes in the gut.

❑❑ **Are there any useful therapies for the rapid renal failure that can complicate cirrhosis?**

Unfortunately not. The hepatorenal syndrome still has a mortality that approaches 100%.

❑❑ **An ascitic patient presents with fever but no localizing signs or symptoms of infection, and a normal WBC. Because you know that spontaneous bacterial peritonitis can be an occult disease, you perform an abdominal paracentesis. What WBC in ascitic fluid suggests SBP?**

Greater than $250/mm^3$. You should also Gram stain the fluid and send at least 10 cc in blood culture bottles for aerobic and anaerobic culture.

❑❑ **The most common organism responsible for SBP?**

E. coli, followed by S. pneumoniae.

❑❑ **So the best therapy is . . .?**

<u>Intravenous</u> Ampicillin **plus** an aminoglycoside is reasonable empiric therapy pending culture results.

❑❑ **What two therapies can reduce the risk of recurrent SBP?**

Diuretics decrease ascitic fluid, and nonabsorbable oral antibiotics decrease the gut bacterial load, limiting bacterial translocation. Both treatments have cut the risk of recurrence in compliant patients.

❑❑ **A non-drinker presents with acute pancreatitis. What conditions may underlie this acute process?**

Biliary tract disease, trauma (blunt or penetrating), ulcers (posterior penetrating duodenal ulcer), diabetes (ketoacidosis), and hypertriglyceridemia.

❑❑ **Which is a more sensitive test for pancreatitis, serum amylase or lipase?**

Amylase elevation is 70-90% sensitive for pancreatitis; lipase is 75-100% sensitive; the combination is up to 95-97% sensitive. Remember that up to 10% of patients with severe acute pancreatitis may have a normal amylase. In chronic pancreatitis, up to 30% may have a normal amylase.

❑❑ **What are Ranson's five predictors of complications from acute pancreatitis <u>upon admission</u>?**

Age over 55, blood glucose >200 mg/dl, WBC > 16,000/mm^3, SGOT (AST) >250 U/l, and LDH > 350 IU/l.

❑❑ **Forty-eight h after admission, what six findings predict poor outcome?**

Hematocrit drop > 10%, rise in BUN > 5 gm/dl, calcium lower than 8 mg/dl, PaO$_2$ < 60 mm Hg, over 6 liter third-space fluid accumulation, and base deficit > 4 mEq/l.

❑❑ **Is a nasogastric tube always indicated in acute pancreatitis?**

Only if nausea and vomiting are severe. One trial showed a worse outcome with NG tubes because of complications, including aspiration.

❑❑ **When are antibiotics useful in acute pancreatitis?**

Pancreatitis is a chemical disease, and antibiotics are only useful for treating complications such as abscess or sepsis. The only exception is in pancreatitis associated with choledocholithiasis, when antibiotics are indicated.

❑❑ **Symptoms that last longer than a week or the presence of an abdominal mass, hyperamylasemia, and leukocytosis suggest what potentially disastrous complications of pancreatitis?**

Pancreatic abscess or pseudocyst.

❑❑ **Are there any useful plain film findings in pancreatitis?**

Right upper quadrant calcifications suggests gallstone pancreatitis, air in the region of the pancreas suggests abscess, and calcific stippling in the epigastrium suggests chronic pancreatitis.

❑❑ **Portal hypertension produces internal hemorrhoids through which veins?**

Internal hemorrhoids are proximal to the fabled dentate line in the **2-**, **5-**, and **9**-o'clock position in the prone patient, and are typically not palpable on rectal exam. They occur in the superior rectal and inferior mesenteric veins.

❑❑ **Are painful hemorrhoids always external hemorrhoids?**

No. Though hemorrhoidal pain is more likely to be due to thrombosed external hemorrhoids, be on the lookout for prolapsed and/or incarcerated internal hemorrhoids.

❑❑ **Distinguish, by location, the following: anal cryptitis, anal fissure, anorectal abscess, and fistula in ano.**

Cryptitis, fissures and perianal abscess typically occur in the posterior midline; deep abscesses can point to areas far from the anus. Goodsall's rule on fistulas: those that open anteriorly go straight to the anal canal, while those that open posteriorly may follow a circuitous route.

❑❑ **T/F - Antibiotics are unnecessary after an uncomplicated perirectal abscess is incised and drained.**

True, assuming the patient has no underlying immunoincompetence (HIV, diabetes, malignancy). Sitz baths beginning the next day are the primary after-care.

❑❑ **Distinguish anal chancres and herpetic ulcers.**

Anal chancres of primary syphilis are painful, symmetric, indurated, and diagnosed by dark-field microscopy.
Herpes simplex produces perianal paresthesias and pruritus, followed by red-haloed vesicles and apthous ulcers (ruptured vesicles); a Tzanck smear is diagnostic. Both cause painful inguinal adenopathy.

❏❏ **A patient presents with proctitis, and a Gram stain of a rectal swab reveals neutrophils with Gram-negative intracellular diplococci. The treatment?**

Ceftriaxone, 250 mg IM, once, with tetracycline, 500 mg qid (or doxycycline 100 mg bid) for 10 days to cover possible Chlamydia co-infection (send a Chlamydia swab and a serologic test for syphilis to the lab, as well). Sexual partners should be notified, and follow-up cultures obtained after therapy. (Note: some authors suggest empiric treatment for Chlamydia in women only, since Chlamydial proctitis is less common in men).

❏❏ **Procidentia in adults mandates what intervention?**

Rectal prolapse can be manually reduced in children with good results; adults typically require proctosigmoidoscopy and surgical repair.

❏❏ **Is it better to have cancer of the anal margin or of the anal canal?**

Anal margin cancer is usually low-grade, and late to metastasize, while anal canal cancers are more aggressive and metastasize early.

❏❏ **Watery diarrhea with profuse rectal discharge and weakness might suggest what uncommon tumor?**

Villous adenoma, with watery diarrhea and hypokalemia.

❏❏ **Do pilonidal abscesses communicate with the anal canal?**

No. They are virtually always midline and overlie the lower sacrum. Posterior-opening, horseshoe-type anorectal fistulas can find their way to the lower sacrum, but are rarely in the midline. Remember Goodsall's rule.

❏❏ **Should pilonidal cysts be excised in the emergency department?**

Probably not. Incision and drainage is OK, followed by a bulky dressing, analgesics, and hot sitz baths beginning the next day; antibiotics are not typically necessary. Excision should be completed in the OR once the acute infection clears up.

❏❏ **In adults, pruritus ani is seen with dietary factors contributing to liquid stool (caffeine, mineral oil), sexually transmitted infections, fecal contamination, overzealous hygiene, and vitamin deficiencies. The most common cause in children?**

Enterobius vermicularis, or pinworm. A cheap and diagnostic test: apply a piece of scotch tape sticky-side down to the perineal area, than smooth it out (with a cotton swab) on a glass slide and examine under low power for eggs. Treatment is mebendazole, 100 mg in a single dose, repeated at 2 weeks.

❏❏ **What stool studies are crucial in evaluating acute diarrhea?**

Statistically speaking, acute diarrhea is so common and typically self-limited that <u>most cases need no testing</u>, just oral rehydration. In sick patients or those at risk for complications (at the extremes of age, recently hospitalized, immunocompromised), <u>enteroinvasive infection should be ruled out</u> with a stool guaiac and test for fecal leukocytes (Gram or methylene blue stains are comparable). Also consider checking for ova and parasites.

❏❏ **Which diarrheal illnesses cause fecal leukocytes?**

Usual culprits:
    Shigella.
    Campylobacter.
    Enteroinvasive E. coli.
Others:
    Salmonella, Yersinia, Vibrio parahaemolyticus, and C. difficile.

Fecal WBCs are absent in toxigenic and enteropathogenic infection, even with such a virulent organism as Vibrio cholera; viral and parasitic infections rarely produce fecal WBCs.

❑❑ **Name the most likely cause of diarrhea in a 6-mo old in day-care.**

Viral diarrhea is most common, with Rotavirus the most common virus; be on the lookout for Giardia and Cryptosporidia, recently added to the list of day-care-associated diarrheal illnesses.

❑❑ **The most common cause of bacterial diarrhea?**

E. coli (enteroinvasive, enteropathogenic, enterotoxigenic).

❑❑ **A former IV drug user with sickle-cell disease and a history of splenectomy presents with unremitting fever, crampy abdominal pain, and meningismus after recently acquiring a pet turtle. He has no diarrhea. What bacteria may be the culprit?**

Salmonella typhi, the causative agent of typhoid fever. The attack rate is remarkably high in patients with HIV, in asplenic patients, and in those with sickle cell disease. Rose spots occur in 10-20%; relative bradycardia in the face of a high fever, and a low or normal WBC with a pronounced left shift are suggestive findings.

❑❑ **The treatment?**

Intravenous Fluoroquinolone, Ceftriaxone, or Chloramphenicol. Make sure to check blood cultures, which may suggest metastatic infection. Avoid antimotility agents.

❑❑ **Match the diarrheal syndrome with the culprit:**

(1) Aeromonas hydrophilia	___Diarrhea on the way to the car after eating fried rice at a Chinese buffet.
(2) Bacillus cereus	___Diarrhea followed by thigh myalgias, perioral dysesthesias, and pruritus.
(3) Campylobacter	___ Profuse, foul-smelling diarrhea with bloating and cramps after a fishing trip.
(4) Clostridium difficile	___Bloody diarrhea and fever in a child.
(5) Clostridium perfringens	___Acute dysentery, fever, and pseudoappendicitis after getting a new puppy.
(6) Vibrio parahaemolyticus	___Rice water diarrhea without fever or constitutional symptoms.
(7) Staph. aureus	___Diarrhea from raw seafood.
(8) Yersinia	___Diarrhea from contaminated meat; no nausea or vomiting.
(9) Giardia	___Diarrhea from antibiotic-associated enterocolitis.
(10) Ciguatera toxin	___Diarrhea (enterocolitis) associated with either antibiotics *or* food.

(Answers: 2, 10, 9, 3, 8, 1, 6, 5, 4, 7)

Diarrhea on the way to the car after eating fried rice at a Chinese buffet - Bacillus cereus; treatment is symptomatic.

Diarrhea followed by thigh myalgias, perioral dysesthesias, and pruritus - Ciguatera toxin; no treatment.

Profuse, foul-smelling diarrhea with bloating and cramps after a fishing trip - Giardia; quinacrine or metronidazole.

Bloody diarrhea and fever in a child - Campylobacter; erythromycin; doxycycline or fluoroquinolone in adults.

Acute dysentery, fever, and pseudoappendicitis - Yersinia; optimal tx unknown, chloramphenicol, tetracycline, TMP/SMX.

Rice water diarrhea without fever or constitutional symptoms - Aeromonas hydrophilia with sx due to enterotoxin; tx primarily symptomatic.

Diarrhea from raw seafood - Vibrio parahaemolyticus; treat symptoms.

Diarrhea from contaminated meat; no nausea or vomiting - Clostridium perfringens; usually no therapy, rarely antitoxin antibodies.

Diarrhea from antibiotic-associated enterocolitis - Clostridium difficile; vancomycin or metronidazole.

Diarrhea (enterocolitis) associated with either antibiotics or food - Staph. aureus; treat symptoms.

❏❏ **What are the symptoms most commonly associated with neuromuscular associated dysphagia?**

Nasopharyngeal Regurgitation and hoarseness.

❏❏ **The most common causes of dysphagia in the elderly population include?**

Hiatal hernia, reflux esophagitis, webs/rings, and cancer.

❏❏ **The most common symptom of esophageal disease is?**

Pyrosis - heartburn.

❏❏ **What are the classical features which distinguish chest pain of esophageal origin from cardiac ischemia?**

There are no classical clinical features which distinguish between these two entities. Exertional pain and palliation with rest or NTG occur in both groups. Pain relief in the GI group usually takes 7-10 min while ischemic pain usually responds in 2-3 minutes.

❏❏ **Radiographs should be performed in all patients suspected of swallowing coins to determine the presence and location of the FB. How will the coin appear on the X-ray in the AP view?**

Coins in the esophagus lie in the frontal plane. Coins in the trachea lie in the sagittal plane.

❏❏ **What is the management of button battery ingestion?**

Button batteries must be removed from the esophagus by endoscopy. One may consider a Foley catheter technique if the battery has been present less that 2 hours.

❏❏ **What is the management of button batteries that have passed the esophagus?**

In the asymptomatic patient - repeat radiographs. The symptomatic patient and those patients where the battery has not passed the pylorus after 48 hours require endoscopic retrieval.

❏❏ **What medical conditions are associated with an increase incidence of PUD?**

COPD, Cirrhosis, and Chronic Renal Failure.

❏❏ **What is the most common location of a perforated peptic ulcer?**

Anterior surface of the duodenum or pylorus and the lesser curvature of the stomach.

❏❏ **What types of patients are at risk for gallbladder perforation?**

Elderly, diabetics, and those with recurrent cholecystitis.

❏❏ **What percentage of patients with a perforated viscus have radiographic evidence of a pneumoperitoneum?**

Sixty to seventy percent will have this finding. Therefore, one-third of patients will not have this sign. keep the patient in either the upright or left lateral decubitus position for at least 10 minutes prior to performing X-rays.

❏❏ **What are the indications for the surgical removal of a GI foreign body?**

GI obstruction; GI perforation; toxic properties of the material, and length, size, and shape that will prevent the object from passing safely.

❑❑ **What size objects rarely pass the stomach?**

Objects longer than 5 cm and wider than 2 cm.

❑❑ **Are gastric and duodenal perforations more common in malignant or benign ulcers?**

Benign ulcerations.

❑❑ **Does significant UGIB accompany perforated ulcers?**

Massive GI bleeding almost rules out the presence of a perforated ulcer. One should consider a secondary penetrating ulcer.

❑❑ **Acalculous cholecystitis commonly occurs in which conditions?**

Post-operative, post-trauma; burn patients secondary to dehydration, and hemolysis secondary to blood transfusions.

❑❑ **What are the most common causes of non-traumatic perforations of the lower GI tract?**

Diverticulitis, carcinoma, colitis, foreign bodies, barium enemas, and endoscopy.

❑❑ **The hallmark of a perforated viscus is?**

Abdominal pain.

❑❑ **Which is one of the earliest signs of sepsis?**

Respiratory alkalosis on an ABG.

❑❑ **What are the more common processes that mimic acute appendicitis?**

Mesenteric lymphadenitis, PID, Mittleshmertz, Gastroenteritis, and Crohn's disease.

❑❑ **What conditions are associated with an atypical presentation of acute appendicitis?**

Situs inversus viscerum, malrotation, hypermobile cecum, long pelvic appendix, and pregnancy (1/2200).

❑❑ **What are the most frequent symptoms of acute appendicitis?**

Anorexia and pain. The classical presentation: anorexia, periumbilical pain with progression to constant RLQ pain is present in only 60% of cases.

❑❑ **What clinical maneuvers may aid in the diagnosis of acute appendicitis?**

The psoas sign and the obturator sign may aid in the diagnosis of an inflamed posteriorly located appendix.

❑❑ **What percentage of acute appendicitis cases have an elevated WBC count?**

An elevated leukocyte count and an elevated absolute neutrophil count are present in 86% and 89% respectively.

METABOLIC AND ENDOCRINE

"Don't confuse me with the facts, Jetson, just get me that cog."

Mr. Spacely (George's boss).

❏❏ **What are the causes of factitious hyponatremia?**

Hyperglycemia, hyperlipidemia, or hyperproteinemia.

❏❏ **How does hyperglycemia lead to hyponatremia?**

Because glucose stays in the extracellular fluid, hyperglycemia draws water out of the cell into the extracellular fluid. Each 100 mg/dL increase in plasma glucose decreases the serum sodium by 1.6 to 1.8 mEq/L.

❏❏ **What is the most common cause of hypovolemic hyponatremia in children?**

Viral gastroenteritis causing vomiting and/or diarrhea.

❏❏ **What is the most common cause of euvolemic hyponatremia in children?**

Syndrome of inappropriate secretion of antidiuretic hormone (SIADH). Causes include CNS disorders, medications, tumors and pulmonary disorders.

❏❏ **What are the signs and symptoms of hyponatremia?**

Weakness, nausea anorexia, vomiting, confusion, lethargy, seizures, and coma.

❏❏ **The most common causes of hypotonic fluid loss leading to hypernatremia are?**

Diarrhea, vomiting, hyperpyrexia, and excessive sweating.

❏❏ **What are the signs and symptoms of hypernatremia?**

Confusion, muscle irritability, seizures, respiratory paralysis, and coma.

❏❏ **What are the ECG findings in a patient with hypokalemia?**

Flattened T-waves, depressed ST segments, prominent P and U waves, and prolonged QT and PR intervals.

❏❏ **What are the ECG findings in a patient with hyperkalemia?**

Peaked T waves, prolonged QT and PR intervals, diminished P waves, depressed T waves, QRS widening, and with levels exceeding 10 mEq/L, a classic sine wave is usually seen.

❏❏ **What is the first ECG finding in a patient with hyperkalemia?**

At levels of 5.6 to 6.0 mEq/L, the development of tall, peaked T waves, best seen in the precordial leads, occur first.

❏❏ **What is the quickest way to treat hyperkalemia?**

Give Calcium gluconate (10%), 10-20 mL, IV with an onset of action of 1-3 min.

❏❏ **What are the causes of hyperkalemia?**

Acidosis, tissue necrosis, hemolysis, blood transfusions, GI bleed, renal failure, Addison's disease, primary hypoaldosteronism, excess po K+ intake, RTA IV, medication (succinylcholine, B-blockers, captopril, spironolactone, triamterene, amiloride, and high dose penicillin).

❏❏ **What are the causes of hypocalcemia?**

Shock, sepsis, multiple blood transfusions, hypoparathyroidism, vitamin D deficiency, pancreatitis, hypomagnesemia, alkalosis, fat embolism syndrome, phosphate overload, chronic renal failure, loop diuretics, hypoalbuminemia, tumor lysis syndrome, and medication (dilantin, phenobarbital, heparin, theophylline, cimetidine, and gentamicin.

❏❏ **What is the most common cause of hyperkalemia?**

Lab error. Chronic renal failure is the most common cause of "true hyperkalemia."

❏❏ **What are the most common causes of hypercalcemia?**

1) Malignancy 2) Primary hyperparathyroidism 3) Thiazide diuretics

❏❏ **What are the signs and symptoms of hypercalcemia?**

A classic mnemonic can be used to remember these:
Stones   renal calculi
Bones   osteolysis
Abdominal groans peptic ulcer disease and pancreatitis
Psychic overtones psychiatric disorders

The most common gastrointestinal symptoms are anorexia and constipation.

❏❏ **What is the initial treatment for hypercalcemia?**

Patients with hypercalcemia are dehydrated because high calcium levels interfere with ADH and the ability of the kidney to concentrate urine. Therefore, the initial treatment is restoration of the extracellular fluid with 5 to 10 L of normal saline in 24 h. Once the patient is rehydrated, give furosemide in doses of 1 to 3 mg/kg.

❏❏ **A patient with a history of alcohol abuse presents after a recent tonic-clonic seizure. Which electrolyte abnormality should be considered and treated during evaluation?**

Malnourished alcoholics are often hypomagnesemic and should be treated with $MgSO_4$ 2 gm IV over 1 h.

❏❏ **What is the most common cause of hyperphosphatemia?**

Acute and chronic renal failure.

❏❏ **What are the two primary causes of primary adrenal insufficiency?**

Tuberculosis and autoimmune destruction account for 90% of cases.

❏❏ **What are the signs and symptoms of primary adrenal insufficiency?**

Fatigue, weakness, weight loss, anorexia, hyperpigmentation, nausea, vomiting, abdominal pain, diarrhea, and orthostatic hypotension.

❑❑ **What are the characteristic lab findings seen with primary adrenal insufficiency?**

Hyperkalemia, hyponatremia, hypoglycemia, azotemia (if volume depletion is present), and a mild metabolic acidosis.

❑❑ **How should acute adrenal insufficiency be treated?**

Hydrocortisone 100 mg IV, and crystalloid fluids containing dextrose.

❑❑ **What are the main causes of death during an adrenal crisis?**

Circulatory collapse and hyperkalemia-induced arrhythmias.

❑❑ **What are the causes of acute adrenal crisis?**

It occurs secondary to a major stress such as surgery, severe injury, myocardial infarction, or any other illness in a patient with primary or secondary adrenal insufficiency.

❑❑ **What is thyrotoxicosis and what are the causes?**

A hypermetabolic state that occurs secondary to excess circulating thyroid hormone caused by thyroid hormone overdose, thyroid hyperfunction, or thyroid inflammation.

❑❑ **What are the hallmark clinical features of myxedema coma?**

Hypothermia (75%) and coma.

❑❑ **What is the most common cause of hypoglycemia seen in the ER.**

Insulin reaction in a diabetic patient.

❑❑ **What is the role of phosphate replacement during the treatment of DKA?**

Phosphate supplementation is not indicated until a serum concentration is below 1.0 mEq/dL.

❑❑ **What is the most important initial step in the treatment of DKA?**

Rapid fluid administration with the first liter given over 30 min to 1 h followed by 3 to 5 liters over the next 3 h.

❑❑ **Why would the nitroprusside test be negative in a patient with alcoholic ketoacidosis?**

This test is used to detect the presence of ketones in the urine and serum. It does not detect ß-hydroxybutyrate which may the predominant ketone in a patient with alcoholic ketoacidosis.

❑❑ **In the first two years of life, what is the most common cause of <u>drug-induced</u> hypoglycemia?**

Salicylates. In the 2-8 y old group, alcohol is the most likely cause, and in the 11 to 30 y old group, insulin and sulfonylureas are the most likely cause.

❑❑ **What is the principle hormone protecting the human body against hypoglycemia?**

Glucagon.

❏❏ What drugs potentiate the hypoglycemic effects of sulfonylurea?

Salicylates, alcohol, sulfonamides, phenylbutazone, and bis-hydroxycoumarin. Chlorpropamide is the sulfonylurea compound most likely to cause hypoglycemic events. It also causes the most prolonged hypoglycemia.

❏❏ How is sulfonylurea-induced hypoglycemia treated?

IV glucose alone may be insufficient. It may require diazoxide 300 mg slow IV over 30 min repeated every four h.

❏❏ What effect does propranolol have on blood sugar in diabetic patients?

Propranolol is thought to precipitate hypoglycemia.

❏❏ What is the most common cause of hypoglycemia in a child?

Ketotic hypoglycemia. Attacks usually occur when the child is stressed with caloric deprivation. Most common in boys, typically between 18 mo and 5 y of age. Attacks may be episodic, vomiting may occur, and are more frequent in the morning or during periods of illness.

❏❏ What are the neurologic signs and symptoms of hypoglycemia?

Hypoglycemia may produce mental and neurologic dysfunction. Neurologic manifestations may include paresthesias, cranial nerve palsies, transient hemiplegia, diplopia, decerebrate posturing, and clonus.

❏❏ What lab findings are expected with diabetic ketoacidosis?

Elevated ß-hydroxybutyrate, acetoacetate, acetone and glucose. Ketonuria and glucosuria are present. Serum bicarbonate level, PCO_2, and pH are decreased. Potassium may be initially elevated but falls if the acidosis is corrected.

❏❏ Outline the basic treatment of DKA.

Fluids, start with normal saline; total deficit may be 5-10 liters. Potassium 100-200 mEq in the first 12-24 h. Insulin 20 unit bolus followed by 5-10 U/h. [Ed. note: many no longer bolus] Add glucose to the IV fluid when glucose levels fall below 250 mg/dl. Phosphate supplement when level drops below 1.0 mg/dl.
Peds : NS 20 ml/kg/h for 1-2 h.
Insulin 0.1 U/kg bolus followed by 0.1 U/kg/h drip.

❏❏ A 42 y old female presents with a history of palpitations, sweating, diplopia, blurred vision, and weakness. The family indicates she has been confused. Symptoms usually occur before breakfast. Diagnosis?

Islet cell tumor of the pancreas can be a cause of a fasting hypoglycemia.

❏❏ What sulfonylurea compound most commonly causes hypoglycemia?

Chlorpropamide.

❏❏ What are the key features of nonketotic hyperosmolar coma?

Hyperosmolality, hyperglycemia, and dehydration. Blood sugar should be greater than 800 mg/dl, serum osmolality should be greater than 350 mOsm/kg, and serum ketones should be negative.

❏❏ What is the treatment of nonketotic hyperosmolar coma?

Fluids (normal saline), potassium 10-20 mEq/h. Insulin 5-10 U/h, and glucose should be added to the IV when the blood sugar drops below 250 mg/dl.

❏❏ **Distinguish between type A and type B lactic acidosis?**

Type A lactic acidosis is often seen in the Emergency Department. It is most commonly due to shock. Type A lactic acidosis is associated with inadequate tissue perfusion and resultant anoxia, with subsequent lactate and hydrogen ion accumulation. Type B lactic acidosis includes all forms of acidosis in which there is no evidence of tissue anoxia.

❏❏ **What are the pathognomonic findings as well as confirmatory lab tests diagnostic of thyroid storm?**

Trick question. Thyroid storm is based on clinical impression. There are no findings or confirmatory tests available.

❏❏ **What is the most common precipitant of thyroid storm?**

Infections, typically pulmonary infections, are the most common precipitating event.

❏❏ **What clinical clues might help in the diagnosis of thyroid storm?**

Eye signs of Graves' disease, a history of hyperthyroidism, widened pulse pressure, and a palpable goiter.

❏❏ **What are the diagnostic criteria for thyroid storm?**

Tachycardia, CNS dysfunction, cardiovascular dysfunction, GI system dysfunction, and temperature greater than 37.8 °C (100 °F).

❏❏ **What are the signs and symptoms of thyroid storm?**

Tachycardia, fever, diaphoresis, increased CNS activity, emotional lability, heart failure, coma, and death.

❏❏ **What are the complications of bicarbonate therapy in DKA?**

Paradoxical CSF acidosis, cardiac arrhythmias, decreased oxygen delivery to tissue, and fluid and sodium overload.

❏❏ **What is the approximate overall mortality of nonketotic hyperosmolar coma?**

Approximately 50%.

❏❏ **What is the most common cause of hypothyroidism?**

Primary thyroid failure. The most common etiology of hypothyroidism in adults is the use of radioactive iodine or subtotal thyroidectomy in the treatment of Graves' disease. The second most common cause is autoimmune thyroid disorders.

❏❏ **In a patient receiving anticoagulation therapy with heparin, when is adrenal hemorrhage most likely to strike?**

Typically between the 3rd and 18th d of anticoagulation. Patients present with sudden hypotension and flank or epigastric pain. Nausea, vomiting, fever, and a change in sensorium may be associated.

❏❏ **What is the most common cause of secondary adrenal insufficiency and adrenal crisis?**

Iatrogenic adrenal suppression from prolonged steroid use. Rapid withdrawal of steroids may lead to collapse and death.

❏❏ An <u>increase</u> of PCO₂ of 10 mmHg will lead to an expected decrease in pH of about:

pH increases 0.08.

❏❏ A <u>decrease</u> of PCO₂ of 10 mm Hg will lead to an expected increase in pH of about:

pH increases 0.13.

❏❏ What is the expected increase in pH associated with a rise in HCO₃ of 5.0 mEq/l?

pH increases 0.08.

❏❏ What is the expected decrease in pH associated with a decrease in HCO₃ of 5.0 mEq/l?

pH decreases 0.10.

❏❏ How is the anion gap calculated from electrolyte values?

Anion gap = Na - Cl - CO₂   The normal gap is 12 ⁺/- 4 mEq/l.

❏❏ Acidosis is closely related to anion gap measurement. Name the causes of an increased anion gap acidosis.

A MUDPILE CAT

A   = alcohol,

M   = methanol,
U   = uremia,
D   = DKA,
P   = paraldehyde,
I   = iron and isoniazid,
L   = lactic acidosis,
E   = ethylene glycol,

C   = carbon monoxide,
A   = aspirin,
T   = toluene.

❏❏ That's a pretty big differential. History and physical can go a long way in narrowing this list down. The magnitude of the anion gap can also be useful; discuss.

Anion gap > 35 mEq/l is usually caused by ethylene glycol, methanol or lactic acidosis.
Anion gap 23 - 30 mEq/l usually also because of increased organic acids.
Anion gap 16 - 22 mEq/l may be due to uremia, which must be quite advanced before it causes an increased gap.

❏❏ There is another "gap" that can aid in diagnosing the cause of an anion gap acidosis - the osmolar gap. Let's distract ourselves for a momentary discussion of the osmolar gap and how it may be useful.

Uh-oh. Osmolality is a measure of the concentration of particles in a solution, its units are osmoles per kg water. Osmolarity is a measure of osmoles per liter of solution - for dilute solutions, like body fluids, these two measures are roughly equivalent. An osmolar gap is a difference between measured osmolality and calculated osmolarity. The osmolar gap is calculated as follows:
    Measured osmolality - calculated osmolarity = osmolar gap.

$$CalculatedOsmol(mOsm/l) = 2(Na) + \frac{glucose}{18} + \frac{BUN}{2.8}$$

(Normal = 275 - 285 mOsm/l)

❏❏ **Different substances contribute to varying degrees to the osmolar gap, these are listed below:**

Substance	mg/dl to increase serum osmol 1 mOsm/l	# mOsm/l increase due to each mg/dl
Methanol	2.6	0.38
Ethanol	4.3	0.23
Ethylene glycol	5.0	0.20
Acetone	5.5	0.18
Isopropyl alcohol	5.9	0.17
Salicylate	14.0	0.07

Thus, small amounts of methanol cause greater increases in osmolality. Large amounts of salicylate will eventually increase osmolar gap.

Note also that the contribution to an osmolar gap due to EtOH may be calculated; this can be useful in when a mixed alcohol ingestion is suspected (and your IM colleagues in the ED will be impressed!).

❏❏ **O.K., with that distraction now behind us, review some other pearls that can help narrow the d/dx of an anion gap acidosis.**

Methanol- visual disturbances and headache common. Can produce quite wide gaps as discussed above.

Uremia- advanced before it causes an anion gap.

Diabetic Ketoacidosis- usually has both hyperglycemia and glucosuria.

Alcoholic Ketoacidosis (AKA)- often has a lower blood sugar and mild or absent glucosuria.

Salicylates- high levels required to contribute to gap.

Lactic Acidosis- can check serum level. Itself has broad differential to be discussed in a question in the random section.

Ethylene glycol- causes calcium oxalate or hippurate crystals in urine.

❏❏ **What are the causes of the oxygen saturation curve shift to the right?**

A shift to the right delivers more O_2 to the tissue.
Right = Release to tissues.

"CADET! Right face!!"

Hyper	Carbia,
	Acidemia,
2,3	DPG,
	Exercise,
increased	Temperature.

The mnemonic CADET helps in remembering causes of an O_2 shift to the right.

❏❏ **When body waste materials (urine & stool) are enterally recycled, they can cause a** normal anion gap **metabolic acidosis. Thus, USED CRAP** does **in fact cause a normal anion gap (hyperchloremic) metabolic acidosis; discuss.**

U = ureteroenterostomy
S = small bowel fistula
E = extra chloride (NH_4Cl or amino acid chlorides 2° TPN)
D = diarrhea

C   = carbonic anhydrase inhibitors
R   = renal tubular acidosis
A   = adrenal insufficiency
P   = pancreatic fistula

❏❏ **What are the two primary causes of metabolic alkalosis?**

Loss of hydrogen and chloride from the stomach.
Overzealous diuresis with loss of hydrogen, potassium and chloride.

❏❏ **What is central pontine myelinolysis, a.k.a. osmotic demyelination syndrome?**

The complication of brain dehydration following too rapid correction of severe hyponatremia. Correct hyponatremia slowly, less than 12 mEq/d in chronic hyponatremia.

PEDI PEARLS

"Somebody BOUNCED me. I was just thinking by the side of the river...when I received a loud BOUNCE."

Eeyore

❏❏ **What is the normal pulse rate of a newborn?**

 120 - 160 bpm.

❏❏ **External chest compressions should be initiated for a newborn with assisted ventilation who has a heart rate less than _____ beats per minute.**

 50 bpm.

❏❏ **Outline the Apgar scoring system.**

Index	0 points	1 point	2 points
Pulse	Ø	< 100	> 100
Resp. effort	Ø	Weak cry	Strong cry
Color	Cyanotic	Extremities cyanotic	Pink
Tone	Flaccid	Weak tone	Strong
Response	Ø	Motion	Cry

❏❏ **A normal appearing term neonate presents with tachypnea and cyanosis. Likely pathology?**

 Congenital cardiac pathology.
 CHF can be presenting symptomatology for VSD, severe aortic coarctation or transposition of the great vessels.
 The "hyperoxia" test may help differentiate cardiac etiology - Place the infant in 100% O_2, the PaO_2 will increase less than 20 mmHg with right to left shunting of cardiac decrease.

❏❏ **Stridor in the neonate is usually caused by congenital anomalies. Is infection also a common cause of neonatal stridor?**

 No.

❏❏ **What is the <u>most common</u> cause of neonatal stridor?**

 Laryngotracheomalacia.

❏❏ **Can the type of stridor localize the level of the obstruction?**

 Yes, Inspiratory stridor points to a site of obstruction above the vocal folds while expiratory stridor points to obstruction below the vocal folds .

❏❏ **Define apnea.**

 No respiration for > 20 s.

❏❏ **Does apnea always indicate a serious problem and require admission?**

True apnea represents serious pathology and always merits immediate appropriate intervention and admission.

❏❏ **Physiologic jaundice occurs at about 2-4 d. How high may the bilirubin level be expected to climb?**

5-6 mg/dl.

❏❏ **A neonate presents with a history of poor feeding, vomiting, respiratory distress, has abdominal distention and is found to have hyperbilirubinemia. What is the likely cause of this complex?**

This neonate is septic!

❏❏ **Name some causes of jaundice occurring at age less than 1 d.**

Sepsis, congenital infections, ABO/Rh incompatibility.

❏❏ **Jaundice due to breast feeding occurs after 7 d and can reach very high levels over weeks; how high?**

Levels of bilirubin near 25 mg/dl can be reached.

❏❏ **Which type of jaundice causes some of the highest levels of bilirubin elevation?**

A-O incompatibility

❏❏ **A cyanotic infant's SaO_2 & PaO_2 do not increase with oxygen therapy. What cause does this suggest?**

Intracardiac (right to left) shunting, not pulmonary disease.

❏❏ **Do not skip to the answer to this question, make a real attempt to answer it - Name 8 clinical presentations of pediatric heart disease.**

1. Cyanosis
2. CHF
3. Pathologic murmur
4. Cardiogenic shock
5. HTN
6. Tachyarrhythmias
7. Abnormal pulses
8. Syncope

❏❏ **Tetralogy of Fallot (TOF) consists of VSD, an "overriding" aorta, pulmonary stenosis and right ventricular hypertrophy. What type of intracardiac shunting occurs?**

Right-to-left shunting whose severity is related to the degree of pulmonary stenosis.

❏❏ **Describe the murmurs of TOF.**

1. Holosystolic murmur of VSD - 3rd ICS @ LSB.
2. Crescendo-decrescendo murmur of pulmonary stenosis - 2nd ICS @ LSB.

N.B. - If you can differentiate these two murmurs in a sick cyanotic infant in a busy ED, go directly to Pediatric Cardiology, do not Pass Go, do not collect $200.

❏❏ **True or False. During childhood symptoms of aortic stenosis are common?**

False, even if severe the left ventricle has the ability to hypertrophy in childhood compensating for many years.

❏❏ **What common physical diagnostic sign in seen in a childhood atrial septal defect?**

A fixed split of S-2 on deep inspiration.

❑❑ **What x-ray findings are often seen in coarctation of the aorta?**

The "3" sign made up of the aortic knob and the dilated post coarctation segment of the descending aorta. The "E" sign is the same thing seen in a negative image on barium esophagram.

❑❑ **Describe the three aspects of acute treatment of TOF.**

Positioning -	Place in knee-chest position. Keep patient unstimulated (i.e., upright on lap in parent's arms).
Oxygenation -	Deliver high FIO_2.
Pharmacologic -	Morphine 0.1 mg/kg or propranolol 0.1 mg/kg

❑❑ **Name three congenital heart lesions with a RIGHT sided aortic arch?.**

Truncus arteriosus, Transposition of the Great Vessels, Tetralogy of Fallot and Tricuspid Atresia

❑❑ **SVT in adults usually occurs with a ventricular rate of about 150 - 200. What is the range of ventricular rates in children?**

220 - 360 bpm.

❑❑ **What is the dose of adenosine given to a pediatric patient with SVT?**

0.1 mg/kg.

❑❑ **Verapamil should not be used to treat infants of less than what age?**

Do not use verapamil in infants less than two years of age (can lead to asystole).

❑❑ **If cardioversion is necessary to treat an infant with unstable SVT, what is the appropriate energy to use?**

0.25 - 1 J/kg.

❑❑ **Differentiate sepsis from bacteremia.**

Bacteremia is the symptom of fever with a positive blood culture; sepsis is bacteremia with focal findings identified.

❑❑ **What are the two <u>most common</u> organisms causing bacteremia in <u>unimmunized</u> children?**

S. pneumoniae, N. meningitidis and H. influenzae.

❑❑ **What are the two <u>most common</u> organisms causing bacteremia in <u>immunized</u> children?**

S. pneumoniae and N. meningitidis.

❑❑ **What are the two <u>most common</u> organisms causing sepsis in the neonate?**

Group B streptococcus and E. coli.

❑❑ **What are the three <u>most common</u> organisms causing sepsis after the newborn period?**

H. influenzae, N. meningitidis and S. pneumoniae.

❑❑ **There is much controversy surrounding the question of when to check a WBC in a pediatric patient with suspected bacteremia and if results of this test should be used to decide whether or not to draw a blood culture or decide to initiate treatment with antibiotics. What is the current recommendation of when to draw a WBC for suspected bacteremia (Tintinalli, 4th Ed.)?**

Draw a WBC for patients 3 mo to 2 y old with temperature > 39.4 °C (102.9 °F) and no clear source. Draw a WBC for patients 3 mo to 2 y old who appear toxic with fever < 39.4 °C.

❑❑ **What is the current recommendation, from the same source, of what level of WBC and absolute polymorphonuclear cell count should then lead to drawing blood for culture?**

WBC > 15,000/mm^3 or absolute polymorphonuclear cell count > 9,000/mm^3 should lead to drawing blood for culture.

N.B. Answers to these two questions are controversial and some sources indicate that greater than 20,000/mm^3 should be used.

❑❑ **A septic pediatric patient is in shock. An initial bolus of normal saline at 20 ml/kg has been given. Urine output should be maintained at what level by delivery of appropriate fluid?**

1-2 ml/kg/h.

❑❑ **What is the appropriate dose of diazepam to be administered to a seizing pediatric patient with suspected meningitis?**

0.3 mg/kg. Load with phenytoin or phenobarbital after termination of seizure activity.

❑❑ **Many authors believe in giving methylprednisolone to pediatric patients with meningitis to decrease sequelae, especially deafness. What is the appropriate dose of methylprednisolone in meningitis?**

30 mg/kg.

❑❑ **What are the two most common organisms causing meningitis in the first month of life?**

Group B streptococci and E. coli.

❑❑ **Describe antibiotic selection to treat meningitis in patients aged < 1 mo.**

Use ampicillin or cefotaxime plus an aminoglycoside*.

❑❑ **What is the most common organism causing meningitis after the second month of life?**

H. influenzae.

❑❑ **Describe antibiotic selection to treat meningitis in patients aged > 1 mo.**

Ceftriaxone

This change in antibiotic choice is due to the increasing rate of H. influenzae as the causative organism during the second mo of life and the resistance of some of these organisms.

*N.B. Answers to above 2 questions on antibiotic choices based on information from Tintinalli, 4th Ed.

❑❑ **What percentage of children with asthma are likely to have symptoms that persist into adulthood?**

50%.

❑❑ **What is the most common cause of bronchiolitis?**

RSV.

❑❑ **What is the most common organism causing epiglottitis?**

H. influenzae.

❑❑ **What is the usual age range for presentation of retropharyngeal abscess?**

6 mo - 3 y.

❑❑ **Surprisingly, extrinsic asthma is the <u>most common</u> form in children. Does extrinsic asthma involve IgE production?**

Yes, extrinsic asthma involves IgE production in response to allergens.

❑❑ **Current recommendations include obtaining a CXR on all pediatric patients with first presentation of symptoms of reactive airway disease or asthma who are less than one y of age. Name some of the etiologies of these symptoms that may be discovered by CXR.**

Foreign body aspiration, bronchiolitis, parenchymal pulmonary disease and heart disease.

❑❑ **What is the common age range for bronchiolitis?**

Though it may occur in patients up to age 2 y, bronchiolitis commonly occurs between ages 2 - 6 months of age as maternal antibody to RSV is waning.

❑❑ **Sympathomimetic agents are used to treat asthma. What enzyme is activated by these agents?**

Adenyl cyclase.

❑❑ **What reaction is catalyzed by adenyl cyclase?**

Adenyl cyclase catalyzes ATP to cyclic AMP.

❑❑ **What effect does increased levels of cyclic AMP have on bronchial smooth muscle and on the release of chemical mediators (histamine, proteases, platelet activation factor and chemotactic factors) from airway mast cells?**

Smooth muscle relaxation and decreased release of mediators.

Recall that the effects of cyclic AMP are opposed by cyclic GMP - this provides another treatment approach by *decreasing* levels of cyclic GMP which is achieved via anticholinergic (antimuscarinic) agents such as ipratropium bromide.

❑❑ **As discussed above, stimulation of ß-adrenergic receptors increases cyclic AMP availability and results in smooth muscle relaxation. Which flavor of ß-adrenergic receptors primarily control bronchiolar and arterial smooth muscle tone?**

ß$_2$-adrenergic receptors.

❑❑ **What is current understanding of the mechanism of action of the methylxanthines?**

The mechanism of action of these agents is not known.

❑❑ **Pediatric patients presenting with severe asthma may be treated with "high-dose" albuterol. What dose of nebulized albuterol is considered "high-dose," and how frequently may it be given?**

<u>0.15 mg/kg</u> (0.03 ml/kg of 0.5%) per dose to a maximum of 5 mg may be provided every 20 min up to six times.

❏❏ **How may albuterol dosing be changed if the patient has not responded to the above 6 doses?**

Consider switching to continuous delivery of albuterol nebulized at 0.5 mg/kg/h up to a rate of 15 mg/h. Monitor heart rate.

❏❏ **What makes albuterol the usual agent of choice?**

Of nebulized ß-adrenergic agonists it has the longest duration of action and the greatest degree of $ß_2$-adrenergic selectivity.

❏❏ **Terbutaline is given SQ for asthma in what dose?**

0.01 ml/kg (of 1 mg/ml) up to 0.25 ml (0.25 mg) which may be repeated once in 20-30 minutes.

❏❏ **Is theophylline of use in the emergency management of severe asthma in pediatric patients?**

No. It has not been shown to cause further bronchodilatation in patients fully treated with ß-adrenergic agents. Theophylline does have a role in inpatient management of asthma and may be started in the ED.

❏❏ **If corticosteroids are given, how should prednisone be dosed?**

1 - 2 mg/kg/d in two divided doses; no tapering is necessary if duration of therapy is 5 d or less.

❏❏ **What effect can acidosis have on treatment with ß-adrenergic agonists?**

Decreased efficacy.

❏❏ **What percentage of aminophylline is theophylline?**

85%.

❏❏ **If one prefers the most simplified algorithm for determining loading dose of theophylline, what are the appropriate doses for:**
  a. A patient who has not taken any theophylline recently,
  b. A patient who has taken a recent theophylline dose?

a. No recent dose - load with 7 mg/kg theophylline.
b. Recent dose - load with 5 mg/kg theophylline.

❏❏ **What is the appropriate parenteral dose of methylprednisolone (Solu-Medrol) to give a pediatric patient with status asthmaticus?**

1 - 2 mg/kg every 6 h.

❏❏ **If mechanical ventilation is required for such a patient, what is an appropriate setting for initial tidal volume?**

10 ml/kg.

❏❏ **Parents of a child who has suffered a febrile seizure often want to know what the risk of a recurrence is. What is it?**

Risk of recurrence is the chance that the same thing will happen again.
About 35%.

❏❏ **Is LP usually an appropriate component of the evaluation of a first febrile seizure?**

Yes. Many clinicians prefer LP in this situation only if a prolonged postictal period or clinical symptoms such as lethargy are present.

❑❑ **Treatment of febrile seizures is primarily directed at gradual cooling and treatment for the source of the fever. If anticonvulsant therapy is begun, which medication is best?**

Diazepam because its pharmacokinetics are such that it is not dependent upon serum concentrations and is therefore more efficacious.

❑❑ **Phenobarbital is also the drug of choice in neonatal seizures. Its half-life in children over one mo of age is about 65 h. The half-life is even longer in newborns up to one week of age. How long is it in this age group?**

100 h.

❑❑ **Neonatal seizures have a broad range of presentations. What are the two frequent causes of myoclonic seizures?**

Metabolic disorders and hypoxia.

❑❑ **The initial treatment of neonatal seizures is directed initially at reversible causes; insure adequate oxygenation, provide pyridoxine (B_6), glucose, calcium and magnesium. Following these measures, pharmacologic intervention can be considered. Outline this treatment.**

Phenobarbital load, 10 - 15 mg/kg IV.
Phenytoin load, 10 - 15 mg/kg IV.
Diazepam, 0.2 mg/kg IV, may repeat.
Lorazepam, 0.05 mg/kg IV, may repeat.
Clonazepam, 0.1 mg/kg NG.

❑❑ **Infantile spasms are usually first noted in children of about 6 months of age. Is it true that these patients have a high rate of developmental disorders, and if so, what percentage of patients have such disorders?**

Yes, it is true; 85%.

❑❑ **Are infantile spasms a form of seizures?**

Yes.

❑❑ **Infantile spasms represent a significant disorder and require aggressive evaluation and management. In addition to anticonvulsants, what hormone plays a role in management of infantile spasms?**

Adrenocorticotropic hormone (ACTH).

❑❑ **Febrile seizures occur relatively commonly; about what percentage of children will experience such a seizure?**

3.5%; about 35% of these patients will experience a recurrence.

❑❑ **Phenobarbital is probably the most efficacious drug used to treat febrile seizures. Should all patients with a febrile seizure receive phenobarbital as prophylaxis against future similar seizures?**

Probably not, though its use may be warranted in patients who are particularly ill, who have had repeated febrile seizures or who have underlying neurologic disease.

❑❑ **Posttraumatic seizures that occur immediately are associated with a very low rate of subsequent epilepsy. About what are the rates of subsequent epilepsy in patients suffering early (within 1 wk) and late (after 1 wk) posttraumatic seizures?**

Early ≈ 25%.
Late ≈ 70%.

❏❏ **For how long must a continuous seizure last to be defined as status epilepticus?**

30 min.

❏❏ **You appropriately elect to administer diazepam to a patient in "status" at a loading dose of 0.3 mg/kg and a rate of 1 mg/min. This dose should be repeated prn up to a total of how many mg/kg?**

2.6 mg/kg maximum dose of diazepam.

❏❏ **The diazepam given above does not break the seizure and phenytoin is appropriately selected as the next agent. Dose and rate of administration?**

Phenytoin load 15 mg/kg at 25 mg/min (cf. adults ≈ 17 mg/kg @ 50 mg/min!).

❏❏ **Your patient is _still_ seizing!@#! What is the dose of phenobarbital to load?**

10 - 15 mg/kg.

❏❏ **The seizure has stopped! What three alternative treatments remained?**

Paraldehyde, lidocaine and general anesthesia.

❏❏ **Hepatic failure is associated with which anticonvulsant?**

Valproic acid.

❏❏ **What antibiotic can cause carbamazepine to accumulate quickly?**

Erythromycin.

❏❏ **Bronchopulmonary dysplasia (BPD) is commonly caused by hyaline membrane disease, prematurity and/or mechanical ventilation. BPD is treated with O_2, hydration and time. Describe the clinical features of BPD.**

Tachypnea, reactive airways, hypoxia, and hypercarbia, on occasion with pulmonary edema and cor pulmonale.

❏❏ **Patients with BPD may have chronic hypercarbia; does administering O_2 blunt respiratory drive in such patients?**

No.

❏❏ **A youngster presents with signs and symptoms that suggest a pneumonia. She describes chest pain that is pleuritic. Is such pain more commonly associated with viral or with bacterial pneumonia?**

Bacterial.

Strep. pneumoniae in particular is the most common cause in this age group, and is often associated with pleuritic pain and a pleural effusion.

❏❏ **The spectrum of likely etiology of a pneumonia changes with patient age. What are likely agents causing pneumonia in neonates?**

Bacterial -
    Group B streptococci (Lancefield group B, mostly S. agalactiae).
    Listeria monocytogenes.
    Enteric Gram negative bacilli.
Chlamydia.
Viral -

Rubella.
CMV.
Herpes.

❑❑ **A neonate presents at 2 wk of age febrile with tachypnea and a history of poor feeding. Your suspicion of a pneumonia is confirmed by a CXR revealing diffuse homogenous infiltrates. You correctly presume a bacterial origin, likely with group B Strep., given the young age and fever (Chlamydia usually presents between about 4 - 10 wk and afebrile, RSV presents between 1 - 6 mo). Though group B Strep. is always susceptible to penicillin G, you are aware that some strains require higher doses of penicillin G and that other less common causes still need to be considered, such as Listeria monocytogenes and Gram negative enteric bacteria. Thus you wish to add a second agent to this patient's treatment, one that is synergistic with penicillin G and will help cover these pathogens. Treat with:**

Penicillin G and gentamycin.

❑❑ **Causes of pneumonia in patients aged 1 mo to 5 y?**

Bacterial - Streptococcus pneumonia and Hemophilus influenzae.
Viral - RSV, parainfluenza, adenovirus. RSV occurs primarily in patients less than 6 mo of age.

❑❑ **Hemophilus influenzae is the second most common cause of pediatric pneumonia; what percentage of cases of H. influenzae occur in patients of less than 1 y of age?**

50%, half of remaining cases occur between ages 1 - 2 y.
H. influenzae pneumonia is common primarily in young infants.

❑❑ **Causes of pneumonia in patients greater than 6 y old?**

Strep. pneumonia, Mycoplasma pneumoniae parainfluenzae virus and influenza virus.

❑❑ **Mycoplasma pneumoniae is the most common cause of non viral pneumonia in children greater than 6 y old. Contrast pneumonia due to Mycoplasma with that due to Strep. pneumoniae.**

Characteristic	S. pneumoniae	M. pneumoniae
Prodrome	Little	Mild fever, malaise, cough, HA.
Onset	Rapid	Gradual
URI sx	Tachypnea, cough, occasional pleuritic pain.	Little
Associated findings	High fever.	Exanthem, arthritis, GI complaints, neurologic complications.
Pleural effusion	Occasional	Rare
Lab	Leukocytosis	WBC normal or sl. elevation.
Tx	Penicillin	Erythromycin

❑❑ **What are the three stages of pertussis?**

Catarrhal stage - rhinorrhea, cough, conjunctivitis.
Paroxysmal stage - after 1 wk of above, paroxysms of continuous coughing. Lasts up to 6 wk.
Convalescent stage - Coughing decreases. (NSS).

Dangerous pneumonias are usually superinfections; treat patient and household contacts with erythromycin (provide broader coverage if pneumonia present), immunize household contacts who are less than 7 y old.

❑❑ SIDS is the <u>most common</u> cause of death of infants between 1 mo and 1 y of age (incidence 2 per 1000 = 10,000/y). What are the four risk factors that increase an infant's risk of SIDS?

Prematurity with low birth weight.
Previous episode of apnea or apparent life threatening event (ALTE).
Mother is a substance abuser.
Sibling of infant who died of SIDS.

❑❑ SIDS has a bimodal distribution. At what ages do the peaks occur?

2.5 & 4 mo.

❑❑ What is the <u>most common</u> cause of neonatal conjunctivitis?

A trick question, as chemical conjunctivitis due to silver nitrate is most common. Chlamydia trachomatis is the <u>most common</u> clinically significant cause in the first 14 d with a usual incubation period of at least 5 d. Gonococcal conjunctivitis has a shorter incubation and may present as soon as 2 d.

❑❑ What is the name of the condition of fluid collected in the middle ear that is usually painless, is without sign of infection and that may result in a hearing deficit?

Serous otitis media, aka otitis media with effusion (OME). An underused diagnosis.

❑❑ Which type of agent is the most common cause of acute otitis media (AOM), found in about 70% of cases, bacteria or viruses?

Bacteria, most commonly S. pneumoniae and H. influenzae.

❑❑ How useful is the light reflex in evaluation of suspected AOM?

It is useless. TM mobility is very valuable.

❑❑ Describe the use of topical steroids, midazolam, antihistamines or decongestants in the management of AOM.

All these agents are of no use in AOM. Antihistamines may decrease Kleenex® use.

❑❑ What solution is appropriate treatment of otitis externa?

Acetic acid ear drops. Treat for ≥ 7 d.

❑❑ Among pediatric emergency patients, what is the <u>most common</u> skin infection?

Nonbullous Impetigo caused by group A, β-hemolytic streptococcus.
Impetigo is a bacterial infection of the dermis, most commonly caused by group A ß-hemolytic streptococcus; it comes in two flavors - impetigo contagiosa and the bullous form.

❑❑ What is the recommended treatment for impetigo?

Erythromycin, 50 mg/kg/d.
Some authors recommend penicillin.
Dicloxacillin and cephalexin in the same dose as erythromycin and topical mupirocin may also be used.

❑❑ What is the recommended treatment for bullous impetigo?

Dicloxacillin and cephalexin in the same dose as erythromycin above since the most common organism causing this type of infection is Staphylococcus aureus.

❏❏ **Impetigo is the most common skin infection affecting children presenting to the emergency department. Honey-colored serous fluid from ruptured vesicles and similarly colored crusts are typical. Erysipelas (St. Anthony's fire) is another pediatric exanthem that represents a primary bacterial infection. What organism causes this uncommon cellulitis that is usually characterized by pain at the affected site, malaise and fever?**

   Erysipelas is also caused by group A, ß-hemolytic streptococci.
   Penicillin or, in penicillin allergic patients, erythromycin usually cause rapid improvement.
   Recurrences are common and can lead to irreversible lymphedema (termed elephantiasis nostras).

❏❏ **"Strawberry tongue" is a physical finding associated with what systemic bacterial infection also caused primarily by group A, ß-hemolytic streptococci?**

   Scarlet fever. Also seek characteristic Pastia's lines found in the antecubital area.
   Recall the scarlet rash that spares the perioral area usually has onset 1 - 2 d after high fever, sore throat, headache and occasional vomiting and abdominal pain.
   Mucocutaneous lymph node syndrome (Kawasaki disease), a disorder of unclear etiology, may also present with this finding.

❏❏ **Speaking of rashes...Dermacentor andersoni is a vector for Rickettsia rickettsii which cause Rocky Mountain spotted fever. The rash of RMSF usually begins on the wrists and ankles and spreads centripetally. What is the underlying pathologic lesion that causes the serious sequelae of this disease, as well as the hemorrhagic rash?**

   Vasculitis 2° to rickettsial invasion of endothelial cells in small blood vessels, including arterioles.

❏❏ **Cellulitis in childhood is <u>most common</u>ly caused by S. aureus. The *least common* causative organism is responsible for most of the dangerous forms of this disease - striking younger children in more dangerous locations (e.g.. periorbital cellulitis), causing fever and bacteremia. What is the *least common* cause (overall) of pediatric cellulitis?**

   H. influenzae.

❏❏ **A pediatric patient presents with cellulitis. As this patient does not have a violaceous lesion, nor a fever, nor a markedly elevated WBC, H. influenzae is not considered likely and discharge is planned. What antibiotic selection is appropriate in such a case?**

   Dicloxacillin or cephalexin.

❏❏ **H. influenzae is the <u>most common</u> cause of periorbital cellulitis. What is the <u>most common</u> cause of *orbital* cellulitis?**

   S. aureus.

❏❏ **Group A ß-hemolytic streptococcus is the most common cause of pharyngitis in older children. About what percentage of such patients with pharyngitis will have GAßHS?**

   ≈ 50 %.

❏❏ **T/F - GAßHS is a *frequent* cause of pharyngitis in patients less than 3 y of age.**

   False.

❏❏ **We all know that the streptococcal antigen sampling tests for pharyngitis have a high false-negative rate (sensitivity variable, generally > 50%). What is the false-negative rate for a single throat culture?**

   ≈ 10 %.

❏❏ **For how long should a school-age child receive antibiotic treatment for GAßHS before being allowed to return to school?**

1 d.

❑❑ **Rheumatic fever is preventable if antibiotic therapy is begun prior to how many days after the start of GAßHS?**

9 d.

❑❑ **Poststreptococcal glomerulonephritis is preventable if antibiotic therapy is begun prior to how many days after the start of GAßHS?**

TRICK QUESTION! Poststreptococcal glomerulonephritis is not an infectious complication of GAßHS and is not preventable with antibiotic therapy.

❑❑ **What are the characteristic findings in measles?**

The three "C's", cough, coryza and conjunctivitis in addition to the characteristic morbilliform rash that begins on the head and spreads downward.

❑❑ **What is the maximum dose of lidocaine for infiltration, a.) without epi and b.) with epi?**

a.) 5 mg/kg without epinephrine.
b.) 7 mg/kg with epinephrine.

❑❑ **Midazolam (Versed) may be given IV, IM, PO, PR and intranasally. The usual IV or IM dose is 0.15 mg/kg. What is a usual PR dose?**

0.25 mg/kg.

❑❑ **A child presents in DKA. On average, how dehydrated is this patient likely to be (give answer in ml/kg)?**

≈ 125 ml/kg average fluid volume deficit.

❑❑ **You are managing a child in DKA. After initial 20 ml/kg bolus with 0.9% NS and careful fluid replacement with 0.45% NS for maintenance and replacement you are considering switching to D$_5$ 0.45% NS. At about what glucose level should this change in fluid selection occur?**

250 mg/dl.

❑❑ **What is the dose of insulin to be used for low-dose continuous infusion therapy?**

0.1 unit/kg/h of regular insulin.

❑❑ **Insulin is usually mixed in NS at 1 unit/5 ml NS. How much of this fluid should be run through the tubing to saturate binding sites in the plastic?**

50 ml = 10 units!

❑❑ **A child known to have IDDM presents unconscious. What is the correct amount of D$_{50}$W (expressed in ml/kg) to administer to this patient?**

0.5 ml/kg.

❑❑ **You have given the dose of medication from the previous question with no real improvement after 5 min. Now what should you do?**

Try to sit tight, clinical response to glucose often takes 10 min. Use the time to think of other causes in this patient's d/dx, including sepsis, meningitis, metabolic abnormalities, poisoning, head injury, postictal state.

❏❏ **Is intestinal intussusception associated with GI bleeding?**

Yes, though the classic history of sudden onset of severe pain that often is relieved as quickly as it arose and is recurrent is more sensitive. The currant jelly stool associated with this disorder is present in about half of cases.

❏❏ **About how old is the average patient presenting with intussusception?**

One year, +/- 6 mo.

❏❏ **Pyloric stenosis usually presents at about what age?**

4 wk.

❏❏ **What is the eponym for congenital aganglionic megacolon (the disease in which a portion of the distal colon lacks ganglion cells impairing the normal inhibitory innervation in the myenteric plexus impairing coordinated relaxation which can in turn cause clinical symptoms of obstruction, and that presents 85% of the time after the newborn period)?**

Hirschsprung's disease.

❏❏ **Acute enterocolitis with development of "toxic" megacolon is the life-threatening complication of Hirschsprung's disease. Between what range of ages does this complication most frequently present?**

2 - 3 mo.

❏❏ **What signs and symptoms are associated with increased probability of a bacterial pathogen causing diarrhea?**

Fever, acute onset of multiple diarrhea stools/day and blood in the stool.

❏❏ **T/F - Antibiotic therapy for gastroenteritis is limited in utility to children with high or prolonged fevers, those with inflammatory cells present in stool, those with protracted diarrhea and infants of less than 6 mo of age.**

True.

❏❏ **Among infants less than 3 mo of age, are UTI's more common in males or in females?**

Males.

❏❏ **Dysuria among female pediatric patients; more common cause - vulvovaginitis or UTI?**

Vulvovaginitis.
Maternally acquired - Candida, Trichomonas, condyloma.
Prepubertal -
    No cause determined (most common).
    Enterobius vermicularis, characterized by nocturnal pruritus.
    Candida, associated with antibiotics, IDDM.
    Foreign body.
    STDs - suggests sexual contact.

❏❏ **About what percentage of injuries in children less than 5 y of age seen in the ED are due to child abuse?**

10%.

❏❏ **Of abused children seen in the ED, about what percentage will be killed by future abuse?**

5%.

What is the most concerning aspect of the definition of Reye's syndrome provided by the CDC?

Two of the criteria required may be determined at autopsy. Mortality is about 25% or less overall and varies with age of patient and clinical stage. The underlying abnormality is one of mitochondrial morphology and function, affecting primarily brain and liver.

Signs and symptoms of Reye's syndrome:

Patient age usually between ages 6 - 11 y with prior viral illness, possible use of ASA, followed by intractable vomiting. Patient may present irritable, combative, or lethargic, and may c/o right upper quadrant tenderness. Seizures may occur, check for papilledema.
Lab findings would include hypoglycemia, and an elevated ammonia level greater than 20 times normal. Bilirubin level is NORMAL.

Describe stage I and stage II of Reye's syndrome.

Stage I -   Vomiting, lethargy and liver dysfunction.
Stage II -   Disorientation, combativeness, delirium, hyperventilation, increased deep tendon reflexes, liver dysfunction, hyperexcitable, tachypnea, fever, tachycardia, sweating and pupillary dilatation.

Treatment of stages I and II?

Supportive.

Describe Stages III, IV, and V of Reye's syndrome.

Stage III -   coma, decorticate rigidity, increased respiratory rate, mortality rate of 50%.
Stage IV -   coma, decerebrate posturing, no ocular reflexes, loss of corneal reflexes, and   liver damage.
Stage V -   loss of DTRs, seizures, flaccid, respiratory arrest, 95% mortality.

Treatment for advanced stages of Reye's syndrome?

Manage ICP - elevate HOB, paralyze, intubate and hyperventilate, furosemide, mannitol, dexamethasone, pentobarbital coma.
Also consider hypertonic glucose and bowel sterilization.

NEURON PEARLS

"Examinations are formidable even to the best prepared, for the greatest fool may ask more than the wisest man can answer."
Unknown

❏❏ **A patient opens his eyes to voice, makes incomprehensible sounds, and withdraws to painful stimulus. What is his GCS?**

9.

❏❏ **What area of the brain is dysfunctional when a patient has Cheyne-Stokes respirations?**

The cortex - the nervous system is relying on diencephalic control.

❏❏ **What is the classic EEG finding associated with petite mal seizures?**

3/second spike and wave pattern.

❏❏ **A patient has an irritative lesion in the left hemisphere. Which way do his eyes deviate?**

To the right.

❏❏ **What motor deficit is seen with an anterior cerebral artery infarct?**

Leg weakness greater than arm weakness on the contralateral side.

❏❏ **What signs are seen in a middle cerebral artery stroke?**

1) Contralateral sensory/motor deficits;
2) Arm/ face weakness greater than leg weakness.

❏❏ **What is the most common neurologic findings in adult botulism?**

Eye and bulbar muscle deficit.

❏❏ **What is the typical presentation of Guillain-Barré syndrome?**

Ascending motor neuron involvement.

❏❏ **What is the most common medication associated with Neuroleptic Malignant Syndrome?**

Haloperidol. Other drugs antipsychotic medications are also causative.

❏❏ **What is the hallmark motor finding in Neuroleptic Malignant Syndrome?**

"Lead-pipe" rigidity.

❏❏ **What neoplastic process is most commonly associated with myasthenia gravis?**

Thymoma.

❏❏ **What is the definition of status epilepticus?**

Continuous seizure activity for greater than 30 min or two or more seizures which occur without full recovery of consciousness between attacks.

❏❏ **What is the significance of bilateral nystagmus with cold caloric testing?**

It signifies that an intact cortex, midbrain, and brainstem are present.

❏❏ **How can upper motor neuron (UMN) lesions of CN VII (facial nerve) be distinguished from peripheral lesions?**

UMN - Unilateral weakness of the lower half of the face.
Peripheral - Involve entire half of the face.

❏❏ **A 35 y old woman with a history of flu like symptoms (URI) one wk ago now presents with vertigo, nausea, and vomiting. No auditory impairment or focal deficits are noted. What is the most likely cause of her problem?**

Labyrinthitis or vestibular neuronitis.

❏❏ **A patient presents with facial droop on the left and weakness of the right leg. What is the most likely site of the lesion?**

Brainstem, specifically the left pons.

❏❏ **A 30 y old presents with progressively severe intermittent vertigo for six mo and progressive unilateral hearing loss for 3 mo. Diagnosis?**

Cerebellopontine angle tumor. Confirm diagnosis with MRI scan.

❏❏ **Describe the key signs and symptoms of classic, common, cluster, ophthalmoplegic, and hemiplegic migraine headache.**

Classic -	Prodrome lasts up to 60 min. Most common symptom is visual disturbance, such as homonymous hemianopsia, scintillating scotoma, and photophobia. Lips, face, and hand tingling as well as aphasia and extremity weakness may occur. Nausea and vomiting may also occur.
Common -	Most common. Slow evolving headache over hours to days. A positive family history as well as two of the following: nausea or vomiting, throbbing quality, photophobia, unilateral pain, and increase with menses. Distinguishing feature from "Classic" migraine is the lack of visual symptoms.
Cluster -	Mostly males. Intense unilateral ocular or retro-ocular pain which lasts less than 2 hours and occurs several times a day for weeks or months. Symptoms include lacrimation, facial flushing, rhinorrhea, sweating, and conjunctival injection. Often awakes patient from sleep.
Ophthalmoplegic -	Most commonly seen in young adults. Patient has an outwardly deviated, dilated eye, with ptosis. The 3rd > 6th > 4th nerves are typically involved.
Hemiplegic -	Unilateral motor and sensory symptoms, mild hemiparesis to hemiplegia.

❏❏ **Treatment of a cluster headache?**

100% O_2 and 4% viscous lidocaine in the ipsilateral nostril +/- 5-10% cocaine solution in same nostril, and a short course of steroids.

❏❏ **A 29 y old drunken male presents after having his head pounded into the concrete by his wife. The patient had a brief episode of LOC, but was then ambulatory and alert. Now he appears drowsy and just threw up on you. Diagnosis?**

Epidural hematoma.

❏❏ **A 25 y old presents with a history of being knocked unconscious for 10 seconds while playing touch football one week ago. Since then he has felt malaise, intermittent vertigo, nausea, vomiting, blurred vision, and a headache. Neuro exam and CT are normal. Diagnosis?**

Post-consussive syndrome. Most recover fully over 2 to 6 wk, few have persistent deficits.

❏❏ **A 64 y old presents with a bilateral "burning" headache. She describes jabs of pain which are worse at night. Treatment?**

Temporal arteritis is treated with long-term steroids. Treatment should begin immediately, do not wait for biopsy confirmation. ESR over 50 mm/h is highly suggestive.

❏❏ **A 53 y old female presents with unilateral right sided sudden-onset lancinating pain in the distribution of the second and third branches of the fifth cranial nerve. Treatment?**

Carbamazepine treats trigeminal neuralgia. An MRI to rule out a brainstem process (tumor) is indicated.

❏❏ **A 28 y old woman raised in Minnesota complains of weakness and tingling in the right arm and leg for 2 d. She reports an episode of right eye pain and blurred vision which resolved over one mo that occurred 2 y ago. She also recalls a two wk episode of intermittent blurred vision one y ago. Diagnosis?**

Presumptive MS. Confirm with MRI and CSF (oligoclonal bands).

❏❏ **What artery is most commonly associated with epidural hematomas?**

Middle meningeal artery.

❏❏ **A 50 y old female presents with acute vertigo, nausea, and vomiting. She reports similar episodes over the last 20 y, sometimes but not always associated with hearing change and/or hearing loss and tinnitus. She has permanent right > left sensorineural hearing loss. Diagnosis?**

Ménière's Disease.

❏❏ **What is the most common cause of a subarachnoid hemorrhage?**

Saccular aneurysm.

❏❏ **For the following clinical presentations identify if each is most consistent with peripheral or central vertigo.**

1. **Intense spinning, nausea, hearing loss, diaphoresis.**
2. **Swaying or impulsion, worse with movement, tinnitus, acute onset.**
3. **Unidirectional nystagmus inhibited by ocular fixation, fatigable.**
4. **Mild vertigo, diplopia, and ataxia.**
5. **Multidirectional nystagmus not inhibited by ocular fixation, nonfatigable.**

    1,2, and 3 -   Peripheral.
    4 and 5 -   Central.

❏❏ **The Nylen-Barany maneuver is performed as follows: the patient is rapidly brought from the sitting to supine position and the head is turned 45°. Match the findings with peripheral and central vertigo:**

1. **Nystagmus is multidirectional, nonfatiguing, has no latent period, and lasts over a minute.**
2. **Vertigo increased. Nystagmus is unidirectional, fatiguing, latent period is 2-20s, with duration less than a minute.**

1 - Central.
2 - Peripheral.

❏❏ **A 42 y old air traffic controller presents with attacks of vertigo whenever he scans the skies for landing airplanes. Symptoms last about a minute. He is worried sick. What do you tell him about his disease?**

The patient has benign positional vertigo. Attacks usually subside in a few weeks.

❏❏ **A 50 y old female presents with hearing loss over the last 6 mo. She now presents at 2 A.M. with vertigo which has progressively become worse over the last 2 months. On exam, she is mildly ataxic. Diagnosis?**

8th nerve lesion, possibly an acoustic schwannoma or meningioma.

❏❏ **Dangerous diagnosis of a purpuric, petechial rash?**

Think meningococcemia. Other causes include Hemophilus influenzae, Streptococcus pneumoniae, and Staphylococcus aureus.

❏❏ **On LP, opening pressure is markedly elevated. What should be done?**

Close 3-way stopcock, remove only a small amount of fluid from manometer, abort LP and initiate measures to decrease intracranial pressure.

❏❏ **A patient presents with acute meningitis; when should antibiotics be initiated?**

Immediately. Do not wait. Patients should receive a CT prior to LP only if papilledema or focal deficit is present.

❏❏ **What is the most common presenting symptom of MS?**

Optic neuritis (about 25%).

❏❏ **A patient with MS presents with a fever. The nurse asks "should I give the patient Tylenol?" What is your response?**

YES! Lowering temperature is important in MS patients as small increases in temperature can worsen existing signs and symptoms.

❏❏ **What rhythm disturbance would make phenytoin relatively contraindicated?**

Second or third degree heart block. If the patient is in status, you may have no choice. Phenytoin is relatively ineffective in seizures due to cyclic antidepressant overdose.

❏❏ **What three bacterial illnesses present with peripheral neurologic findings?**

Botulism, tetanus, and diphtheria.

TOX PEARLS

"Prepare for the difficult while it is still easy.
Deal with the big while it is still small.
Difficult undertakings have always started with what is easy,
And great undertakings have always started with what is small....
He who takes things too easily will surely encounter much difficulty.
For this reason even the sage regards things as difficult,
And therefore he encounters no difficulty."

Tao-te Ching, 63; Lao Tzu

❏❏ **Name some primary actions of cyclic antidepressants in overdose.**

1. Inhibition of amine reuptake.
2. Sodium channel blockade (causes negative inotropy).
3. Anticholinergic effects, primarily antimuscarinic.
4. CNS depression.
5. Alpha adrenergic antagonism (contributes further to hypotension).
6. GABA antagonism (.

■❏ **What is the appropriate treatment of QRS widening in a TCA poisoning?**

$NaHCO_3$ is administered intravenously for patients with a QRS > 100 ms. 1-2 meq/kg are initially administered and repeated until the blood pH is between 7.50 and 7.55. A continuous infusion of $NaHCO_3$ (3 Amps in 1 L of D5W) may then be initiated; run in over 4-6 h titrating to maintain appropriate pH. Potassium levels are closely monitored; supplementation may be required to prevent hypokalemia.

■❏ **What is the appropriate treatment of TCA induced seizures?**

Benzodiazepines and barbiturates are the agents of choice, phenytoin is not generally effective. Bicarbonate and alkalosis is mainstay of treatment.

❏❏ **Which TCA may induce seizures without concomitant cardiac toxicity?**

Amoxapine.

❏❏ **What is the treatment for TCA induced hypotension?**

Isotonic saline is initially administered. If the patient is resistant to fluid resuscitation, a directly acting alpha agonist should be started such as norepinephrine. Dopamine and dobutamine administration are contraindicated as these agents may increase hypotension through beta adrenergic stimulation. Further, dopamine acts in part by releasing norepinephrine; this agent may already be depleted by the reuptake inhibition of the CA and by stress.

■❏ **What is the clinical presentation of anticholinergic poisoning?**

Mydriasis, tachycardia, hypoactive bowel sounds, urinary retention, dry axilla, hyperthermia, and mental status changes.

■❏ **An observation period of what time length is required prior to medically clearing a TCA overdose?**

6 h.

❏❏ **What signs and symptoms are typical for the serotonin syndrome?**

Agitation, anxiety, sinus tachycardia, shivering, tremor, hyperreflexia, myoclonus, muscular rigidity, and diarrhea.

❏❏ **A 32 y old female is given meperidine (Demerol) for an open fracture. The patient is chronically on fluoxetine (Prozac). What is a potential complication?**

The serotonin syndrome.

❏❏ **What are potential pharmacological treatment modalities for the serotonin syndrome?**

Serotonin antagonists such as methylsergide and cyproheptadine. Benzodiazepines and propranolol have also been successfully employed.

❏❏ **A patient chronically on Nardil drinks a glass of red wine. What potential toxicity may result?**

The tyramine reaction.

❏❏ **A patient who ingests a toxic quantity of an MAOI presents to the ED in a hyperadrenergic state with a blood pressure of 240/160. What is the appropriate treatment of the patient's hypertension?**

Short acting antihypertensives such as phentolamine and nitroprusside should be employed as the patient may soon develop refractory hypotension.

❏❏ **What are the major pharmacological effects of neuroleptics?**

Blockade of dopamine, alpha adrenergic, muscarinic, and histamine receptors.

❏❏ **What constellation of findings occur with the neuroleptic malignant syndrome?**

Altered mental status, muscular rigidity, autonomic instability, hyperthermia, and rhabdomyolysis.

❏❏ **What lithium level is generally considered toxic?**

2.0 meq/L.

❏❏ **Does charcoal bind lithium?**

No.

❏❏ **What are the signs and symptoms of lithium toxicity?**

Neuro: Tremor, hyperreflexia, clonus, fasciculations, seizures, coma. GI: Nausea, vomiting, diarrhea. CV: ST-T wave changes, bradycardia, conduction defects and arrhythmias.

❏❏ **What is the treatment of lithium toxicity?**

Supportive care, normal saline diuresis, hemodialysis for patients with clinical signs of severe poisoning (seizures, arrhythmias etc.), renal failure, or decreasing urine output.

❏❏ **A patient who is chronically on lithium for bipolar disease becomes depressed. Prozac is added to the patient's therapeutic regiment. What adverse effect may occur?**

Serotonin syndrome.

❏❏ **What is the pharmacological effect of barbiturates and benzodiazepines?**

Both enhance chloride influx through the GABA receptor associated chloride channel. Benzodiazepines increase the frequency of channel opening whereas barbiturates increase the duration of channel opening.

❏❏ **Alkalinization of the urine is beneficial in the management of which barbiturates?**

Long acting barbiturates such as phenobarbital.

■❏ **The administration of flumazenil to acutely poisoned patients has resulted in what adverse effect?**

Seizures. Flumazenil has induced seizures in patients status post ingestion of potential seizure-inducing agents particularly TCAs. Flumazenil may induce withdrawal seizures in patients chronically on benzodiazepines.

❏❏ **Why are patients status post halogenated hydrocarbon exposure are susceptible to cardiac arrhythmias?**

Myocardial sensitization.

❏❏ **Which syndrome is atypical for the sedative hypnotics but unique to glutethimide?**

Anticholinergic poisoning syndrome.

❏❏ **The mixture of alcohol and chloral hydrate is referred to as:**

A "Mickey Finn."

❏❏ **Why may a chloral hydrate ingestion result in hematemesis?**

Chloral hydrate is corrosive with a pH of 3.5-4.4 as a 10% solution in water.

■❏ **Ethanol is metabolized at what rate in an intoxicated patient?**

About 20 mg/dl/hr.

■❏ **What is the pharmacological treatment of alcohol withdrawal?**

Benzodiazepines or barbiturates.

❏❏ **Isopropanol is metabolized via which enzyme to which metabolite?**

Isopropanol is metabolized by alcohol dehydrogenase in the liver to acetone.

■❏ **What is a normal osmolar gap?**

Less than 10 mOsm.

❏❏ **What is the toxic metabolite in methanol poisoning?**

Formic acid.

❏❏ **What cofactor is needed to convert formic acid to carbon dioxide and water?**

Folate. Leucovorin (folinic acid, the active form of folate) is preferentially administered at 1 mg/kg. Folate may be substituted at the same dose if leucovorin is not available.

❏❏ **Is NaHCO₃ beneficial in the management of methanol poisoning?**

Yes. In animal models maintenance of a normal pH through bicarbonate administration decreased toxicity including visual impairment.

❏❏ **What is the methanol level that warrants dialysis?**

50 mg/dl. Other indications include visual impairment, severe metabolic acidosis, and ingestion of greater than 30 cc.

❏❏ **What two cofactors are administered to the patient with ethylene glycol poisoning?**

Thiamine and pyridoxine. These cofactors will aid in transforming glyoxylic acid to nontoxic metabolites. Both are administered intravenously in 100 mg increments.

❏❏ **Isopropanol, ethylene glycol, and methanol are all metabolized by alcohol dehydrogenase. Is an alcohol drip beneficial to all of these poisonings?**

No. Isopropanol is converted via alcohol dehydrogenase to the nontoxic acetone.

❏❏ **What are the three clinical phases of ethylene glycol poisoning?**

Stage I: Neurological symptomatology i.e., inebriation.
Stage II: Metabolic acidosis and cardiovascular instability.
Stage III: Renal failure.

❏❏ **When should dialysis be initiated in ethylene glycol poisoning?**

Serum level greater than 25 mg/dl, renal insufficiency, or severe metabolic acidosis.

❏❏ **What valve is most commonly infected in an intravenous drug abuser?**

The tricuspid valve, usually with Staph aureus.

❏❏ **What is the toxic dose of naloxone?**

There is none. Narcan is a safe drug and may be given in large quantities. The usual adult dosage is 2 mg iv, 0.01 mg/kg in a child. Narcan may precipitate acute withdrawal and may therefore be titrated to effect.

❏❏ **What is the etiology of noncardiogenic pulmonary edema after heroin injection?**

Unknown. May be delayed 24 to 48 h after injection although most present immediately after injection. Treatment is the same as any patient with ARDS.

❏❏ **What is the urinary metabolite tested for in cocaine exposures?**

Benzoylecgonine.

❏❏ **How does treatment of a cocaine induced MI differ from a typical MI?**

Both are treated the same except that ß-blockers are not used in a cocaine induced MI secondary to unopposed alpha adrenergic activity. The tachycardia of a cocaine associated MI is first treated with benzodiazepine sedation.

❏❏ **What is the difference between a body packer and a body stuffer?**

The body packer has instilled packets of cocaine in his body in an attempt to evade customs officials. The packets are generally well sealed and contain lethal quantities of drugs if rupture occurs. The body stuffer will eat packets of cocaine upon police arrest in order to conceal evidence.

❏❏ **An employee claims that he has been using Vick's Nasal Spray and this is the reason for his urine GC/MS to be positive for methamphetamine. How can we determine if the patient is telling the truth.**

Vick's Nasal Spray contains the l-isomer of methamphetamine whereas street methamphetamine is a racemic mixture. Isomerization studies need to be performed on the patient's urine.

❏❏ **What syndrome is associated with Jimson Weed?**

Anticholinergic poisoning.

❏❏ **What is the mechanism of salicylate toxicity?**

Salicylates uncouple oxidative phosphorylation and therefore halt cellular ATP production.

❏❏ **Metabolic acidosis favors which form of salicylate: ionized or un-ionized?**

Un-ionized. Patients with salicylate poisoning should have arterial pH maintained at or greater than 7.4 so that salicylate is in the ionized form and therefore unable to cross the blood brain barrier. Urinary alkalinization promotes the formation of the ionized form of salicylate which is unable to be reabsorbed by the tubules thereby enhancing excretion.

❏❏ **What is the acid-base disturbance typical for salicylate poisoning?**

Mixed respiratory alkalosis (secondary to central respiratory center stimulation) and metabolic acidosis (secondary to uncoupling of oxidative phosphorylation).

❏❏ **T/F: A patient who ingests enteric coated aspirin and is asymptomatic for 6 h in the ED may be safely discharged home.**

False. Enteric coating allows for delayed absorption. Any patient who by history has ingested 150 mg/kg of enteric coated aspirin should be admitted to the hospital for serial salicylate levels and observation.

❏❏ **Arterial pH is 7.5 through alkalinization but urine pH is still low. What electrolyte is probably responsible?**

Potassium. When reabsorbing sodium, the renal tubules will preferentially excrete hydrogen ions into the tubular lumen rather than potassium ions thus, potassium should be maintained at 4.0 mmol/L.

❏❏ **What is the treatment of a prolonged prothrombin time in salicylate poisoning?**

Parenteral Vitamin K1 administration. Salicylates inhibit Vitamin K1 epoxide reductase in poisoning resulting in an ability for the inactive vitamin K1 epoxide to be regenerated into the active Vitamin K1.

❏❏ **What are the indications for dialysis in salicylate poisoning?**

1. Persistent CNS involvement. 2. ARDS. 3. Renal failure. 4. Severe acid-base disturbance despite appropriate care. 5. Acute salicylate level > 100 mg/dl.

❏❏ **Can a patient present with salicylate poisoning and a therapeutic level?**

Yes. Patients with chronic salicylate poisoning have a large Vd and thus may present with mental status changes and a therapeutic level.

❏❏ **What are the four stages of acetaminophen (APAP) poisoning?**

I.   1/2-24 h.   Nausea, vomiting.
II. 24-48 h.   Abdominal pain, elevated LFTs.
III. 72-96 h.   LFTs peak, nausea, vomiting.
IV. 4d-2 wk.   Resolution or fulminant hepatic failure.

❏❏ **APAP poisoning produces what type of hepatic necrosis?**

Centrilobular necrosis. The toxic metabolite of APAP is generated in the liver via the P450 system, located in the centrilobular region.

❏❏ **What is the toxic metabolite of APAP?**

NAPQI. When the glucuronidation and sulfation pathways are saturated, APAP is metabolized by the P450 system to the toxic metabolite N-acetyl-para-benzoquinoneimine (NAPQI).

❏❏ **What hepatic laboratory parameter is the first to become abnormal in APAP poisoning?**

The prothrombin time (PT).

❏❏ **An acutely intoxicated, nonalcoholic, otherwise healthy patient ingests APAP. Is this patient more or less likely to develop hepatotoxicity?**

Less likely. An acute ingestion of alcohol will inhibit the P450 system thereby inhibiting the formation of NAPQI. A chronic alcoholic has an induced P450 system and will suffer greater APAP hepatic toxicity through increased NAPQI formation.

❏❏ **What is the minimum dose of APAP in a child and an adult that is capable of causing hepatotoxicity?**

Child 140 mg/kg. Adult 7.5 g.

❏❏ **Per the Rumack-Matthew nomogram, which 4 h APAP level requires treatment?**

150 µG/ml.

❏❏ **How is the nomogram utilized in a patient who ingests an Extended Relief formulation of APAP?**

A four h and an eight h level are obtained. If either level is in the "Possible" hepatotoxic range, the patient should be treated.

❏❏ **What is the proposed mechanism of theophylline induced seizures?**

Adenosine antagonism. Adenosine is released into the synaptic cleft from presynaptic terminals along with excitatory neurotransmitters, binds to presynaptic adenosine receptors resulting in inhibition of further excitatory neurotransmitter release.

❏❏ **What is the appropriate initial treatment of theophylline induced seizures?**

Benzodiazepines and barbiturates. Theophylline induced seizures warrant hemodialysis or hemoperfusion.

❑❑ **What is the treatment of theophylline induced hypotension?**

Fluid administration and beta blockers. Theophylline induced cardiovascular instability is secondary to beta agonist effects therefore beta blockers are beneficial in the treatment of arrhythmias and hypotension.

❑❑ **What are absolute indications for hemodialysis or hemoperfusion in theophylline toxicity?**

Seizures or arrhythmias that are unresponsive to conventional therapy.

❑❑ **Why is multidose activated charcoal administration advocated for theophylline poisoning?**

Theophylline undergoes enterohepatic circulation.

❑❑ **What abnormal laboratory parameters are typical in the patient with acute theophylline poisoning?**

Hypokalemia, hyperglycemia, and leukocytosis. The beta agonist properties of theophylline produce these abnormalities.

❑❑ **What are absolute indications for Digibind administration in digoxin poisoning?**

Ventricular arrhythmias, hemodynamically significant bradyarrhythmias unresponsive to standard therapy, and a potassium level greater than 5.0 meq/L.

❑❑ **Why is calcium chloride administration contraindicated in digoxin poisoning?**

Digoxin inhibits the Na-K-ATPase, resulting in an increased intracellular concentration of sodium. The sodium-calcium exchange pump is then activated leading to high intracellular concentrations of calcium. Calcium chloride administration would further increase intracellular calcium leading to increased myocardial irritability.

❑❑ **What is the correct dose of Digibind in a patient with life threatening digoxin poisoning and an unknown level?**

Ten vials.

❑❑ **What is the appropriate treatment of hyperkalemia in digoxin poisoning?**

1. Digibind. 2. Insulin and glucose. 3. Sodium bicarbonate. 4. Potassium resin binder (Kayexalate). 5. Hemodialysis.

❑❑ **Can a digoxin level be followed after the administration of Digibind?**

No. Digibind administration will lead to falsely elevated digoxin levels.

❑❑ **A patient on Digoxin presents bradycardic and hypotensive with significantly peaked T waves. What would be your initial line of treatment?**

Administer 10 vials of Digibind intravenously and simultaneously treat the presumed hyperkalemia with insulin and glucose, sodium bicarbonate, and Kayexalate. Once the Digibind is administered hyperkalemic induced arrhythmias may be safely treated with calcium chloride.

❑❑ **What is the antidote for beta blocker poisonings and what is the biochemical rational?**

Glucagon. Glucagon receptors, located on myocardial cells, are G protein coupled receptors which activate adenylate cyclase leading to increased levels of intracellular cAMP. Thus glucagon administration leads to the same intracellular effect as beta agonist.

■❑ A child presents to the Emergency Department status post ingestion of a sustained release calcium channel blocker. What is the disposition?

Hospital admission to a monitored setting. Sustained release preparations have the capability of producing delayed toxicity.

■❑ What are potential treatment modalities for a calcium channel blocker poisoning?

Symptomatic patients are admitted to an intensive care unit and treatment is best guided by Pulmonary Artery Catheter hemodynamic measurements. Therapeutic interventions include intravenous calcium, isoproterenol, glucagon, transvenous pacers, atropine, and vasopressors such as norepinephrine, epinephrine, or dopamine.

❑❑ What is the mechanism and treatment of clonidine induced hypotension?

The mechanism is decreased cardiac output secondary to decreased sympathetic outflow from the CNS. Treatment is with intravenous fluid administration and dopamine.

■❑ Clonidine poisoning presents with what typical eye finding?

Pinpoint pupils.

❑❑ At which adrenergic receptor is clonidine active?

Clonidine is an alpha 2 agonist.

❑❑ Can clonidine lead to hypertension in the acute overdose setting?

Yes. Clonidine acts on peripheral post synaptic alpha 2 receptors resulting in initial vasoconstriction and hypertension. The drug will then cross the blood brain barrier and suppress sympathetic outflow leading to hypotension.

■❑ Does oral phenytoin poisoning require cardiac monitoring in an otherwise healthy patient?

No. Oral phenytoin poisoning has resulted in arrhythmias in only two case reports. These two individuals had previous underlying cardiac abnormalities.

❑❑ What is the pharmacological basis of the anticonvulsant effect of phenytoin?

Sodium channel blockade.

■❑ Why does intravenous phenytoin administration lead to cardiovascular toxicity?

The propylene glycol diluent is a myocardial depressant and vasodilator.

■❑ What are the four stages of iron poisoning?

I. (Initial h) Gastrointestinal symptomatology. Abdominal pain, vomiting, and diarrhea secondary to the corrosive effects of iron.
II. (6 to 24 h) Quiescent period during which iron is being absorbed.
III. (> 12 h) Shock, metabolic acidosis, hepatic dysfunction, heart failure, cerebral dysfunction, and renal failure.

IV. (d to wk) Gastric outlet or small bowel obstruction secondary to scarring.

■❑ What dose of iron is expected to produce clinical toxicity?

20 mg/kg of elemental iron. A toddler ingests 10 tablets of 324 mg ferrous sulfate (20% elemental iron). This equals 648 mg of elemental iron. This would be a toxic dose of 32.4 mg/kg in a 20 kg child.

■❑ What 4 h iron level is generally considered toxic?

300-350 μg/dl.

❑❑ What are indications for deferoxamine therapy?

1. All symptomatic patients exhibiting more than merely transient symptomatology. 2. Patients with lethargy, significant abdominal pain, hypotension, or metabolic acidosis. 3. Patients with a positive KUB. 4. Any symptomatic patient with a level greater than 300 μG/dl.

❑❑ What is the standard dose of deferoxamine?

15 mg/kg/hr continuous intravenous infusion.

❑❑ What are the criteria for stopping deferoxamine therapy?

1. The patient must be asymptomatic. 2. A KUB must be negative. 3. The serum iron concentration must be normal or low. (Most laboratories cannot accurately measure serum iron in the presence of deferoxamine. Therefore, the iron level should be less than 100 μG/dl in these facilities.) 4. The vin rose urine should clear.

❑❑ Which oral chelator has proven to reduce iron absorption in animal models?

Magnesium hydroxide or Milk of Magnesia.

❑❑ Which hydrocarbons carry the greatest risk of aspiration?

Those with a low viscosity < 60 SSU.

❑❑ What historical disclosure warrants ED evaluation after a hydrocarbon ingestion?

Coughing. Any patient who coughs after ingesting a hydrocarbon has the potential to develop chemical pneumonitis.

❑❑ When may a hydrocarbon ingestion be discharged safely to home?

After a six h asymptomatic period patients with a normal chest x-ray and pulse ox may be discharged to home.

❑❑ Chronic solvent abusers develop what metabolic complication?

Renal tubular acidosis.

❑❑ Is the urine acidic or alkaline in renal tubular acidosis?

Alkaline. Distal tubules are unable to secrete hydrogen ions; therefore, the blood is acidotic and the urine is alkalemic. Potassium ions are secreted as hydrogen ions are not capable of excretion; hypokalemia results. Chloride ions are reabsorbed to preserve electroneutrality in the extracellular fluid. Result: Non-anion gap hyperchloremic metabolic acidosis.

❏❏ **Carbon tetrachloride poisoning produces what type of liver damage?**

Centrilobular necrosis.

❏❏ **Methylene chloride is metabolized to which toxin?**

Carbon monoxide.

❏❏ **A two year old child is asymptomatic after ingestion of a button battery. KUB reveals the foreign body in the stomach. What is the disposition of this patient?**

Discharge to home. If the battery is lodged in the esophagus urgent endoscopy is mandatory; otherwise, reassure and check stools.

❏❏ **Oral hydrofluoric acid exposure may result in which life threatening electrolyte abnormalities?**

Hyperkalemia and hypocalcemia.

❏❏ **What is the antidote for cutaneous hydrofluoric acid exposures?**

Intradermal injection or intraarterial infusion of calcium gluconate.

■❏ **What enzyme is inhibited by organophosphates?**

Cholinesterase.

■❏ **What are the two principle antidotes used for organophosphate poisoning?**

Atropine and Pralidoxime.

❏❏ **Is pralidoxime administration beneficial in carbamate poisoning?**

No. Carbamates bind reversibly to cholinesterases whereas organophosphates bind irreversibly. Pralidoxime is used to reactivate cholinesterase molecules phosphorylated by an organophosphate molecule. Pralidoxime should be administered prior to the onset of irreversible aging of the enzyme.

❏❏ **What is the mechanism of cyanide toxicity?**

Electron transport inhibition through cyanide binding to the ferric ion in cytochrome oxidase.

❏❏ **What does the Lilly Cyanide Antidote Kit contain and what is the mechanism of action?**

Amyl nitrite for inhalation, sodium nitrite for intravenous infusion, and sodium thiosulfate for infusion. The nitrites induce methemoglobinemia and thereby displace cyanide from cytochrome oxidase. Thiosulfate enhances rhodanese activity and accelerates the conversion of cyanide to thiocyanate for excretion.

■❏ **What antihypertensive agent may induce cyanide poisoning?**

Nitroprusside. One molecule of sodium nitroprusside contains 5 molecules of cyanide. In order to prevent toxicity, sodium thiosulfate should be infused with sodium nitroprusside at a ratio of 10:1 (thiosulfate:nitroprusside). Beware of thiocyanate toxicity!

❏❏ **What is arterialization of venous blood?**

High partial pressure of oxygen in venous blood. In cyanide poisoning, electron transport is inhibited leading to an inability to utilize oxygen as an electron acceptor. Therefore, venous blood will contain a high partial pressure of oxygen.

❏❏ **A semiconductor employee presents to the ED with a triad of abdominal pain, hematuria, and jaundice. To which toxic gas was this patient exposed?**

Arsine. Toxic arsine gas exposure results in intravascular hemolysis and this classic triad.

❏❏ **A patient chronically on an oral hypoglycemic agent presents to the ED with a depressed mental status. Accucheck is 20 mg/dl. An amp of D_{50} is administered with rapid return of a normal mental status. What is the disposition of this patient.**

Hospital admission with serial glucose level determination. Oral hypoglycemic agents are long acting thus, patients must be admitted and observed for recurrent hypoglycemia.

❏❏ **What is the antidote for Isoniazid induced seizures?**

Pyridoxine. Dose intravenously gram for gram or in unknown overdoses administer 5 grams.

❏❏ **A patient is administered topical Cetacaine spray prior to endoscopy. The patient then complains of shortness of breath and is noted to be cyanotic. What is the antidote?**

Methylene Blue 1 mg/kg intravenously. Methemoglobinemia developed secondary to the local anesthetic.

❏❏ **A 32 yo female presents to the ED with the chief complaint of vomiting and diarrhea which developed 8 h after ingesting mushrooms. Is the mushroom potentially hepatotoxic?**

Yes. The hepatotoxic cyclopeptide containing mushrooms induce a delayed onset of gastrointestinal symptomatology, generally occurring 6 h after ingestion. The benign mushrooms with gastrointestinal toxins induce symptomatology within 0.5-3 h.

❏❏ **A patient presents with seizures 6 h status post mushroom ingestion. What is the antidote?**

Pyridoxine. The Gyromitra mushrooms contain monomethylhydrazine which inhibits GABA production similarly to isoniazid through pyridoxine kinase inhibition.

❏❏ **A two y old child is found with Brodifacoum rat poison pellets in his mouth. The patient is asymptomatic. What is the disposition?**

Discharge to home with a follow up PT at 24 and 48 h. Brodifacoum is a superwarfarin. Toxicity is generally only seen with massive intentional or chronic overdoses.

❏❏ **What iron level is toxic?**

Moderate OD is considered with serum level 350 µg/dl, measured 4 h after ingestion.
Alternatively, try to determine the amount of <u>elemental</u> iron ingested, 20-40 mg elemental iron/kg is toxic.
Treat symptomatic patients without waiting for lab test results.

❏❏ **What is the treatment for cyanide overdose?**

Oxygen, CPR prn.
Amyl nitrite perle inhaled.
Sodium nitrite 10 ml of 3% solution in an adult which is 300 mg, or 0.2 - 0.33 ml/kg in a child.

Sodium thiosulfate - give 5 times the volume of sodium nitrite; 12.5 mg in an adult which is 50 ml of a 25% solution or 1.0 - 1.5 ml/kg in a child.

❏❏ **Interesting treatment! The mechanism of action of nitrites is not completely clear, though formation of methemoglobin is probably important. Methemoglobin rapidly combines with cyanide to form cyanomethemoglobin. O.K., so now you've stripped the cyanide off it's binding to cytochrome A_3, but how is the cyanomethemoglobin handled?**

The intrinsic enzyme rhodanase catalyzes the transport of cyanide from cyanomethemoglobin to sulfur forming thiocyanate. This reaction is limited by sulfur availability. Sodium thiosulfate is given to act as a sulfur donor. Thiocyanate is excreted by the kidney.

❏❏ **What order are the kinetics of elimination of ASA overdose?**

Zero-order elimination with hepatic enzymatic clearance saturated and renal clearance becoming important.

❏❏ **We all remember to think of ASA poisoning when a patient presents with mental status changes associated with respiratory alkalosis and metabolic acidosis. Many of us may recall that salicylate toxicity may be associated with elevated, normal, or decreased glucose levels. By what mechanisms are hyperglycemia and hypoglycemia caused?**

Hyperglycemia is caused by salicylate induced mobilization of glycogen.
Hypoglycemia is caused by salicylate inhibition of gluconeogenesis.

❏❏ **Is ARDS more likely to be a complication of acute or chronic ASA poisoning?**

Chronic.

❏❏ **ARDS is <u>not</u> a common complication of acute ASA OD. However, with acute ingestion, does ARDS occur more often in adults or children?**

Adults.

❏❏ **What is the "magic number" for the dose of non-enteric coated ASA which must be exceeded to cause toxicity (mg/kg)?**

150 mg/kg.

❏❏ **What is the "magic number" for the dose of enteric coated ASA which must be exceeded to require admission for observation and serial salicylate levels?**

150 mg/kg.

❏❏ **Metabolic acidosis favors formation of what form of salicylate, ionized or un-ionized?**

UN-IONIZED.
This is a KEY point because:
    a.) It is the reason to therapeutically produce an alkaline urine which then makes more of the free salicylate ionized, not reabsorbed by tubules, and excreted.
    b.) It is the reason for the large changes in amount of free drug able to diffuse into tissue. Small decreases in pH result in decreased protein binding and more salicylate in the un-ionized form able to diffuse into tissue thereby increasing its volume of distribution. [Thus, always treat the patient and not the level - serum levels can decrease as salicylate moves into tissue!!].

❏❏ **Under what circumstances is use of A.D. Done's nomogram O.K.?**

Only when the patient has an acute, single ingestion of non-enteric coated ASA without recent prior use.

❏❏ Can a patient who is symptomatic with mental status changes from chronic salicylate poisoning have a level in the therapeutic range?

Yes! Interestingly, patients taking acetazolamide are at particular risk for chronic salicylate poisoning because the carbonic anhydrase inhibitor results in acidified plasma (leading to increased V_d) and more alkalotic CSF, thereby encouraging salicylate concentration in the CNS.

❏❏ Is hemodialysis used to treat salicylate toxicity?

Yes, in severe poisoning (coma, ARDS, cardiac toxicity, serum level > 100 mg/dl), and for patients who are unresponsive to maximal therapy.

❏❏ What is the "magic number" for the minimum ingestion of acetaminophen (N-acetyl-para-aminophenol, APAP) necessary to cause hepatic toxicity in an adult?

7.5 gm.

❏❏ In a child?

140 mg/kg.

❏❏ What region of liver lobules contains the greatest amount of P_{450} related mixed-function oxidases ($P_{450}MFO$)?

The centrilobular regions, accounting for primarily centrilobular necrosis.

❏❏ How is APAP usually metabolized under non-overdose conditions?

Most APAP metabolism is by glucuronidation.
Some APAP metabolism is by conjugation with sulfate. This percentage increases with decreasing age. 4% or less is transformed into an extremely toxic intermediary compound by $P_{450}MFO$'s. This toxic metabolite is likely immediately conjugated with glutathione and harmlessly excreted in the urine.

❏❏ How does N-acetylcysteine (NAC, Mucomyst) work?

Precise mechanism is still unknown. We know that NAC enters cells and is metabolized to cysteine which serves as a glutathione precursor.

❏❏ Which measures of hepatic function are better indicators of prognosis, liver enzyme levels or bilirubin level and prothrombin time?

Bilirubin level and prothrombin time.

❏❏ Clonidine is a centrally acting presynaptic a_2-adrenergic agonist that results in decreased central sympathetic outflow. While its primary use is to treat hypertension, it has additional emergency utility in blunting withdrawal symptoms from opiates and EtOH. Clonidine overdose closely resembles OD with what other class of drugs?

Opiates.

❏❏ Can clonidine ever cause hypertension?

Yes; high serum levels can result in direct peripheral α-adrenergic stimulation. Such hypertension usually yields to ensuing hypotension.

❏❏ Toxicity from clonidine (Catapres) usually occurs within what time period?

4 h.

❏❏ **What agent may be useful as an "antidote" for clonidine OD.**

Naloxone.

❏❏ **Name a few substances that have anticholinergic properties.**

Antihistamines, cyclic antidepressants, phenothiazines, atropine, amanita sp., Jimson weed.

❏❏ **Sure, patients who suffer anticholinergic toxicity have mental status changes, mydriasis, urinary retention, cardiogenic pulmonary edema, dry skin, tachycardia and decreased salivation, but what is the most common ECG abnormality?**

Sinus tachycardia. Other, dangerous, arrhythmias include conduction problems and V-Tach.

❏❏ **What is "cornpicker's pupil?"**

Mydriasis from contact of Jimson weed with the eye. Jimson weed contains atropine, scopolamine and hyoscyamine. It is a common plant and is available through health food stores.

❏❏ **Intermediate-chain aliphatic hydrocarbons are responsible for most of the exposures to hydrocarbons. What is the most common complication from these liquids?**

Chemical pneumonitis caused by direct injury to pulmonary parenchyma after aspiration.

❏❏ **Which hydrocarbons carry the greatest risk of aspiration?**

Those with low viscosity, less than 60 SSU.
(We'll return to the SSU in the random question section.)

❏❏ **Aromatic hydrocarbons, such as toluene present in glue, may be sniffed. Resulting effects most closely resemble those of what other class of compounds?**

Effects are similar to those of inhalational anesthetic agents: initial excitatory response gives way to CNS depression.

❏❏ **Can solvent abusers be scared to death?**

Yes. Halogenated hydrocarbons can "sensitize" myocardium to catecholamines, thus exertion or fright can lead to fatal arrhythmias.

❏❏ **What is the relationship between toluene and A MUDPILE CAT?**

Toluene is the "T"!

❏❏ **Is charcoal useful in hydrocarbon ingestions?**

No.

❏❏ **For what period of time should an asymptomatic patient with hydrocarbon ingestion be observed prior to discharge?**

6 h.

❏❏ **Sure, digitalis increases myocardial inotropy by inhibiting Na^+-K^+-ATPase, thereby allowing intracellular Na^+ to increase providing more substrate for the Na^+-Ca^{2+} membrane exchange that leads to increased intracellular (sarcoplasmic) Ca^{2+} concentration, but does it also increase vagal tone and slow conduction through the AV node?**

Yes.

❑❑ **Serum potassium can soar to very high levels with acute digitalis toxicity; is this also true for chronic digitalis poisoning?**

No, not really.

❑❑ **T/F- A patient with acute digitalis OD presents with frequent multifocal PVC's, peaked T-waves and a K^+ of 6.2 mEq/l; correct treatment is to first administer $CaCl_2$ as this is the fastest acting agent for reducing hyperkalemia.**

No, no, this is a trick question! Yes, $CaCl_2$ is the fastest acting agent for decreasing hyperkalemia, but you don't want to give any more Ca^+ to a patient with digitalis induced cardiac toxicity.

❑❑ **Signs and symptoms of phenytoin toxicity?**

Seizure, heart blocks, bradyarrhythmias, hypotension, coma. All dangerous cardiovascular complications of phenytoin OD result from parenteral administration; high levels after PO doses do not cause such signs in a stable patient.

❑❑ **Treatment of phenytoin overdose?**

Systemic support, charcoal, atropine for bradyarrhythmias, and phenobarbital 20 mg/kg IV for seizures.

❑❑ **At what serum level of phenytoin do nystagmus, ataxia, and lethargy generally occur?**

Nystagmus -   20 μg/ml.
Ataxia -   30 μg/ml.
Lethargy -   40 μg/ml.

❑❑ **What rhythm and ECG findings are expected with phenytoin toxicity?**

Bradycardia, AV block, ventricular tachycardia, VF, and asystole. ECG findings might include increased PR interval and a wide QRS.

❑❑ **What is the treatment of phenytoin toxicity?**

Charcoal. Seizures are treated with benzodiazepine or phenobarbital. Extravasation may be limb threatening, consult an orthopedic or plastic surgeon. Hemodialysis and hemoperfusion are not helpful.

■❑ **How many vials of digoxin-specific Fab should be administered to a patient in critical condition from digitalis toxicity in whom neither the ingested dose nor the serum level is known?**

10 vials = 400 mg Fab.

❑❑ **ß-adrenergic antagonists have 3 main effects on the heart - name them.**

Negative chronotropy.
Negative inotropy.
Decrease AV nodal conduction velocity.

❑❑ **T/F - ß-adrenergic antagonists can cause mental status changes and seizures.**

True.

■❑ **What is the agent of choice to counteract the effects of ß-adrenergic antagonists, and how does it work?**

Glucagon should be given in boluses of 3 - 5 mg q 5 min until response is obtained or 10 -15 mg has been administered. It has rapid onset and short-lived effect (≈ 15 min), therefore administer a continuous infusion at the same number of mg/hr as the number of mg initially provided in boluses to obtain a response. The initial dose is 50 - 150 µg/kg in children.

Glucagon works by increasing intracellular cAMP by direct glucagon (non-adrenergic) receptors, bypassing ß-adrenergic receptors.

❏❏ **What is the <u>most common</u> cause of acute heavy metal poisoning?**

    a.) Twisted Sister
    b.) Metallica
    c.) Arsenic

❏❏ **Arsenic is initially housed in RBC's, WBC's and bound to serum proteins. From there it is distributed to major organs, bone, hair and nails. What is the primary mechanism of toxicity of arsenic?**

It blocks the conversion of a cofactor necessary for oxidative phosphorylation (Krebs cycle).
Arsenic also substitutes for phosphate, disrupting high-energy phosphates.

❏❏ **What is the resultant pathology of arsenic intoxication?**

N, V, D, cerebral edema, cerebral hemorrhage, arrhythmias, encephalopathy associated with mental status changes, and seizures, pulmonary edema, ARF, rhabdomyolysis.

❏❏ **T/F- Chronic arsenic poisoning tends to present less dramatically with constitutional symptoms and peripheral neuropathy.**

True.

❏❏ **Charcoal probably doesn't absorb arsenic much. What chelating agents are appropriate?**

Play BAL with a DMSAl named MAG!

This means that Mercury, Arsenic and Gold (MAG) can be chelated with BAL and with DMSA. D-Penicillamine can also be used.

❏❏ **Arsine is a gaseous form of arsenic; is chelation also used to treat arsine?**

No.

❏❏ **What are the effects of arsine poisoning?**

Binds to hemoglobin; causes anemia with jaundice, ARF.
Manage with transfusions and dialysis for ARF.

❏❏ **A patient with a history of CA overdose is found by paramedics awake and alert. Prognosis?**

25% - 50% of patients who die from cyclic overdose are awake and alert at the scene.

❏❏ **Is degree of toxicity in CA overdose closely related to QRS duration?**

QRS > 100 ms has a specificity of 75 percent and a sensitivity of 60% for serious complications. A normal ECG will not rule out serious overdose! Of those with QRS > 100 ms, 30% will seize; of those with QRS > 160 ms, 50% will develop arrhythmias.

❏❏ **How is pulmonary edema associated with heroin use treated?**

Naloxone and ventilatory support. Diuretics, digitalis, and rotating tourniquets are not effective.

❏❏ **What valve is most commonly infected in narcotic IV drug abusers?**

Tricuspid valve, usually with Staphylococcus aureus.

❑❑ What is the treatment of narcotic overdose?

Naloxone, 0.4 to 2.0 mg in an adult, and 0.01 mg/kg in a child. Naloxone's duration of action is about 1 h.

❑❑ A cocaine addict presents with chest pain. The ECG is normal. What are the odds they will have abnormal CPK and CPK-MB isoenzymes?

6 - 19%.

❑❑ What type of nystagmus is expected with PCP overdose?

Vertical, horizontal, and rotary. Vertical nystagmus is not common with other conditions/ingestions. The most common findings of PCP overdose are hypertension, tachycardia, and nystagmus.

❑❑ What are the two most common complications of PCP intoxication?

Hyperpyrexia and rhabdomyolysis. Urine acidification as a treatment is no longer recommended.

❑❑ What is the most common cause of chronic heavy metal poisoning?

Lead.

❑❑ A patient presents with neurologic dysfunction and abdominal complaints. Lab studies reveal a hemolytic anemia. Diagnosis?

Lead toxicity. Diagnosis is confirmed by finding an elevated PbB level. If indication of PB are found on abdominal x-ray, initiate whole-bowel irrigation with Golytely. Chelate with BAL followed by EDTA. Oral chelating agents , D-penicillamine and DMSA, may also be considered.

ID PEARLS

"Nobody will fly for a thousand years!"

Wilbur Wright, 1901, in a fit of despair.

❏❏ **Describe the pathophysiologic features of HIV:**

HIV attacks the T4 helper cells. HIV genetic material consists of single-stranded RNA. HIV has been found in semen, vaginal secretions, blood and blood products, saliva, urine, cerebrospinal fluid, tears, alveolar fluid, synovial fluid, breast milk, transplanted tissue and amniotic fluid. There as not been documentation of infection from casual contact.

❏❏ **How quickly do patients infected with HIV become symptomatic?**

5-10% develop symptoms within three years of seroconversion. Predictive characteristics include low T4 count, and hematocrit less than 40. Mean incubation time is about 8.23 y for adults and 1.97 y for children less than 5 y. When AIDS develops, survival is about 9 months. New treatments may improve survival.

❏❏ **Name the most common causes of fever in HIV infected patients:**

HIV-related fever, Mycobacterium avium-intracellular. CMV, non-Hodgkin's and Hodgkin's lymphoma.

❏❏ **An HIV positive patient presents with a history of weight loss, diarrhea, fever, anorexia, and malaise. They are also dyspneic. Lab studies reveal abnormal LFTs and anemia. Diagnosis?**

Mycobacterium avium-intracellular. Lab confirmation is made by acid-fast stain of body fluids or by blood culture.

❏❏ **What is the <u>most common</u> cause of retinitis in AIDS patients?**

CMV. GI involvement is also common.

❏❏ **What is the second <u>most common</u> complication of AIDS?**

Kaposi's sarcoma. PCP is the most common.

❏❏ **What drugs are used to treat CNS toxoplasmosis in AIDS patients?**

Pyrimethamine plus sulfadiazine.

❏❏ **What is the <u>most common</u> cause of focal encephalitis in AIDS patients?**

Toxoplasmosis. Symptoms include focal neurologic deficits, headache, fever, altered mental status, and seizures. Ring enhancing-lesions are seen on CT.

❏❏ **The differential diagnosis of ring-enhancing lesions in AIDS patients is:**

Lymphoma, cerebral tuberculosis, fungal infection, CMV, Kaposi's sarcoma, toxoplasmosis. and hemorrhage.

❏❏ **What are the signs and symptoms of CNS cryptococcal infection in an AIDS patient?**

Headache, depression, lightheadedness, seizures, and cranial nerve palsies.
Diagnosis is made by India ink prep, fungal culture, or by cryptococcal antigen in the CSF.

❏❏ **Presentation of an AIDS patient with tuberculous meningitis:**

Fever, meningismus, headache, seizures, focal neurologic deficits, and altered mental status.

❏❏ **On physical exam, what is the most common eye finding in AIDS patients?**

Cotton-wool spots thought to be associated with PCP. These may be hard to differentiate from fluffy-white, often perivascular retinal lesions that are associated with CMV.

❏❏ **An AIDS patient presents with complaints of decreased visual acuity, photophobia, redness, and eye pain. Diagnosis?**

Retinitis or malignant invasion of the periorbital tissue or eye.

❏❏ **What is the most common cause of retinitis in AIDS patients?**

Cytomegalovirus.
Findings include photophobia, redness, scotoma, pain, or change in visual acuity. On exam, findings include fluffy white retinal lesions.

❏❏ **Most common opportunistic infection in AIDS patients?**

PCP.
Symptoms may include non-productive cough and dyspnea. Chest x-ray may show diffuse interstitial infiltrates or be negative. Gallium scanning is more sensitive but results in false positives. Initial treatment includes TMP-SMX. Pentamidine is an alternative.

❏❏ **How is Candida of the esophagus diagnosed in the ED?**

Air-contrast barium swallow will show ulcerations with plaques. In contrast, herpes esophagitis will produce punched-out ulcerations with no plaques.

❏❏ **What is the most common gastrointestinal complaint in AIDS patients?**

Diarrhea. Hepatomegaly and hepatitis are also common. Jaundice is an uncommon finding.
Cryptosporidium and Isospora are the common causes of prolonged watery diarrhea.

❏❏ **What is the risk of contracting HIV infection after occupational exposure?**

0.32%. 80% of the occupational exposure related infections are from needle sticks.

❏❏ **A patient is infected with Treponema pallidum, what is the treatment?**

Depends on the stage (1°, 2°, 3°), 1°& 2° syphilis is treated with benzathine penicillin G, 2.4 million units IM X 1 dose or doxycycline 100 mg bid po for 14 d . 3° syphilis benzathine penicillin G, 2.4 million units IM X 3 doses 3 wk apart.

❏❏ **Describe lesions associated with lymphogranuloma venereum:**

LV caused by Chlamydia presents as painless skin lesions with lymphadenopathy. Lesions may be papular, nodular or herpetiform vesicles. Sinus formation involving the vagina and rectum are common in women.

❏❏ **What is the cause of chancroid? Describe the lesions.**

Hemophilus ducreyi.
Presents with one or more painful necrotic lesions. Suppurating inguinal lymphadenopathy may also be present.

❏❏ **What is the cause of granuloma inguinale; describe the lesions?**

Calymmatobacterium granulomatis.
Typically begins with small papular, nodular, or vesicular lesions that develop slowly into ulcerative or granulomatous lesions. Lesions are PAINLESS and are located on mucous membranes of the genital, inguinal, and anal areas.

❏❏ **What is the causative agent in tetanus?**

Clostridium tetani, gram-positive rod, vegetative and spore form.
C. tetani produces tetanospasmin an endotoxin. This produces disinhibition of motor and autonomic nervous system, thus tetanus clinical symptoms.

❏❏ **What is the incubation period in tetanus?**

Hours to over one mo. The shorter the incubation the more severe the disease. Most patients in the US who get the disease are over 50.

❏❏ **What is the most common presentation of tetanus?**

"Generalized tetanus" with pain and stiffness in the trunk and jaw muscles. Trismus develops and results in risus sardonicus (sardonic smile).

❏❏ **What cranial nerve is most commonly involved in cephalic tetanus?**

Cephalic tetanus usually occurs after injuries to the head and typically involves the 7th cranial nerve.

❏❏ **Outline tetanus treatment**

1. Respiratory	Succinylcholine for immediate intubation if required.
2. Immunotherapy	Human tetanus immune globulin will neutralize circulating tetanospasmin and toxin in the wound (it will not neutralize toxin fixed in the nervous system). Dose TIG 3000 to 5000 units. Tetanus toxoid, 0.6 ml IM at 1 and 6 wk and 6 month
3. Antibiotics	Clostridium tetani is sensitive to cephalosporins, tetracycline, erythromycin, and penicillin. Pen G is the drug of choice.
4. Muscle Relaxants	Diazepam or dantrolene.
5. Neuromuscular block	Pancuronium bromide, 2 mg plus sedation.
6. Autonomic dysfunction.	Labetalol 0.25-1.0 mg/min IV or magnesium sulfate 70 mg/kg IV load then 1-4 g/h continuous infusion is used to treat autonomic dysfunction. MS, 5-30 mg IV infusion q 2-8 h. Clonidine, 300 µG q8h per NG.

NOTE: FATAL CARDIOVASCULAR COMPLICATIONS HAVE OCCURRED IN PATIENTS TREATED WITH B-ADRENERGIC BLOCKING AGENTS ALONE. ADRENERGIC BLOCKING AGENTS USED TO TREAT AUTONOMIC DYSFUNCTION MAY PRECIPITATE MYOCARDIAL DEPRESSION.

❏❏ **What is the most common tapeworm in the U.S.?**

Hymenolepis nana. Infections occur in institutionalized patients.

❏❏ **A patient presents with fever, dyspnea, cough, hemoptysis and eosinophilia Diagnosis?**

Ascaris lumbricoides. This helminth is a roundworm. Serologic tests: ELISA, bentonite flocculation, and indirect hemagglutination. Treat with pyrantel pamoate (pyrimidine pamoate) or mebendazole. Obstruction of the intestine may require surgery.

❏❏ **How is hookworm (Necator americanus) infection acquired?**

In areas where human fertilizer is used and people don't wear shoes. Patients present with chronic anemia, cough, low-grade fever, diarrhea, abdominal pain, weakness, weight loss, eosinophilia and guaiac positive stools. Diagnosis is made by finding ova in the stool. Treatment is mebendazole or pyrantel pamoate [This is not a zebra - SHP].

❏❏ **What are the signs and symptoms of Trichuris trichiura?**

This hookworm lives in the cecum. Complaints include anorexia, abdominal pain especially RUQ, insomnia, fever, diarrhea, flatulence, weight loss, pruritus, eosinophilia, and microcytic hypochromic anemia. Diagnosis is made by ova in the stool. Mebendazole is the treatment.

❏❏ **A patient presents with a history of attending a walrus, bear and pork roast. He now has N/V/D/F, urticaria, myalgia, splinter hemorrhages, muscle spasm, headache, and a stiff neck. What physical finding will clinch the diagnosis?**

Trichinella spiralis
Periorbital edema is pathognomonic of the infection.
Patients may have acute myocarditis, nonsuppurative meningitis, catarrhal enteritis bronchopneumonia.
Lab studies may reveal leukocytosis, eosinophilia, ECG; changes, and elevated CPK
Diagnosis is confirmed with latex agglutination, skin test, complement fixation or
bentonite flocculation test.
Stool exam is not helpful after the initial GI phase in confirming the diagnosis.

❏❏ **List 3 common protozoa that can cause diarrhea.**

Entamoeba histolytica. Occurs worldwide. Half of the infected patients are asymptomatic. Symptoms: N/V/D/F, anorexia, abdominal pain, leukocytosis. Diagnosis by stool tests, ELISA for extraintestinal infections. Treatment is metronidazole or tinidazole followed by chloroquine phosphate.

Giardia lamblia. Occurs worldwide. One of the most common intestinal parasites in the United States. Symptoms: explosive watery diarrhea, flatus, abdominal distention, fatigue, fever. Diagnosis by stool examination. Treatment is metronidazole.

Cryptosporidium parvum. Occurs worldwide. Symptoms: profuse watery diarrhea, cramps, N/V/F, weight loss. Treatment is supportive care. Medications may be needed for immunocompromised patients.

❏❏ **Explain the pathophysiology of rabies:**

Infection occurs within the myocytes for the first 48 to 96 h. It then spreads across the motor endplate, ascends and replicates along peripheral nervous, axoplasm into the dorsal root ganglia, the spinal cord, and CNS. From the gray matter, the virus, spreads by peripheral nerves to tissues and organ systems.

❏❏ **What is the characteristic histologic finding in rabies?**

Eosinophilic intracellular lesions found within cerebral neurons called Negri bodies are the site of CNS viral replication. They are found in 75% of rabies cases; although pathognomonic for rabies. their absence does not rule out rabies.

❏❏ **What are the signs and symptoms of rabies?**

Incubation period of 12 to 700 d, average 20 to 90 d.

Initial - fever, headache malaise, anorexia, sore throat, nausea, cough, and pain or paresthesias at the bite site.

CNS stage - agitation, restlessness, altered mental status, painful bulbar and peripheral muscular spasms, bulbar or focal motor paresis, and opisthotonos. Similar to Landry-Guillain-Barré syndrome, 20% develop ascending, symmetric flaccid and areflexic paralysis. Hypersensitivity to water and sensory stimuli (light, touch, and noise) may occur.

Progressive stage - lucid and confused intervals with hyperpyrexia, lacrimation, salivation? and mydriasis may occur along with brainstem dysfunction, hyperreflexia and extensor planter response.

Final stage - coma, convulsions, and apnea, followed by death at d 4 to 7 in the untreated patient.

❏❏ **What is the diagnostic procedure of choice in rabies?**

Fluorescent antibody testing (FAT).

❏❏ **How is rabies treated?**

Prevention is the most effective treatment. Wound care of suspected rabies bite should include debridement, irrigation and leaving the wound open (not sutured). This will decrease rabies infection by 90%.
RIG 20 IU/kg, half at wound site and half in the DELTOID muscle. HDCV 1-ml doses IM on days 0,3,7,14, and 28 also in the DELTOID muscle.

❏❏ **What is the second most common tick borne disease?**

Rocky Mountain spotted fever. Causative agent - Rickettsia rickettsii. Vector - Female Ixodi ticks, Dermacentor andersoni (wood tick) and D. variabilis (American dog tick). Lyme disease is the most common.

❏❏ **A patient presents with fever up to 40 ∞C followed by a rash which is erythematous, macular, and blanching. The rash progresses to deep red, dusky, papular and becomes petechial. The patient also complains of a headache, vomiting, myalgias, and cough. Where did the rash begin?**

RMSF rash typically begins on the flexor surfaces of the ankles and wrists and spread centripetally and centrifugally.

❏❏ **Test to confirm RMSF?**

Immunofluorescent antibody staining of skin biopsy or serologic fluorescent antibody titer. The Weil-Felix reaction and complement fixation tests are no longer recommended.

❏❏ **Antibiotics for RMSF?**

Tetracycline or chloramphenicol. Antibiotic therapy should not be withheld pending serologic confirmation.

❏❏ **What is the most deadly form of malaria?**

Plasmodium falciparum.

❏❏ **What is the vector for malaria?**

The female anopheline mosquito.

❏❏ **What lab findings are expected in a patient with malaria?**

Normochromic normocytic anemia, normal or depressed leukocyte count, thrombocytopenia, an elevated sed rate, abnormal kidney and LFTs, hyponatremia, hypoglycemia, and false-positive VDRL.

❏❏ **How is the definitive diagnosis of malaria established?**

Visualization of parasites on Giemsa-stained blood smears. In early infection, especially with P. falciparum, parasitized erythrocytes may be sequestered and be undetectable

❏❏ **How is P. falciparum diagnosed on blood smear?**

1. Small ring forms with double chromatin knobs within the erythrocyte. 2. Multiple rings infected within red blood cells. 3. Rare trophozoites and schizonts on smear. 4. Pathognomonic crescent-shaped gametocytes. 5. Parasitemia exceeding 4%.

❏❏ **What is the drug of choice for treating P. vivax, ovale, and malariae?**

Chloroquine.

❏❏ **How is uncomplicated chloroquine-resistant P. falciparum treated?**

Quinine + pyrimethamine-sulfadoxine + doxycycline or mefloquine.

❏❏ **How is complicated chloroquine-resistant P. falciparum treated?**

Quinidine gluconate IV + doxycycline IV.

❏❏ **What complication of quinine and quinidine therapy should be considered?**

Insulin release which may result in hypoglycemia.

❏❏ **What are the adverse effects of chloroquine?**

N/V/D/F, pruritus, headache, dizziness, rash, and hypotension.

❏❏ **What type of parasitic infection commonly presents with a papular pruritic rash?**

Schistosoma.

❏❏ **What type of parasite infections do not typically result in eosinophilia?**

Protozoa infections such as amebas, Giardia, Trypanosoma, and Babesia.

❏❏ **What is the most common intestinal parasite in the U.S.?**

Giardia. Cysts are obtained from contaminated water or passed by hand-to-mouth transmission. Symptoms include explosive foul smelling diarrhea, abdominal distention, fever, fatigue, and weight loss. Cysts reside in the duodenum and upper jejunum.

❏❏ **How is Chagas disease transmitted?**

The blood-sucking Reduviid (kissing) bug, blood transfusion, or breast feeding. A nodule or chagoma develops at the site of the bite.
Symptoms include fever, headache, conjunctivitis, anorexia, and myocarditis. CHF and ventricular aneurysms can occur. The myenteric plexus is involved and may result in megacolon.
Lab findings include anemia, leukocytosis, elevated sed rate, and ECG changes (PR interval, heart block, T-wave changes, and arrhythmias).

❏❏ **What two diseases does the deer tick, Ixodes dammini transmit?**

Lyme disease and Babesia.

❏❏ **How do patients present with Babesia infection?**

Intermittent fever, splenomegaly, jaundice, and hemolysis. The disease may be fatal in patients without spleens. Treatment is with clindamycin and quinine.

❏❏ **What is the most frequently transmitted tick-borne disease?**

Lyme disease. Causative agent - spirochete Borrelia burgdorferi.
Vector - Ixodes dammini (deer tick) also I. pacificus, Amblyomma americanum, and Dermacentor variabilis.

❏❏ **When are patients most likely to acquire Lyme disease?**

Late spring and late summer, peaks in July.

❏❏ **How is Lyme disease diagnosed?**

Immunofluorescent and immunoabsorbent assays diagnose the antibodies to the spirochete.
Treatment includes doxycycline or tetracycline, amoxicillin, IV penicillin V in pregnant patients, or erythromycin.

❏❏ **What type of paralysis does tick paralysis cause?**

Ascending paralysis. The venom which causes paralysis is probably a neurotoxin which causes a conduction block at the peripheral motor nerve branches. This prevents acetylcholine release at the neuromuscular junction, 43 species of ticks are implicated as causative agents.

❏❏ **What is the most common sign of tularemia?**

Lymphadenopathy, usually cervical in children and inguinal in adults. It is caused by Francisella tularensis and is transmitted by the vectors Dermacentor variabilis and A. americanum.

❏❏ **What two tick born diseases are transmitted by the tick vector I. dammini? FEEL the Force, Luke...**

Lyme disease and babesiosis.

❏❏ **A patient presents with sudden-onset of fever, lethargy, headache, myalgias, anorexia, nausea and vomiting. They describe the headache as retro-orbital and are extremely photophobic. They have been on a camping trip in Wyoming. What tick borne disease might cause these symptoms?**

Colorado tick fever is caused by a virus of the genus Orbivirus of the family Reoviridae. The vector is the tick D. andersoni. The disease is self-limited and treatment is supportive.

RHEUM/IMMUNOLOGY

"SUCCESS FOUR FLIGHTS THURSDAY MORNING ALL AGAINST TWENTY ONE MILE WIND STARTED FROM LEVEL WITH ENGINE POWER ALONE AVERAGE SPEED THROUGH AIR THIRTY ONE MILES LONGEST 57 SECONDS INFORM PRESS HOME CHRISTMAS."

Telegram from Orville Wright to his father, 12/17/1903

❏❏ **What class of immunoglobulins is responsible for urticaria (hives) and angioedema?**

Urticaria and angioedema both are mediated by IgE.

❏❏ **What class of immunoglobulins is responsible for food allergies?**

Food allergies are mediated by IgE.

❏❏ **What are the most common food allergies?**

Dairy products, eggs, and nuts are the most common food allergies.

❏❏ **When do the clinical manifestations of a new drug allergy usually first become apparent?**

1 - 2 weeks after starting the drug.

❏❏ **What class of drugs is commonly associated with angioedema?**

Severe and refractory angioedema of the face, lips, and tongue can occur from use of angiotensin-converting-enzyme (ACE) inhibitors. A patient who has suffered angioedema from one ACE inhibitor should not be tried on another ACE inhibitor, because the complication can result from any member of this class of antihypertensive agents.

❏❏ **What drug is the most common pharmaceutical cause of true allergic reactions?**

Penicillin accounts for approximately 90 percent of true allergic drug reactions, and for more than 95 percent of fatal anaphylactic drug reactions. Parenterally administered penicillin is more than twice as likely to cause a fatal anaphylactic reaction as is orally administered penicillin.

❏❏ **How long after exposure to an allergen does anaphylaxis (a severe hypersensitivity reaction characterized by cardiovascular collapse and respiratory compromise) occur?**

The symptoms of anaphylaxis may occur within seconds or may be delayed up to one hour.

❏❏ **A patient who is on beta blockers and who develops anaphylactic cardiovascular collapse may not respond to epinephrine or dopamine infusions. What drug can be used in this setting?**

Glucagon (5 to 15 micrograms per minute intravenously) may be useful for refractory hypotension associated with beta blocking agents.

❏❏ **Penicillin is the most common cause of death due to anaphylaxis. What is the second most common?**

Insect stings are the second most common cause of death due to anaphylaxis, and are responsible for approximately 100 deaths annually in the United States.

❏❏ **Most children with mucocutaneous lymph node syndrome are below what age?**

MLNS, or Kawasaki disease, is predominantly found in children under 9 years of age.

❏❏ **Are the nodules of Erythema Nodosum most often symmetrically or asymmetrically distributed?**

E. Nodosum presents a distinctive appearance, with bilateral tender nodules underlying red or purple shiny patches of skin in a symmetric distribution along the shins, arms, thighs, calves, and buttocks.

❏❏ **What therapy is effective for erythema nodosum?**

There is no therapy known to alter the course of the disease, which usually lasts several weeks. Non-steroidal antiinflammatory agents are usually recommended to relieve the pain associated with the tender lesions.

❏❏ **What percentage of patients with MLNS will develop an acute carditis?**

50 percent will develop carditis, usually myocarditis with mild to moderate congestive heart failure. Pericarditis, conduction abnormalities, and valvular disturbances may be seen, but are less common.

❏❏ **A patient presents with fever, acute polyarthritis, or migratory arthritis a few weeks after a bout of streptococcal pharyngitis. What disease should be suspected?**

Acute rheumatic fever. Although the early symptoms may be nonspecific, physical exam eventually reveals signs of arthritis (60 - 75 percent of cases), carditis (30 percent of cases), choreiform movements (10% of cases), erythema marginatum, or subcutaneous nodules.

❏❏ **What treatment should be started when the diagnosis of acute rheumatic fever has been made?**

Penicillin or erythromycin should be given even if cultures for group A streptococcus are negative. High-dose aspirin therapy is used at an initial dose of 75 - 100 mg/kg/day. Carditis or congestive heart failure is treated with prednisone in a dose of 1 - 2 mg/kg/day.

❏❏ **Rheumatic fever is associated with migratory arthritis. What other diseases commonly cause migratory arthritis?**

Diseases other than rheumatic fever that may be associated with migratory arthritis include subacute bacterial endocarditis, Henoch-Schönlein purpura (HSP), drug sensitivity reactions, septicemia (especially gonococcemia, meningococcemia, and staphylococcal or streptococcal septicemia), Lyme disease, and prodromal pulmonary infections with Mycoplasma, coccidiomycosis, or histoplasmosis.

❏❏ **What is Lhermitte sign in ankylosing spondylitis, and what other diseases may produce it?**

A sensation of electric shock that radiates down the back when the neck is flexed. This is a sign that atlantoaxial subluxation and cervical spine instability may be present. This sign may also be seen in patients with rheumatoid arthritis and in those with multiple sclerosis.

❏❏ **What rheumatic syndrome may lead to corneal irritation, ulceration, and infection?**

Sjogren's syndrome. This syndrome, in which the mouth and eyes are dry due to lymphocytic infiltration of the lacrimal and salivary glands, may occur as an independent entity or as an accompaniment to other rheumatologic diseases.

❏❏ **What are the most common organisms responsible for septic arthritis and osteomyelitis of the foot in an immunocompetent adult?**

Staphylococcus and Pseudomonas.

❏❏ **How can gout and pseudogout be distinguished using a microscope with a polarizing filter?**

When the plane of polarization is perpendicular to the crystal, pseudogout (calcium pyrophosphate) crystals appear yellow and rhomboidal, while gout (uric acid) crystals appear blue and needle-shaped. The mnemonic CUB, or 'crossed urate blue' is a reminder.

❏❏ **Give an example of each of the 4 major types of allergic reaction listed below.**

Type I: (immediate hypersensitivity)
Type II: (cytotoxic)
Type III: (arthus reaction)
Type IV: (delayed hypersensitivity)

Type I: Asthma and food allergies (IgE)
Type II: Transfusion reaction (IgG & IgM)
Type III: Serum sickness; post-streptococcal glomerulonephritis (complex activates complement)
Type IV: Skin testing (Activated T-lymphocytes)

❏❏ **Which of the four types of allergic reaction can be caused by drug allergy?**

Drug allergy can produce all four types of allergic reaction.

❏❏ **In which disease is the onset of pain more rapid: gout, or pseudogout?**

Gout. The onset of pain in acute gouty arthritis occurs over a few hours, while pain in pseudogout usually evolves over a day or more.

❏❏ **What is the common name for granulomatous arteritis of the thoracic aorta and its branches? What are its common symptoms?**

Temporal arteritis. Symptoms include tender scalp, headache, fluctuating vision, reduced brachial pulse, and jaw or tongue pain.

❏❏ **What is the normal atlantodental distance on lateral flexion views of the cervical spine?**

3.5 mm in adults and 4 mm in children under 12 years of age.

❏❏ **Myocardial Infarction can be related to which two rheumatic diseases?**

Kawasaki disease (mucocutaneous lymph node syndrome) and polyarteritis nodosa (PAN)

❏❏ **What diagnostic procedure is indicated for a patient with rheumatoid arthritis who presents with dysphagia, hoarseness, and stridor?**

Urgent laryngoscopy to assess the paired cricoarytenoid joints, which can cause airway compromise if they become fixed in a closed position.

❏❏ **What is the most common cause of anaphylactoid reactions?**

Radiographic contrast media.

❏❏ **A bacterial infection and an allergic phenomenon both can cause a generalized confluent exfoliation of skin. What are the two diseases, and what test can tell the two apart?**

Ritter's disease, or dermatitis exfoliativa neonatorium is caused by infection with staphylococcus, and thus is also known as the 'staphylococcal scalded-skin syndrome' (SSSS). It causes exfoliation at the superficial granular layer of the epidermis. Toxic epidermal necrolysis (TEN) looks very similar, but is an allergic phenomenon. Skin biopsy can tell the two apart, because in TEN the exfoliative cleavage plane is deeper, at the dermal-epidermal junction or lower.

❏❏ **What is needed to make a diagnosis of mucocutaneous lymph node syndrome, or Kawasaki disease in a young patient with prolonged fever?**

The diagnosis requires four of these five common clinical findings: (1) conjunctival inflammation, (2) rash, (3) adenopathy, (4) strawberry tongue and injection of the lips and pharynx, and (5) erythema and edema of extremities. Desquamation of fingers and toes may be striking, but it is a late finding and is not one of the key clinical features of the disease.

❏❏ **What is the likely diagnosis in an adolescent girl with unexplained pain and tenderness at the head of the second metatarsal? What clinical and x-ray findings are likely?**

Frieberg's infarction is an avascular necrosis of a metatarsal head, most often the second metatarsal, and occasionally occurring bilaterally. Typical findings include local swelling and tenderness, restricted range of motion at the MTP joint, and x-ray evidence of sclerosis, flattening, or irregularity of the metatarsal head.

❏❏ **What is the treatment of choice for the patient in anaphylactic shock?**

Epinephrine in a dose of 0.3 - 0.5 mg intravenously. If there is no IV access, inject into the venous plexus at the base of the tongue.

❏❏ **How long should a patient with a generalized anaphylactic reaction be observed?**

Because recurrence of hemodynamic collapse and airway compromise is common within the first 24 hours, patients should be observed for that period of time. Treatment with antihistamines and steroids should be continued for 72 hours.

❏❏ **How does relapsing polychondritis affect the airway?**

Approximately 50% of patients with relapsing polychondritis have airway involvement, and may present with pain and tenderness over cartilaginous structures of the larynx, as well as with dyspnea, stridor, cough, hoarseness, and erythema and edema of the oropharynx and nose.

❏❏ **How should a patient with airway involvement from relapsing polychondritis be managed?**

Admit these patients for high-dose steroids and close observation. Repeated exacerbations may lead to severe airway compromise and asphyxiation.

❏❏ **How common is pleurisy in patients with systemic lupus erythematosus, and what should be the diagnostic approach?**

Approximately half of patients with SLE will develop symptoms of pleurisy at some time. All pleural effusions in patients with rheumatic disease require thoracentesis to distinguish inflammatory from infectious effusions. Pulmonary embolism is common in patients with SLE, thus a nuclear ventilation-perfusion (V/Q) scan is also indicated.

❏❏ **What percentage of patients with Kawasaki disease who do not receive proper therapy will develop coronary artery aneurysms?**

Without treatment, approximately 20% will develop coronary artery aneurysms, and 1% - 2% of patients with an aneurysm will die of acute myocardial infarction during the resolution phase of the illness.

❏❏ **A patient who is on chronic steroids presents with weakness, depression, fatigue, and postural dizziness. What pathological process should be suspected, and what is the treatment?**

Adrenal insufficiency should be suspected. The treatment is to administer large doses ('stress doses') of steroids.

❏❏ **If adrenal insufficiency is suspected, what test should be performed and what drug should be given?**

A serum cortisol level should be drawn before administering a large dose of steroids. Dexamethasone is the preferred agent because it does not interfere with subsequent tests that may be indicated.

❏❏ **What cardiac complication is commonly seen in systemic lupus erythematosus as well as in juvenile rheumatoid arthritis and rheumatoid arthritis?**

Pericarditis.

❏❏ **What is the normal atlantodental distance on lateral flexion views of the cervical spine, and what rheumatologic diseases commonly alter this?**

The normal atlantodental space is up to 3.5 mm in an adult and up to 4 mm in a child. Ankylosing spondylitis and rheumatoid arthritis can destroy ligamentous supporting structures and produce atlantoaxial subluxation with widening of this space.

❏❏ **What are the symptoms of atlantoaxial subluxation?**

Patients with this syndrome may present with changes in bowel of bladder function, limb paresthesias, or new weakness.

❏❏ **What vascular disease is accompanied by polymyalgia rheumatica in 10% to 30% of cases?**

Temporal arteritis.

❏❏ **What is the most pressing priority in a patient suspected of having new onset of acute gouty arthritis?**

The exclusion of a septic arthritis must assume top priority when new gout is suspected, because the signs and symptoms of the two diseases may be indistinguishable.

❏❏ **What complication of rheumatoid arthritis may produce signs and symptoms that mimic those of deep vein thrombosis?**

Rheumatoid arthritis (and other chronic inflammatory arthritides) may be associated with the formation and rupture of a Baker's cyst. A Baker's cyst can occasionally be distinguished clinically from DVT when deep hemorrhage from the ruptured cyst produces bruising or staining in a purple crescent below the malleoli, or when localized swelling at the site of the ruptured popliteal cyst spares the more distal parts of the leg and the foot.

❏❏ **Arthritis of the elbow joint causes limitation of all motion at the joint. In what way does olecranon bursitis differ?**

Pain from olecranon bursitis may limit flexion and extension at the elbow, but it usually does not affect pronation and supination.

❏❏ **How should a potentially septic olecranon bursitis be treated?**

As much fluid as possible should be aspirated from the bursa via a large-bore needle, and antibiotics should be started immediately.

❑❑ **How do the white blood cell counts in fluid aspirated from septic bursitis differ from those found in septic arthritis?**

The white blood cell count in fluid from a septic joint is usually 10 times higher than the white blood cell count in fluid from a septic bursitis.

❑❑ **What are the articular symptoms of disseminated (stage II) Lyme disease?**

Migratory arthritis (with attacks that are typically brief) along with bursitis and tendonitis.

❑❑ **What are the articular symptoms of late (stage III) Lyme disease?**

Chronic arthritis, especially in the knee, along with periostitis and tendonitis.

❑❑ **In a patient with rheumatoid arthritis, how should a new monarthritis be approached?**

The risk of infection is increased in a joint that has been previously injured or affected by arthritis, thus a new monarthritis in a patient with known rheumatoid arthritis should be considered to be septic until proven otherwise.

❑❑ **What painful bone abnormality often complicates steroid therapy in patients with rheumatoid arthritis or systemic lupus erythematosus?**

Avascular necrosis of the femoral head, femoral condyles, or bones of the feet.

❑❑ **A 10-year-old child presents limping, complaining of several weeks of groin, hip, and knee pain, worse with activity. What diseases should be considered?**

Transient tenosynovitis of the hip, slipped capital femoral epiphysis, Legg-Calvé-Perthes, suppurative arthritis, rheumatic fever, juvenile rheumatoid arthritis, and tuberculosis of the hip.

❑❑ **What is Legg-Calvé-Perthes disease, how does it present, and who is affected?**

Legg-Calvé-Perthes disease is avascular necrosis of the femoral head, presenting in a child between 2 and 13 years of age as subacute groin, hip, and knee pain, worse with activity. The disease is also known as 'Coxa Plana'.

❑❑ **What is the diagnosis in a preadolescent child with activity-related knee pain and a thickened and tender patellar tendon?**

Osgood-Schlatter disease, an inflammatory repetitive-injury process in which cartilaginous fragments are pulled loose from the tibial tuberosity by the ligamentum patellae of the quadriceps tendon. Treatment is by several months of restriction from excessive physical activity.

❑❑ **What disease is suspected in an adolescent with a tender, purpuric dependent rash, colicky abdominal pain, migratory polyarthritis, and microscopic hematuria?**

Henoch-Schonlein purpura, a leukoclastic vasculitis. Intestinal or pulmonary hemorrhage may occur, and 7 to 9 percent will develop chronic renal sequelae. Salicylates are effective for the arthritis. Other treatment is directed at the symptoms. Steroids are not particularly effective.

❑❑ **A child has painful swollen joints along with a spiking high fever, shaking chills, signs of pericarditis, and a pale erythematous coalescing rash on the trunk, palms, and soles. Hepatosplenomegaly is found. What is suspected?**

Systemic juvenile rheumatoid arthritis. Arthrocentesis is necessary to rule out septic arthritis. Rheumatoid factor and antinuclear antibody usually are negative, and one fourth of patients will proceed to have joint destruction. This is the least common of the three types of JRA.

❏❏ **What treatment besides aspirin has been shown to be effective in preventing the complications of Kawasaki disease?**

Intravenous immunoglobulin can reduce the incidence of coronary artery aneurysms to less than 5 percent.

❏❏ **What joint is most commonly involved in the most common form of juvenile rheumatoid arthritis?**

The most common of the three forms of JRA usually involves the knee and does not lead to joint destruction. Reiter's syndrome, iridocyclitis, and inflammatory bowel disease all may be associated with this 'pauciarticular' form of the disease.

❏❏ **A child has post-traumatic tenderness at the end of a long bone, and a joint effusion is the only radiographic finding. What management is appropriate?**

Immobilization and subsequent orthopedic evaluation for possible separation of the epiphysis from the metaphysis (Salter-Harris type I fracture).

❏❏ **A patient presents with pain along the radial aspect of the wrist, extending into the forearm. What test can make the diagnosis?**

Finkelstein's test can make the diagnosis of DeQuirvain's tenosynovitis (overuse inflammation of the extensor pollicis brevis and the abductor pollicis where they pass along the groove of the radial styloid). The patient makes a fist with the thumb tucked inside the other fingers, and pain is reproduced when the examiner gently deviates the fist in the ulnar direction.

❏❏ **In carpal tunnel syndrome, Tinel's sign is produced by tapping the volar wrist over the median nerve. If the test is positive, what does the patient experience?**

Paresthesias extending into the index and long fingers.

❏❏ **A patient with shoulder pain radiating to the medial forearm also has a reduction in the radial pulse upon passive abduction of the shoulder. What is the diagnosis?**

Thoracic outlet syndrome. Compression of the brachial plexus can cause pain and paresthesias that sometimes radiate all the way down to the ring and small fingers.

❏❏ **What is suspected when a patient with shoulder pain has a palpable fullness in the supraclavicular fossa?**

Pancoast's tumor in the superior sulcus of the lung.

❏❏ **What are the three most common cervical problems that cause pain radiating to the shoulder?**

Degenerative disease of the cervical spine, degenerative disc disease, and herniated nucleus pulposus.

❏❏ **Which herniated cervical disc can cause pain mimicking the pain of a rotator cuff injury?**

C5 - C6.

❏❏ **A 70-year-old patient complains of progressive pain and restriction of motion at the shoulder for several months. On examination, there is minimal tenderness to palpation, but active and passive range of motion are limited in abduction and in rotation. What is the likely diagnosis?**

114

Adhesive capsulitis. The pain is usually a poorly localized diffuse aching, often worse at night. The etiology is unclear, but the condition commonly follows injury or chronic inflammation, particularly after immobilization.

❏❏ **A 40-year old patient reports the sudden spontaneous onset of shoulder pain while at rest. Any shoulder movement reproduces the pain. There is crepitus with motion, and the point of maximum tenderness is over the proximal humerus at the insertion of the rotator cuff. What is the diagnosis and what will be seen on x-ray?**

The x-ray will reveal calcified deposits in the rotator cuff, typical of calcific tendonitis. The cause is unknown, but the calcific deposits are painless until they begin to undergo spontaneous resorption. The symptoms are self-limited.

❏❏ **What autoimmune disease produces lesions that are sometimes urticarial in appearance, yet are not pruritic?**

Erythema multiforme

❏❏ **What disease classically produces erythematous plaques with dusky centers and red borders, resembling a bulls-eye target?**

Erythema multiforme. This disease can also produce non-pruritic urticarial lesions, petechiae, vesicles, and bullae,

❏❏ **What drugs are most commonly implicated in toxic epidermal necrolysis?**

Sulfonamides and sulfones, phenylbutazone and related drugs, barbiturates, other antiepileptic drugs, and antibiotics.

❏❏ **What is the appropriate management of TEN?**

Admit for management similar to that for extensive second-degree burns. The mortality of TEN can be as high as 50% due to fluid loss and secondary infections.

❏❏ **What can cause erythema multiforme?**

EM can be triggered by viral or bacterial infections, drugs of nearly all classes, and by malignancy.

❏❏ **What is the most common cause of allergic contact dermatitis?**

Toxicodendron species (poison oak, poison ivy, and poison sumac) are responsible for more cases of contact dermatitis than all other allergens combined.

❏❏ **Why does scratching cause poison oak or poison ivy to spread?**

The antigenic resin contaminates the hands and fingernails, and is spread by rubbing or scratching. A single contaminated finger can produce more than 500 reactive groups of lesions.

❏❏ **How can the antigen of poison oak or poison ivy be inactivated?**

Careful washing with soap and water destroys the antigen. Special attention must be paid to the fingernails, which otherwise can carry the antigenic resin for weeks.

❏❏ **What underlying illnesses should be considered in a patient with nontraumatic uveitis?**

Collagen vascular diseases, sarcoid, ankylosing spondylitis, Reiter syndrome, tuberculosis, syphilis, toxoplasmosis, juvenile rheumatoid arthritis, and Lyme disease.

❏❏ **What is the difference between episcleritis and scleritis?**

Both are associated with collagen vascular disorders, but episcleritis is a benign superficial inflammation of the tissues between the sclera and the conjunctive, while scleritis is a more severe and more painful inflammation of the deep sclera that can sometimes result in visual loss.

❏❏ **Which cervical radiculopathy can produce pain mimicking the pain of cardiac ischemia?**

C6-C7.

❏❏ **What anatomic fact makes cervical radiculopathies so often confusing?**

Motor and sensory roots are separate at the neural foramina, so severe sensory complaints and findings often lack a motor component.

❏❏ **Where does cervical disc prolapse most often occur?**

At C6 - C7 on the left and at C5 - C6 on the left.

❏❏ **Neck pain and upper-extremity hyperreflexia suggest a cervical lesion at what level?**

Above C5.

❏❏ **Which cervical root is nearly always involved when radiculopathy causes bilateral shoulder pain?**

C6. This myotome encompasses most of the proximal shoulder muscles, and the C6 nerve root is the earliest and most commonly affected by cervical disc syndromes.

❏❏ **What bony abnormality can produce Horner's syndrome, radicular symptoms without neck pain, vertebral-basilar insufficiency, and painless weakness in an upper-extremity myotome?**

Osteophytes encroaching on cervical neural foramina.

❏❏ **A patient presents with acute lower back pain. What are the criteria for admission?**

Paralysis, paraparesis, loss of bowel or bladder function, inability to stand or sit, need to sleep in an upright position, intractable pain and spasticity, or metastatic cancer.

❏❏ **What type of spinal lesion is suspected when back pain forces a patient to sleep in an upright position?**

The pain from thoracic root lesions is usually worse when reclining.

❏❏ **In what way can trochanteric bursitis mimic lumbar radiculopathy?**

Both can produce pain that involves the hip and radiates along the iliotibial band to the lateral knee.

❏❏ **A patient with sudden, symmetric, multilevel areflexia, lower extremity muscle weakness, and bowel or bladder incontinence may have what lesion?**

A midline herniation of a lumbar disk with compromise of the distal cauda equina. Emergency decompression may restore function and prevent permanent paraparesis.

❑❑ **What spinal lesion can produce 'shin splints'?**

Compromise of the L5 and S1 nerve roots. This lesion may also produce calf pain mimicking the symptoms of deep vein thrombosis.

❑❑ **A patient with back pain who cannot walk on the toes has a lesion at what level?**

S1.

❑❑ **A patient with back pain who cannot walk on the heels has a lesion at what level?**

L5.

❑❑ **What is wrong with a patient who has back pain when the hip and knee are flexed and the sciatic nerve is 'plucked' or 'strummed' in the popliteal fossa?**

Disc herniation with nerve root impingement produces this 'strum sign'

❑❑ **What is the likely diagnosis in a patient with myalgias, arthralgias, headache, and an annular erythematous lesion with central clearing?**

Stage I Lyme disease, with the classic lesion of Erythema Chronicum Migrans (ECM). The primary lesion occurs at the site of a tick bite.

❑❑ **What rheumatologic ailments produce pulmonary hemorrhage?**

Goodpasture's disease, systemic lupus erythematosus, Wegener's granulomatosis, and nonspecific vasculitides.

❑❑ **What rheumatologic ailments produce pulmonary fibrosis?**

Ankylosing spondylitis, scleroderma, and rheumatoid arthritis (less common).

❑❑ **What rheumatologic ailments can produce respiratory muscle failure?**

Dermatomyositis and polymyositis.

❑❑ **What rheumatologic ailments can produce acute airway obstruction?**

Relapsing polychondritis and rheumatoid arthritis.

❑❑ **What infectious agents may produce a chronic smoldering arthritis with sterile aspiration cultures?**

Tuberculosis and fungal infections. Synovial biopsy may be required to make the diagnosis.

❑❑ **How is septic bursitis contracted?**

A puncture wound or an overlying cellulitis are the most common sources for septic bursitis.

❑❑ **What rheumatologic ailments produce valvular heart disease?**

Ankylosing spondylitis, relapsing polychondritis, and rheumatic fever.

PSYCHOSOCIAL PEARLS

"It is difficult to say what is impossible, for the dream of yesterday is the hope of today and the reality of tomorrow."

Robert H. Goddard, at his high school
graduation, 1904.

❏❏ **Name some over the counter and street medications that may produce delirium or acute psychosis.**

Salicylates, antihistamines, anticholinergics, alcohols, phencyclidine, LSD, mescaline, cocaine and amphetamines.

❏❏ **You are considering chemical restraint. List your options.**

Benzodiazepines: lorazepam, (Ativan), 1-2 mg IV, 2-6 mg orally every 30 min
midazolam, (Versed), 2-4 mg IV every 30 min
diazepam, (Valium), 5 mg IV or orally every 30 min.

Sedative hypnotics: haloperidol, (Haldol), 1-5 mg IM/IV, titrate to clinical response
droperidol, (Inapsine), 1-2 mg IV every 30 min.

Benzodiazepines may be given in combination with sedative hypnotics above to both hasten and potentiate their effect. Titrate to effect and monitor appropriately, of course.

❏❏ **A patient has ingested a phenothiazine and arrives hypotensive. What intervention(s) may be considered?**

IV crystalloid boluses usually suffice. Severe cases are best managed with norepinephrine, (Levophed), or metaraminol, (Aramine). These pressors stimulate alpha adrenergic receptors preferentially. Beta agonists such as isoproterenol, (Isuprel), are contraindicated due to the risks of beta receptor stimulated vasodilation.

❏❏ **List some potential complications of clozapine therapy.**

Clozapine appears to stimulate limbic rather than striated dopaminergic receptors preferentially, reducing the incidence of extrapyramidal symptoms. Well documented complications include oversedation, hypotension, anticholinergic symptoms, EKG changes and agranulocytosis.

❏❏ **Why are Type 1A antiarrhythmics best avoided in clozapine or risperidone ingestion?** ·

These medications prolong the QT interval as well as widen the QRS complex. Agents such as procainamide, quinidine and disopyramide can further prolong the QT interval, raising the risk of refractory SVT, VT and cardiovascular collapse.

❏❏ **What is Wellbutrin?**

Bupropion, (Wellbutrin), is an aminoketone, a different chemical structure than other antidepressants. Mechanism of action remains unknown. Its effect on serotonin and norepinephrine reuptake is minimal as are its anticholinergic effects. It is best avoided in patients with seizure disorder or taking medications known to lower seizure threshold. Use with MAO inhibitors is contraindicated.

❏❏ **List some common pathophysiology associated with eating disorders?**

Hyponatremia, hypokalemia, hypocalcemia, hypophosphatemia, anemia, hypoglycemia, starvation ketoacidosis, abnormal glucose tolerance, hypothyroidism due to low T3 levels, persistently elevated cortisol due to starvation, low FSH, LH and estrogens, and elevated growth hormone.

❏❏ **What are characteristics of failure to thrive syndrome in infants?**

Body mass index (BMI) < 5%, irritable, hard to console behavior, increased muscle tone in the lower extremities or hypotonia, and subsequent weight gain in the hospital.

❏❏ **When considering failure to thrive syndrome which historical features are important to assess?**

History of prematurity, birth weight, maternal use of cigarettes, alcohol, and or drugs during the pregnancy, previous hospitalizations, and parental stature.

❏❏ **In what percentage of cases of child sexual abuse is the abuser known by the child?**

90%.

❏❏ **In what percentage of cases of child abuse is the mother also abused?**

50%.

❏❏ **What is involved in the genital examination with a history of child sexual abuse?**

Unless there is a suspicion of perforating vaginal trauma, genital examination should be confined to an examination of the external genitalia and perianal area. There is no need for a speculum exam unless the victim is an older adolescent.

❏❏ **In the case of child sexual assault, what laboratory tests should be done?**

As indicated, oral, rectal, vaginal or urethral swabs for GC and Chlamydia. Serological tests for syphilis or HIV testing should be done if there is a history of, or clinical evidence of infection in the assailant or the victim. Urine or plasma ß-HCG should be checked in girls beyond age of menarche.

❏❏ **What is considered physical evidence of acute ano-genital trauma in the genital exam of a child?**

With acute sexual abuse you may see fissures, abrasions, hematomas, changes in tone (either dilation or spasm), or discharges (semen fluoresces with a woods light, or examine under microscope). Erythema is a sign of inflammation, irritation or manipulation and is not specific for abuse.

❏❏ **What is considered physical evidence of chronic ano-genital trauma in the genital exam of a child?**

With chronic sexual abuse signs of an STD such as vaginal or anal discharge, venereal warts or vesicles may be observed. Injuries can heal without residual scarring and a lack of physical changes in no way rules out child sexual abuse.

❏❏ **In addition to the history, physical, laboratory tests and collection of physical evidence, what else needs to done in the case of child sexual abuse?**

File a report with child protective services and law enforcement agencies. Provide emotional support to the child and family. Give a return appointment for follow-up of STD cultures and testing for pregnancy, HIV, Syphilis as indicated. Assure follow up for psychological counseling by connecting the family/child to the appropriate services in your area.

❏❏ **What are the most common ages for child physical abuse?**

Two thirds of physically abused children are under the age of three and one third are under the age of 6 months.

❑❑ In cases where the mother is abused how often are the children also abused?

Approximately 40% of cases.

❑❑ In addition to an evaluation for child abuse, what laboratory studies should be done in the child with multiple bruises?

CBC with differential, platelet count, PT, and UA.

❑❑ An infant with mental status changes and retinal hemorrhages and/or subdural hematomas who has no evidence of external head injury may be a victim of what type of child abuse?

"Shaken baby syndrome."

❑❑ What is our best knowledge about the frequency of rape?

According to the 1987 Uniform Crimes Report at least one in eight women have been raped and it is estimated that only 25% of all rapes are reported.

❑❑ What is the definition of domestic abuse?

A pattern of assaultive and coercive behaviors including physical, sexual, and psychological abuse designed to gain power and control over an intimate partner.

❑❑ What is the epidemiology of domestic violence?

95% of the victims are women. An estimated 4 million women are battered each year. The life time prevalence of abuse for adult women is about 10%. Domestic abuse is the number one cause of injuries to women. More than half of all women murdered in the U.S. are killed by a current or intimate partner.

❑❑ What are the rates of domestic abuse in the acute care setting?

In an ED, trauma or acute psychiatric setting, prevalence rates of domestic abuse have been reported to range from 15 to 25% with appropriate screening protocols. In the absence of screening protocols, physicians identify less than 5% of cases of domestic abuse.

❑❑ What are characteristics of an abusive relationship?

The abusive relationship evolves over time usually escalating from jealousy and a desire to control a partner's behavior into humiliation, degradation, and use of the fear of physical violence. He may or may not have to actually hit her if she knows that he is capable of hurting her or her children. The end result is low self-esteem, control, isolation and entrapment.

❑❑ What are the socio-economics of domestic abuse?

Anyone can be involved in an abusive relationship, including men and women in same-sex relationships. Domestic abuse crosses all socio-economic, religious, and racial lines.

❑❑ What historical factors have been reported to be associated with a history of domestic abuse?

Young, pregnant, unmarried or separated women appear to be at greater risk. There has also been high prevalence reported in women with HIV, anxiety disorders, substance abuse, chronic pain syndromes (headaches, functional GI complaints, pelvic pain) and mental illness.

❑❑ In what percentage of domestic abuse are the children also abused?

In 33 - 50% of the families in which the mother is battered, the partner also abuses the children. An abused mother is also 7 times more likely to abuse her children.

❑❑ What are clinical clues of domestic violence?

Any evidence of injury during pregnancy or late entry into prenatal care. Injuries presenting after significant delay or in various stages of healing especially to the head, neck, breasts, and abdomen or those suggesting a defensive posture such as forearm bruises. Vague complaints or unusual injuries such as bites, scratches, burns, and rope marks. Suicide attempts and rapes.

❑❑ What is the standard of care for victims of domestic violence currently recommended by JCAHO, the AMA, and the CDC?

Establish an effective confidential system of identification of DV victims. Documentation of the abuse. Collection of physical evidence. Evaluation of the safety issues, potential for lethality, or suicide. Formulation of a safety plan with the victim. Advising the victim of all her options and resources. Referrals for counseling and other services including legal assistance. Coordination with law enforcement. Transportation to a shelter if desired or needed. Appropriate follow-up by a domestic violence advocate.

❑❑ What are reasons some women stay with abusers?

Real fear of escalation of the violence. Economics/Lack of resources. Low self-esteem. Feelings of isolation. Love for the abuser. Belief that the violence is her fault. Hope that he'll change. Psychological immobilization, depression, substance abuse. Concern about being able to provide for the children. Cultural or religious beliefs in the maintenance of the family at all costs.

❑❑ What helps an abused woman leave an abusive relationship?

Leaving is a process. Extrication from an abusive intimate relationship usually takes place over a period of time as the woman ideally builds a network of support, accesses needed resources, and regains confidence in her own strengths. Women leave when they know they have adequate resources. Most women test out those resources several times first before leaving for good.

❑❑ What is the problem with the medical model in dealing with victims of domestic abuse?

The medical model of diagnosing, prescribing, treating symptoms has traditionally been paternalistic and controlling. Patients who do tell physicians about abuse have described experiences with physicians who ignore or minimize their feelings, "prescribe" leaving, are judgmental and abandon her if she is not ready. This desire to control her behavior, mirrors her experience with the abuser. A more therapeutic response would include validating her experience, expressing concern for her safety and that of her children and empowering her by providing access to the resources she needs to escape an unhealthy situation when it is safe for her to do so.

❑❑ What factors contribute to violence in the ED work setting?

High patient volumes, long waiting times, substance abuse, and lack of adequate security.

❑❑ What are predictors of a potentially violent patient?

Male gender, a history of being violent, and a history of substance abuse are the only reliable predictors. Cultural, educational, economic, and language barriers to effective patient/staff communication as well as trivializing a patient or family member's concerns can increase frustrations and lower the threshold for violent episodes.

❑❑ **What are important clinical considerations in handling an intoxicated violent, psychotic, or threatening patient?**

These patients require a careful history and physical with attention to the mental status exam, looking for evidence of trauma, toxic ingestion, or metabolic derangement. Historical sources such as family, paramedics, mental health workers, police, or medical records may need to be accessed. The patient may need to be physically and at times chemically restrained to obtain an adequate examination and for the safety of the patient and ED staff.

❑❑ **What organic problems are associated with violence?**

Organic problems associated with violent behavior include but are not limited to: delirium, dementia, head trauma, CNS infection, seizures, neoplasm, CVA, hypoglycemia, hypoxia, hyperthermia, anemia, AIDS psychosis, electrolyte abnormalities, vitamin deficiencies, endocrinopathies, toxic ingestion of aromatic hydrocarbons, drug reactions, steroids, alcohol and sedative/hypnotic intoxication and withdrawal, anticholinergics, PCP, cocaine, LSD, and amphetamines.

❑❑ **What psychiatric problems are associated with violence?**

Acute schizophrenia, paranoid ideation, catatonic excitation, mania, borderline and antisocial personality disorders, delusional depression, post-traumatic stress disorder, and decompensating obsessive/compulsive disorder.

❑❑ **What are the prodromes of violent behavior?**

Anxiety, defensiveness and volatility, and physical aggression.

❑❑ **What are the best strategies for prevention of violence in the emergency department setting?**

The physical plan in the ED should be one of controlled access with a reasonable but enforced visitation policy. Isolation rooms should be quite and calm settings, safe for both the patient and the staff, with accessible panic buttons and large enough for a team of security guards, should a "show of force" or use of force be necessary. The training of all ED personnel to recognize and defuse potentially violent situations with cooperation and fast response times from security is critical to staff and patient safety.

❑❑ **What is the number one cause of death for African-American males between the ages of 10 and 24 y?**

Firearm injury. The overall homicide rate for young men in the US is over 7 times that of the next developed country. For Hispanic males this rate is 10 times more and for African American males the rates are over 30 times higher than comparable countries.

❑❑ **Which accounts for more firearm related deaths, intentional or unintentional causes?**

Intentional causes account for 94% of firearm deaths - suicide 48% ad homicide 46%. Unintentional firearm injuries account for about 4%. Only 1% of firearm deaths occur as a result of legal intervention. The number of firearm related fatalities has more than doubled over the last 30 years.

❑❑ **What are risk factors for homicide?**

Most homicide victims are killed by someone they know, someone of the same race, and usually during an argument or fight. Drugs and alcohol are important co-factors as is the presence of a handgun.

❏❏ **What are the relative risks for suicide and homicide if a gun is kept in the home?**

If there is a gun in the home, a suicide is 5 times more likely to occur (9 times more likely if a loaded handgun is available). A homicide is 3 times more likely to occur and the victim is 43% more likely to be a member of the family than an intruder. In the case of domestic violence, a gun at home increases the risk of homicide 20 fold.

❏❏ **What is the clinical significance of the increased availability of semi-automatic weapons?**

Between 1982 and 1992 the percentage of gunshot victims with multiple gunshot wounds increased from 5% to 20%. The rate of spinal cord injuries from GSWs quadrupled. This trend has resulted in an increased numbers of major organ injuries, complications, surgeries, severity of injury and probability of death.

❏❏ **Describe a patient with generalized anxiety disorder.**

Patients appear apprehensive, restless, irritable and easily distracted. Patients may experience muscle tension and fatigue as well as various autonomic symptoms such as palpitations, shortness of breath, chest tightness, nausea or diffuse weakness and numbness.

❏❏ **Name a few substances that may mimic generalized anxiety when ingested.**

Nicotine, caffeine, amphetamines, cocaine, anticholinergics; alcohol and sedative withdrawal.

❏❏ **What is the epidemiologic difference between those who attempt and those who complete suicide?**

Suicide completers tend to be older males with medical problems, living alone or with a poor social network.

❏❏ **Name 2 Axis I disorders commonly associated with suicidal ideation.**

Alcohol abuse and affective (mood) disorder.

❏❏ **What happens when one combines EtOH with an anxiolytic (benzodiazepine)?**

Death! (Due to their combined respiratory depressive effects).

❏❏ **Name another contraindication to benzodiazepine use.**

Known hypersensitivity, acute narrow angle glaucoma, pregnancy especially 1st trimester.

❏❏ **Why have mono-amine oxidase (MAO) inhibitors been prescribed less frequently?**

Why don't you try a tyramine-free diet sometime! Mmm Mmm good!
Tyramine containing substances can cause hypertensive crisis - such foods include pickled herring, snails, chicken liver, beer, red wine and cheese.

❏❏ **Name some drugs <u>contraindicated</u> for a patient taking MAO inhibitors.**

Toxic reactions that include excitation and hyperpyrexia can occur with meperidine (Demerol) and with dextromethorphan. The effects of indirect acting adrenergic drugs are potentiated, including ephedrine, sympathomimetic amines in cold remedies, amphetamines, cocaine and methylphenidate (Ritalin).

❏❏ **Name the three common MAO inhibitors (chemical and Brand name).**

Phenelzine (Nardil).
Isocarboxazid (Marplan).
Tranylcypromine (Parnate).

❏❏ **How does one treat hypertensive crisis caused by combining MAO inhibitors with a known toxin, cheese pizza?**

An α- and ß-adrenergic antagonist such as labetalol.
Also consider nifedipine or nitroglycerin. If unsuccessful, consider IV phentolamine or sodium nitroprusside.

❑❑ **A 27 y old male arrives somnolent with vitals of P 130, R 26, BP 170/80 T of 105 °F. You note diffuse muscular rigidity and intermittent focal muscle twitching/jerking lasting 1-2 seconds. As you 'work him up', your faithful nurse returns from the waiting area with news from the family that the patient has had a progressive decline of mental status for 2 d after seeing his psychiatrist. The patient has had a history of 'psychosis' for almost one year. What process should be included in your differential diagnosis at this time?**

Neuroleptic malignant syndrome.

❑❑ **Psychiatrists use a multiaxial diagnostic system to describe a particular patient's medical problem list; discuss.**

Axis I: Symptoms and syndromes comprising a mental disorder, includes substance abuse/addiction.
Axis II: Personality and developmental disorders (underlying the Axis I diagnosis).
Axis III: Physical medical problems/conditions which may or may not contribute to Axis I diagnosis.
Axis IV: Psychosocial factors.
Axis V: Adaptive ability/disability.

❑❑ **What is organic brain syndrome?**

Reversible or non-reversible mental condition thought to be caused by disease process or substance use which interrupts normal anatomical, physiological or biochemical brain functions.

❑❑ **Describe dementia.**

Disturbed cognitive function resulting in impaired memory, personality, judgment and/or language. Insidious onset, but may present as acute worsened mental state while facing other physical or environmental stressors.

❑❑ **Describe delirium.**

"Clouding of consciousness" resulting in disorientation, decreased alertness and impaired cognitive function. Acute onset, visual hallucinosis, fluctuating psychomotor activity; all symptoms variable and may change over hours.

❑❑ **Neuroleptic medications come in three flavors: low, medium and high potency. Can you name some of these meds and their category?**

Low potency: Chlorpromazine (Thorazine).
Medium potency: Perphenazine (Trilafon).
High potency: Haloperidol, droperidol (Inapsine), thiothixene (Navane), fluphenazine (Prolixin), trifluoperazine (Stelazine).

❑❑ **So, what's the big deal?**

Neuroleptics act to block dopamine receptors. Receptor blockade within the mesolimbic area of the brain provides their antipsychotic effect. Dopaminergic receptor blockade throughout the CNS and anticholinergic effect produce many side effects observed in the ED.

❑❑ **Which neuroleptics produce which side effects?**

Low potency: Sedative, orthostatic hypotension, anticholinergic effects.

High potency: Less sedating, profound extrapyramidal reactions.

❏❏ **What are extrapyramidal reactions?**

Dopamine receptor blockade within the nigrostriatal system results in involuntary and spontaneous motor responses including: dystonia, akathisia and Parkinson's-like syndrome.

❏❏ **What is a dystonic reaction?**

Very common side effect of neuroleptics seen in the ED. Muscle spasm of tongue, face, neck and back are seen. Severe laryngospasm and extraocular muscle spasm may occur also. Patients may bite the tongue leading to potential airway compromise either by inability to open the mouth or by tongue edema or hemorrhage.

❏❏ **How do you treat a dystonic reaction?**

Diphenhydramine (Benadryl), 25-50 mg IM or IV or benztropine (Cogentin), 1-2 mg IV or PO. Remember that dystonias can recur acutely.

❏❏ **Describe symptoms of alcohol withdrawal.**

Autonomic hyperactivity: tachycardia, hypertension, tremors, anxiety, agitation; 6-8 h after drinking.

Hallucinations: auditory, visual, tactile; 24 h after drinking.

Global confusion: 1-3 d after drinking.

❏❏ **List some life-threatening causes of acute psychosis.**

WHHHIMP: Wernicke's Encephalopathy, Hypoxia, Hypoglycemia, Hypertensive encephalopathy, Intracerebral hemorrhage, Meningitis/Encephalitis, and Poisoning.

❏❏ **Characteristics of schizophrenia?**

Delusional disorder, hallucinations, (usually auditory), disorganized thinking, loosening of associations, disheveled appearance, lack of insight in realizing thoughts and behavior are abnormal, onset age usually less than 40, and duration of symptoms longer than 6 mo.

❏❏ **What is the difference between schizophrenia and schizophreniform disorder?**

Very little. In schizophreniform disorder, schizophrenic symptoms have lasted less than 6 mo.

❏❏ **What is a brief reactive psychosis?**

Acute psychotic break, usually after an emotional or traumatic event. Short duration, usually less than 2 wk.

❏❏ **Signs and symptoms suggestive of organic source of psychosis.**

Acute onset, disorientation, visual or tactile hallucinations, evidence suggesting overdose or acute ingestion, such as abnormal vital signs, pupil size and reactivity, nystagmus, and age less than 10 or older than 60.

❏❏ **Name some symptoms of major depression.**

In sad cages: Interest, sleep, appetite, depressed mood, concentration, activity, guilt, energy, suicide.

❏❏ **Name some vegetative symptoms.**

Loss of appetite, lack of concentration, chronic fatigue, agitation, restlessness, inability to sleep, weight loss.

GU PEARLS

"Honesty is the first chapter in the book of wisdom."

Thomas Jefferson

❑❑ **What are the clinical findings suggestive of acute glomerulonephritis (GN)?**

Oliguria
Hypertension
Pulmonary edema
Urine sediment containing: red blood cells, white blood cells, protein, and red blood cell casts.

❑❑ **What is the most common cause of intrinsic renal failure?**

Acute tubular necrosis (80% - 90% of cases) resulting from an ischemic injury (the most common cause of ATN) or a nephrotoxic agent.

The less frequent causes of intrinsic renal failure (10% - 20% of cases) are vasculitis, malignant hypertension, acute GN, or allergic interstitial nephritis.

❑❑ **Which syndrome is characterized by rapidly progressive antiglomerular basement membrane antibody induced GN that is preceded by pulmonary hemorrhage and hemoptysis?**

Goodpasture's Syndrome.

❑❑ **What is the <u>most common</u> cause of postinfectious GN?**

Post-streptococcal (group A, β-hemolytic) although other infections may be the cause. The GN is due to immune complex deposition in glomeruli. Most patients recover renal function spontaneously within a few weeks.

❑❑ **What is the differential diagnosis for rapidly progressive GN?**

Polyarteritis Nodosa (PAN) - A systemic necrotizing vasculitis affecting primarily medium and small caliber arteries that can occur from infancy to old age. The peak incidence is at approximately 60 y of age. 90% of patients with PAN will have renal involvement.

Systemic Lupus Erythematosus - An autoimmune disorder resulting, in part, in necrotizing vasculitis of primarily small vessels complicated by direct immunoglobulin deposition in glomeruli. The mortality rate is 18% - 58% depending on the histologic type.

Henoch-Schönlein Purpura - Another systemic necrotizing vasculitis of small vessels. Patients present with a nephritic syndrome without edema or hypertension, or with hematuria.

Hemolytic Uremic Syndrome (HUS) - Patients present with microangiopathic hemolytic anemia, thrombocytopenia, and renal dysfunction. The onset is rapid. It occurs in children about one week after a gastroenteritis or a URI. HUS may occur in adults, most commonly complicating pregnancy or postpartum period. Acute renal failure develops in 60% of children with HUS, and usually resolves in weeks with only supportive therapy.

Thrombotic Thrombocytopenic Purpura - This is closely related to HUS with higher occurrence in young adults. It is associated with fevers, more neurologic problems, and less renal involvement (usually with hematuria and proteinuria). The prognosis is much worse than HUS with a 75% three-month mortality rate.

❏❏ **Name some common nephrotoxic agents/substances.**

Aminoglycosides, NSAIDs, contrast dye, and myoglobin.

❏❏ **Which patients with a UTI are candidates for single dose or short-course (three d) antibiotic therapy with trimethoprim-sulfamethoxazole (TMP-SMX)?**

Nonpregnant adult women without risk factors for subclinical pyelonephritis such as prolonged symptoms, recurrent UTIs, diabetes mellitus, urinary tract abnormalities, or recurrent pyelonephritis. These patients must be able to follow up within one week.

❏❏ **Outpatient management of pyelonephritis should be reserved for which patients?**

Young, otherwise healthy patients who are not vomiting, are hemodynamically stable, who defervesce with antipyretics, and are able to drink fluids. These patients should be treated with intravenous fluids, antipyretics, and a dose of intravenous antibiotics (gentamycin, a third-generation cephalosporin, or TMP-SMX).

❏❏ **What is the eponym for idiopathic scrotal edema, and how is this disease treated?**

Fournier's gangrene is a polymicrobial infection of the subcutaneous tissue that is characterized by widespread tissue necrosis. Treatment consists of broad-spectrum parenteral antibiotics and immediate surgical debridement.

❏❏ **What is the significance of the "blue dot" sign?**

This is pathognomonic of torsion of the appendix testis or epididymis. With transillumination of the testis, a blue reflection is seen. When seen early, the patient with torsion of the appendages will have pain that is more intense near the head of the epididymis or testis that is frequently associated with a palpable tender nodule. If this diagnosis can be confirmed by testicular ultrasound that documents normal flow to the affected testis, immediate surgery can be avoided since most appendages will calcify or degenerate within 10 to 14 d, without harm to the patient.

❏❏ **How does the pain associated with epididymitis differ from that of prostatitis?**

Epididymitis - The pain begins in the scrotum or groin and radiates along the spermatic cord. It intensifies rapidly, is associated with dysuria, and is relieved with scrotal elevation (Prehn's sign).

Prostatitis - Patients will have frequency, dysuria, urgency, bladder outlet obstruction, and retention. They may have low back pain, perineal pain associated with fever, chills, arthralgias, and myalgias.

❏❏ **How does the treatment of epididymitis differ according to age?**

In patients less than 40 years old, the most common pathogens are Chlamydia and gonorrhea that are treated with ceftriaxone IM and doxycycline PO

In patients over 40 years of age, the common causes are urinary pathogens such as Escherichia coli (E. coli) and Klebsiella that are treated with TMP-SMX.

❏❏ **What percentage of patients with epididymitis will have pyuria?**

24%.

❑❑ **What are the causative organisms of prostatitis?**

E. coli in 80% and Klebsiella, Enterobacter, Proteus, or Pseudomonas in 20%.

❑❑ **What is the outpatient treatment of prostatitis?**

TMP-SMX DS PO BID for 30 d or
Ciprofloxacin 500 mg PO BID for 30 d or
Norfloxacin 400 mg PO BID for 30 d.

Great quote series:

"Two things are infinite: the universe and human stupidity, and I'm not so sure about the universe."

Albert Einstein

❑❑ **When are the two peaks in the incidence of testicular torsion?**

The first year of life and at puberty.

❑❑ **True or false- Testicular torsion frequently follows a history of strenuous physical activity or occurs during sleep.**

True.

❑❑ **True or false- 40% of patients with testicular torsion have a history of similar pain in the past that resolved spontaneously?**

True.

❑❑ **What is the definitive diagnostic test for testicular torsion?**

Emergent surgical exploration. Although radionuclide imaging and doppler ultrasonography may be helpful, they are time-consuming and their accuracy is operator dependent. The warm ischemia time for testicular salvage may be as short as four h. Therefore, once the diagnosis is entertained, immediate urologic consultation and surgical exploration are necessary.

❑❑ **When is a retrograde urethrogram necessary in the evaluation of a patient with a penile fracture?**

A penile fracture is rupture of the corpus cavernosum with tearing of the tunica albuginea that results from blunt trauma to the erect penis. Urethral injury occurs in approximately 10% of patients with a penile fracture. Patients with hematuria, blood at the urethral meatus, or inability to void should undergo retrograde urethrography to rule out a urethral injury.

❑❑ **What is the initial treatment of priapism?**

Terbutaline 0.25 mg - 0.5 mg subcutaneously.

❑❑ **What are most urinary calculi made of?**

75% are composed of calcium (calcium oxalate or calcium phosphate).

❑❑ **What percent of urinary calculi are radiopaque?**

90%.

❑❑ **What percent of urinary calculi will pass spontaneously?**

90%.

❑❑ **What are admission criteria for patients with renal calculi?**

Patients should be admitted if they have infection with concurrent obstruction, a solitary kidney and complete obstruction, uncontrolled pain, intractable emesis, large stones (only 10% of stones > 6 mm pass spontaneously). Other indications for admission and urologic consultation include renal insufficiency, and complete obstruction or urinary extravasation demonstrated by the IVP.

❑❑ **What percent of patients with urinary calculi will not have hematuria?**

10%.

Great quote series:

"Space is almost infinite. As a matter of fact, we think it is infinite."

Dan Quale, VP, head of the Space Council

❑❑ **Describe acute glomerulonephritis (GN).**

Hematuria.
Proteinuria.
Oliguria or Anuria.
Edema.
Hypertension.

❑❑ **Can a selected group of women with a UTI probably be treated safely with single dose or short-course (3 d) antibiotic therapy with TMP/SMX?**

Yes; those with few "priors", short period of UTI symptoms and no risk factors for subclinical pyelonephritis.

❑❑ **What are the risk factors for subclinical pyelonephritis?**

Those are the things that make someone more likely to have it. They include multiple prior UTIs, longer duration of sx, recent pyelonephritis, diabetes, anatomic abnormalities, immunocompromised patients and in those who are indigent.

❑❑ **The "rule of twos" is a wonderful pearl described by Dr. David S. Howes of the University of Illinois in Tintinalli, 4th Ed. which explains outpatient management for appropriate women who present at that institution with uncomplicated pyelonephritis. Outline the "rule of twos."**

Give 2 L of IV fluid.
Give 2 Tylenol #3.
Give 2 g ceftriaxone.
If patient can tolerate 2 glasses of water and fever decreases by 2 degrees:
Give TMP/SMX Double strength bid for 2 weeks, plan f/u in 2 d for progress check.

Ed. note: Gotta love that one!! We give one g ceftriaxone or use other IV abx.

❑❑ **About what percentage of patients with epididymitis will have pyuria?**

24%.

❏❏ **Contrast the pain associated with epididymitis to that of prostatitis.**

Epididymitis -pain begins in scrotum or groin radiates along spermatic cord, often intensifies quickly after onset, may be associated with dysuria and may be relieved by scrotal elevation.
Prostatitis -acute prostatitis is associated with more frequency, dysuria and urgency, bladder outlet obstruction and retention, low back and perineal area pain associated with fever and chills, and with arthralgias and myalgias.

Patients with either of these disorders may become toxic and require admission.

❏❏ **What is the initial treatment for priapism?**

Terbutaline 0.25-0.5 mg SQ q 4 - 6 h.

❏❏ **What are most renal calculi made out of?**

70% of renal calculi are composed of calcium oxalate.

❏❏ **About what percentage of renal stones are radiopaque?**

90%.

❏❏ **About what percentage of renal calculi will pass spontaneously?**

90%.

EMS PEARLS

"Houston, Tranquillity Base here. The Eagle has landed."

Neil Armstrong, radio transmission to Mission Control, at the moment of the first manned landing on the moon, 7/20/1969.

❑❑ **What two events in 1966 heralded the birth of pre-hospital medical services?**

1) The publication of national report, Accidental Death and Disability: the Neglected Disease of Modern Society which emphasized the scope of preventable death and injury from trauma.
2) The passage of the National Highway Safety Act which forced states to develop systems for the provision of pre-hospital medical care.

❑❑ **Which federal law delineated the components of an EMS system?**

Public Law 93-154 (the Emergency Medical Services Systems Act) defined fifteen elements of an EMS system.

❑❑ **Describe the three levels of recognized EMS providers and estimate the h of training necessary to achieve that level:**

EMT-Basic: 100 h. These EMTs can apply perform CPR, do basic airway management, perform spinal immobilization, control hemorrhage, extricate and transport patients.
EMT-Intermediate: 100-200 h. An intermediate level of provider that adds several specific skills to those of EMT-Bs: defibrillation, IV access, invasive airway management.
EMT-Paramedic: 1000-2000 h. The most sophisticated level of prehospital care; EMT-P's provide definitive airway management (including needle cricothyroidotomy), defibrillation, needle thoracostomy, intraossoeus infusions and most importantly, intravenous drug administration.

❑❑ **Describe the difference between a regular and enhanced 911 system?**

Enhanced 911 will give the public service access point (fire/EMS/police) the caller's address and telephone number via a computer screen should the caller be unable to give such information.

❑❑ **Describe three key components of an effective emergency medical dispatch center?**

1) Tiered dispatch: To get the appropriate level of provider to a scene based on presentation of symptoms. To decrease deployment of unnecessary resources.
2) Pre-arrival instructions: To give specific first aid instructions to the caller prior to the arrival of EMS providers.
3) CPR: Dispatchers will instruct the caller in CPR.

❑❑ **What are the two ways in which physicians can provide oversight to EMS systems?**

On-line and Off-line medical control.

❑❑ **True or False: Physicians are the only personnel that may provide on-line medical control.**

False. In 14 states, physician surrogates (Mobile Intensive Care Nurses (MICN's) or paramedic communicators) may provide direction that is concurrent with the provision of prehospital medical care.

❏❏ **What are three duties of an Off-line (indirect) medical director?**

1) Prospective medical control: The development of protocols, establishment of training regimens and the implementation of operating policies.
2) Immediate medical control: Differing from on-line medical control; this oversight evaluates components of in-field care not related to medical decision-making (i.e. ride alongs, turnaround times).
3) Retrospective medical control: Review of system components to ensure quality care (i.e. chart review, QI analysis).

❏❏ **Name one difference between a VHF and an UHF EMS radio system?**

VHF radio systems are simplex: can only broadcast messages one way at a time; UHF communications can be sent and received simultaneously. Other differences include UHF's ability to better penetrate buildings and ability to support repeaters that increase broadcast distance.

❏❏ **What percentage of an EMS system's call volume do cardiac arrests comprise?**

Approximately 5%.

❏❏ **What recent development has been shown to increase survival from out-of-hospital cardiac arrest?**

The Automatic External Defibrillator (AED).

❏❏ **In which city would you want to have an out-of-hospital cardiac arrest and explain why?**

Seattle. From the earliest research in cardiac arrest, Seattle has shown excellent overall (approx. 25%) and neurologic survival in those people with cardiac arrests secondary to ventricular arrhythmias.

❏❏ **What percentage of an EMS system's call volume do pediatric runs comprise?**

10-15%. A majority of these runs are related to respiratory emergencies.

❏❏ **What is the proper position to transport a pregnant trauma patient?**

With spinal backboard tilted 30 degrees to the left in order to prevent the supine hypotension syndrome.

❏❏ **Identify three elements that distinguish the provision of EMS in rural settings from that in urban areas?**

Low call volumes that make maintenance of skills (for primarily volunteer departments) difficult;
Long transport times to facilities without specific expertise (i.e. trauma or cardiac centers);
Rural EMS systems deal with more elderly patients with the concomitant increase in the number of cardiac and medical cases (70% (rural) to 30% (urban)).

❏❏ **Define a medical disaster.**

A medical disaster is defined by ACEP as a situation where the destructive effects of natural or manmade forces overwhelm the ability of a community to meet the demands for health care. Thus a MVA with many victims in a small community may be as much a disaster as a large earthquake.

❏❏ **Describe two components of the National Disaster Medical System (NDMS).**

The first are the participating community hospitals that have committed to receiving disaster victims from other communities. The second is the development of Disaster Medical Assistance Teams (DMATs) to respond to the site of a civilian disaster.

❏❏ **When responding to a HAZMAT incident, what must EMS providers do to prevent becoming a victim?**

EMS providers must wear appropriate protective clothing and assure proper decontamination procedures.

❏❏ **About what percentage of normal <u>coronary</u> blood flow is achieved during CPR?**

5%.

❏❏ **About what percentage of normal cardiac output is achieved during CPR?**

20-25%.

❏❏ **What is the currently favored theory explaining how CPR works?**

The thoracic pump theory - that blood flow is induced by a pressure gradient between the intrathoracic and extrathoracic compartments.

❏❏ **What is the favored theory explaining how MAST works?**

MAST increases peripheral vascular resistance (PVR).

❏❏ **What is the absolute contraindication to using MAST?**

Pulmonary edema.

❏❏ **Name relative contraindications to MAST.**

Pregnancy.
Impaled objects.
Evisceration.
Thoracic/diaphragmatic injuries.

❏❏ **About what percentage of patients who undergo cardiac resuscitation attempts recover and are neurologically intact?**

10%.

❏❏ **About what percentage of patients who undergo cardiac resuscitation attempts survive, but are not functionally and neurologically intact?**

25%.

❏❏ **Intracellular accumulation of what electrolyte is currently thought to initiate a cascade of events that lead to cell death?**

Calcium.

❏❏ **EOA is contraindicated in patients less than how old?**

16 y.

❏❏ **Catheter over needle puncture/ventilation, rather than cricothyroidotomy is recommended for patients under how many years of age?**

10 y.

❏❏ **Uncuffed ET tubes should be selected for patients under how old?**

6 y.

❏❏ **What is the most common complication of EOA use?**

Insertion into the trachea (about 10%).

❏❏ **T/F- When a patient arrives in the ED with an EOA the first thing the ED physician should do is remove the EOA and replace it with an endotracheal tube.**

False - an endotracheal tube should be placed with the EOA still in position.

❏❏ **What recent development, in the pre-hospital setting, has been documented to show improvement in cardiac arrest outcome?**

Automatic External Defibrillator.

❏❏ **EMS systems had an emphasis in their development of managing cardiac arrests. What percent of EMS calls are cardiac arrests?**

<5%.

❏❏ **What percent of an EMS system's call are pediatric?**

10%.

ENVIRONMENTAL PEARLS

"He who possesses virtue in abundance may be compared to an infant.
Poisonous insects will not sting him. Fierce beasts will not seize him.
Birds of prey will not strike him....
He may cry all day without becoming hoarse,
This means that his natural harmony is perfect."

Tao-te Ching, 55; Lao Tzu

❏❏ **Above what altitude does acute mountain sickness typically develop?**

8,000 feet.

❏❏ **What organ is most commonly affected in a radiation accident?**

The skin. Burns may take up to two weeks to become clinically apparent.

❏❏ **What is the LD_{50} for a radiation victim?**

The dose causing death in 50% of patients at 60 days is 450 rads; the LD_{90} is 700 rads.

❏❏ **What is the clinical significance of fixed and dilated pupils in a drowning victim?**

Don't give up the ship! 10% to 20% of patients presenting with coma and fixed and dilated pupils recover completely. Asymptomatic patients should be observed for a minimum of 4 to 6 hours.

❏❏ **What blood gas findings are expected in a drowning victim?**

Poor perfusion and hypoxia result in metabolic acidosis.

❏❏ **Are abdominal thrusts (Heimlich maneuver) indicated in a drowning victim?**

No. Drowning victims usually aspirate small quantities of water and no drainage procedure has been found helpful.

❏❏ **What percentage of dog and cat bites become infected?**

About 10% of dog and 50% of cat bites become infected. Pasteurella multocida infects 30% of dog and 50% of cat bites.

❏❏ **A six year old child presents with headache, fever, malaise, and tender regional lymphadenopathy about a week after a cat bite. A tender papule develops at the site. Diagnosis?**

Cat-scratch disease. Usually develops 3 days to 6 weeks following a cat bite or scratch. The papule typically blisters and heals with eschar formation or a transient macular or vesicular rash may develop.

❏❏ **What is the most likely cause of an infection from an animal bite that develops in less than 24 hours? More than 48 hours?**

Less than 24 hours is typically P. multocida or streptococci. More than 48 hours is usually S. aureus.

❑❑ **A patient presents with two minute puncture wounds, a halo lesion is present with a circular area of pallor surrounded by a ring of erythema. Diagnosis?**

Black widow spider envenomation.

❑❑ **Describe the presentation of a black widow spider versus a scorpion envenomation.**

Black widow victims typically stay in one position for a few seconds to minutes before moving, they also have a halo lesion. Scorpion victims present with a constant writhing and abnormal eye movements.

❑❑ **What are the indications for giving antivenin in a black widow spider envenomation?**

Severe pain, dangerous hypertension, pregnant women with moderate to severe envenomations, and pregnant women threatening abortion who are mildly symptomatic after an envenomation. Antivenin should be avoided in patients taking β-adrenergic blocking agents as if anaphylaxis occurs, it will be difficult to treat.

❑❑ **When is calcium used in the treatment of black widow envenomations?**

Recent literature suggests that calcium provides little if any benefit.

❑❑ **What is the recommended treatment for brown recluse spider envenomations?**

Benign neglect. Dapsone 25-100 mg orally for 1-2 weeks may prevent ulceration if started early; especially useful if face or digits are involved. Dapsone is contraindicated if pregnant and in patients with G-6-PD deficiency. Steroids, vasodilators, and antibiotics are not generally helpful. Avoid NSAIDs as they may induce bleeding. Early wide excision is ineffective, unnecessary, and expensive, it may result in increased disability or worsen scarring.

❑❑ **Can a scratch from a rattlesnake result in a serious envenomation?**

A single puncture wound or scratch has resulted in serious envenomation. Up to 25% of bites do not result in envenomation.

❑❑ **At what point should fasciotomy be considered in a rattlesnake bite victim?**

Only after documented increased compartment pressure unresponsive to limb elevation, antivenin (5-10 vials), and mannitol (1-2 g/kg IV).

❑❑ **Which rattlesnake patients will develop serum sickness following antivenin administration?**

Most patients who receive more than five vials will develop serum sickness. Symptoms may range from a mild viral-like to severe urticarial rash and arthralgias. Treatment includes antihistamines, corticosteroids, and analgesics.

❑❑ **Is horse serum allergy an absolute contraindication to antivenin administration in a rattlesnake victim?**

No.

❑❑ **A patient is brought to the ED with a history of a bite wound inflicted at a mental ward. What bacterium is likely?**

Eikenella corrodens is more common in hospitalized and institutionalized patients. Most human bite infections are due to staphylococcus aureus or streptococcus.

❑❑ **What is the frequency of eye injuries in lightning strike victims?**

Half develop structural eye lesions. Cataracts is the most common and develops within days to years. Unreactive dilated pupils may not equal death as transient autonomic instability may occur.

❑❑ **What is the most common otologic injury in a lightning strike victim?**

50% have tympanic membrane rupture. Hemotympanum, basilar skull fracture, and acoustic and vestibular deficits may also occur.

❑❑ **What is the most common arrhythmia found in a patient with hypothermia?**

Atrial fibrillation. Other ECG findings include PAT, prolongation of the P-R, QRS, or Q-T, decreased P-wave amplitude, T-wave changes, PVCs, or humped ST segment adjacent to the QRS complex (Osborn wave).

❑❑ **What is the first-line treatment of ventricular fibrillation in a hypothermic patient?**

Bretylium NOT lidocaine.

❑❑ **A near-drowning victim presents to the ED. What electrolyte abnormalities are expected?**

Electrolyte abnormalities are usually not significant.

❑❑ **What antibiotics and what steroid dose are indicated in the ED for a near-drowning victim?**

Trick question. Prophylactic antibiotics and steroids are not useful for preventing aspiration pneumonia or pulmonary edema. Steroids may be used for increased ICP.

❑❑ **A 14 y old football player presents to the ED with a history of light-headedness, headache, nausea, and vomiting. On exam, the patient has a HR of 110, RR 22, BP of 90/60, and is afebrile. Profuse sweating is noted. Diagnosis?**

Heat exhaustion. Treat with .9 NS IV fluid.

❑❑ **A 23 y old marathon runner presents confused and combative. Temperature is 105° C. Why must renal function be monitored?**

Patient has heatstroke. Rhabdomyolysis may occur 2-3 d post-injury. Recall that in heatstroke volume depletion and dehydration may not always occur.

❑❑ **Treatment of heatstroke?**

Cool sponging, ice packs to groin and axilla, fanning, and iced gastric lavage. Antipyretics are not useful.

❑❑ **A 12 y old male presents with complaints of fatigue, fever, headache, itching rash, and joint aches. Exam reveals multiple sites of lymphadenopathy. The patient cannot recall any past medical problems. Just as you are about to leave the room, scratching your head, mom says "Oh doctor, he was stung by a bee 2 wk ago. Is that important?" Diagnosis?**

Serum-sickness-like delayed reaction.

❑❑ **How should a honeybee's stinger be removed?**

Scrape it out. Squeezing with a tweezers or finger may increase envenomation.

❑❑ **A 4 y old presents with an itching lesion on the legs and waist. On exam, you find hemorrhagic puncta surrounded by urticarial and erythematous patches following a zig-zag pattern. Treatment?**

Starch baths at bedtime are used to treat pruritus of flea bites.

❑❑ **A 16 y old presents with intense itching of the penis and the web spaces of his hands. Diagnosis?**

Scabies frequently attacks the web spaces of the hands and feet. Small vesicles and papules may be present.

❏❏ **A 6 y old in Texas presents with a history of being bitten by a caterpillar. The child has tense rhythmic pain. Edema and a red blotchy rash are apparent at the site as well as a white vesicle. Diagnosis and treatment?**

Megalopyge opercularis larva (puss caterpillar) sting.   Remove remaining spines with sticky-tape and treat with 10 ml of 10% calcium gluconate IV.

❏❏ **A color blind 36 y old Texan presents with a history of snake bite. He says the snake was as big as a telephone pole, had fangs like a lion, and was striped like a zebra. On exam, you find ptosis, slurred speech, dysphagia, myalgia, and dilated pupils. What snake bit this man?**

Most likely a coral snake (Micrurus sp.).

❏❏ **Should blisters be débrided for a burn victim?**

YES. They contain vasospastic agents and should be drained.

❏❏ **An Osborn (J) wave seen on ECG is associated with what disorder?**

Hypothermia.

❏❏ **Hypothermia is defined as a core temperature below:**

35 °C.

❏❏ **Heat loss can occur via radiation, convection, conduction and evaporation. Which of these accounts for the greatest loss?**

Radiation, followed by convection when not perspiring.
If immersed, conduction causes the greatest heat loss.

❏❏ **A 4 y old bites into an extension cord and receives a burn on the lips. What specific concern do you have?**

Delayed rupture of the labial artery may occur 3-5 d post-injury.

❏❏ **Compare the entrance and exit wounds of AC and DC.**

AC -   Entrance and exit wounds same size.
DC -   Small entrance and large exit.
NB. -   Not all texts agree!

❏❏ **How is a sodium metal wound débrided?**

Cover with mineral oil and excise retained metal fragments.

❏❏ **Is lightning AC or DC?**

DC. May cause asystole and respiratory arrest.

❏❏ **What type of arrhythmia is expected with AC shock?**

V-fib.

❏❏ **Can lightning strike twice in the same place?**

Yes. Yes.

❏❏ **Why should the ears be examined in a lightning strike victim?**

TM rupture (50%). Associated with basilar skull fracture.

❏❏ For how long should an asymptomatic lightning strike victim be monitored?

Several hours as CHF may be delayed. Serial enzymes if EKG changes or chest pain.

❏❏ What neurologic injury may be expected in a lightning injury?

Lower and upper extremity paralysis due to vascular spasm.

❏❏ What lab work-up should be considered in a lightning victim?

CBC, BUN/Cr, UA (Check myoglobin), CPK -MM & MB, EKG, and CT if change in sensorium.

❏❏ What eye finding is associated with lightning strike?

Cataracts.

❏❏ A patient presents with a history of headache, nausea, vomiting, and weakness. They also feel lightheaded. In addition to gastroenteritis, what other diagnosis should always be considered?

CO poisoning.

❏❏ What is the most common cause of death with CO poisoning?

Cardiac arrhythmias.

❏❏ How is topical phenol exposure treated?

Water and olive oil can be useful in the field. Isopropyl alcohol, glycerol, or polyethylene glycol mixture in the ED for carbolic acid exposure.

❏❏ In what two plant ingestions is ipecac contraindicated?

Jequirity bean (alkaline) and hemlocks sp. (may induce seizures).

HEM/ONC PEARLS

"Nature does nothing without a purpose."

Aristotle

❏❏ **What types of blood loss are suggestive of a bleeding disorder?**

Spontaneous bleeding from many sites.
Bleeding from non-traumatic sites.
Delayed bleeding several h after trauma.
Bleeding into deep tissues or joints.

❏❏ **What common drugs have been implicated in predisposing to acquired bleeding disorders?**

Ethanol, ASA, NSAIDs, warfarin, antibiotics.

❏❏ **Mucocutaneous bleeding, including petechiae, ecchymoses, epistaxis, GI, GU or menorrhagia is indicative of what coagulation abnormality?**

Qualitative or quantitative platelet disorders.

❏❏ **Bleeding into joints or potential spaces, (i.e. retroperitoneum) as well as delayed bleeding, suggests what type of bleeding disorder?**

Coagulation Factor Deficiency.

❏❏ **What is primary hemostasis?**

It is the platelet interaction with the vascular subendothelium that results in the formation of a platelet plug at the site of injury.

❏❏ **What components are required for primary hemostasis?**

Normal vascular subendothelium (collagen).
Functional platelets.
Normal von Willebrand factor (connects the platelet to the endothelium via glycoprotein Ib).
Normal Fibrinogen (connects platelets to each other via glycoprotein IIB-IIIA).

❏❏ **What is the final end-product of secondary hemostasis (coagulation cascade)?**

Cross-linked fibrin.

❏❏ **What mechanism limits the size of the fibrin clots that are formed?**

The fibrinolytic system.

❏❏ **What is the principle physiologic activator of the fibrinolytic system?**

Tissue plasminogen activator (tPA). tPA is released from endothelial cells, converts plasminogen (adsorbed in the fibrin clot) to plasmin. Plasmin degrades fibrinogen and fibrin monomer into fibrin degradation products (FDPs [once called fibrin split products]) and cross-linked fibrin into D-dimers.

❏❏ **Below what platelet count is spontaneous hemorrhage likely to occur?**

< 10,000/mm^3.

❏❏ **It is generally agreed that most patients with active bleeding and platelet counts < 50,000/mm^3 should receive platelet transfusion. How much will the platelet count be raised for each unit of platelets infused?**

10,000/mm^3.

❏❏ **What groups of patients with thrombocytopenia would be unlikely to respond to platelet infusions?**

Those with platelet antibodies (ITP or hypersplenism).

❏❏ **How can an overdose of warfarin be treated? What are the advantages and disadvantages of each treatment?**

Treatment depends on the severity of symptoms, not the degree of prolongation of the prothrombin time (PT); if there are no signs of bleeding, temporary discontinuation may be all that is necessary; if bleeding is present, treatment can be initiated with fresh frozen plasma (FFP) or Vitamin K.

FFP: Advantages: rapid repletion of coagulation factors and control of hemorrhage. Disadvantages: volume overload, possible viral transmission

Vitamin K: Advantages: ease of administration. Disadvantages: possible anaphylaxis when given IV; delay in onset of 12-24 h; effects may last up to 2 wk making anticoagulation of the patient difficult or impossible.

❏❏ **What is the only coagulation factor not synthesized by hepatocytes?**

Factor VIII.

❏❏ **What hemostatic alterations are seen in patients with liver disease?**

Decreased protein synthesis leading to coagulation factor deficiency.
Thrombocytopenia.
Increased fibrinolysis.
Vitamin K deficiency.

❏❏ **What treatment options are available for patients who are bleeding and have liver disease?**

Transfusion with PRBCs (maintains hemodynamic stability).
Vitamin K.
Fresh frozen plasma.
Platelet transfusion.
DDAVP (Desmopressin).

❏❏ **Which test of hemostasis is most often prolonged in uremic patients?**

Bleeding time.

❏❏ **What options are available for treatment of patients with renal failure and coagulopathy?**

Dialysis.
Optimize hematocrit
　　-recombinant human erythropoietin

-transfusion with PRBCs.
Desmopressin.
Conjugated estrogens.

Cryoprecipitate and platelet transfusions if hemorrhage is life-threatening.

❏❏ **What are the clinical complications of DIC?**

Bleeding.
Thrombosis.
Purpura fulminans.

❏❏ **What three laboratory studies would be most helpful in establishing the diagnosis of DIC?**

Prothrombin time - Prolonged.
Platelet count - Usually low.
Fibrinogen level - Low.

❏❏ **What are the most common hemostatic abnormalities in patients infected with HIV?**

Thrombocytopenia
Acquired circulating anticoagulants (causes prolongation of aPTT)

❏❏ **What is the pentad of Thrombotic Thrombocytopenic Purpura (TTP)?**

Fever.
Thrombocytopenia.
Neurologic symptoms.
Renal insufficiency.
Microangiopathic hemolytic anemia (MAHA).

❏❏ **What is the leading cause of death in hemophiliacs?**

AIDS.

❏❏ **How much will one unit of Factor VIII concentrate raise the circulating Factor VIII level?**

2%.

❏❏ **How much will one unit of Factor IX concentrate raise the circulating Factor IX level?**

1%.

❏❏ **What is the most common inherited bleeding disorder?**

von Willebrand Disease.

❏❏ **70-80% of patients with von Willebrand disease have Type I. What is currently the approved mode of therapy for bleeding in these patients? What is the dose?**

DDAVP
0.3 µg/kg IV or sc q 12h for 3-4 doses.

❏❏ **What is the most common hemoglobin variant?**

Hemoglobin S (Valine substituted for glutamic acid in the sixth position on the ß-chain).

❏❏ **What types of clinical crises are seen in patients with sickle cell disease?**

Vasoocclusive (Thrombotic).
Hematologic
    -Sequestration
    -Aplastic.
Infectious.

❏❏ **What is the most common type of sickle cell crisis?**

Vasoocclusive (Average: 4 attacks/y).

❏❏ **What percentage of patients with sickle cell disease have gallstones?**

75% (only 10% are symptomatic).

❏❏ **What is the only type of vasoocclusive crisis that is painless?**

CNS crisis (most commonly cerebral infarction in children and cerebral hemorrhage in adults).

❏❏ **What are the mainstays of therapy for a patient in sickle cell crisis?**

Hydration.
Analgesia.
Oxygen (only beneficial if patient is hypoxic).
Cardiac monitoring (if patient has history of cardiac disease or is having chest pain).

❏❏ **What is the most commonly encountered sickle hemoglobin variant?**

Sickle cell trait.

❏❏ **What is the most common human enzyme defect?**

Glucose-6-Phosphate Dehydrogenase Deficiency (G-6-PD).

❏❏ **What drugs should be avoided in patients with G-6-PD Deficiency?**

Drugs that induce oxidation.
Sulfa.
Antimalarials.
Pyridium.
Nitrofurantoin.

❏❏ **What is the single most useful test in ascertaining the presence of hemolysis and a normal marrow response?**

The reticulocyte count.

❏❏ **What is the most common morphologic abnormality of red cells in hemolytic states?**

Spherocytes.

❏❏ **What is the most common clinical presentation of TTP (Thrombotic thrombocytopenic purpura)?**

Neurologic symptoms: headache, confusion, cranial nerve palsies, coma, seizures.

❏❏ **In a child 6 mo to 4 y of age with an antecedent URI, the findings of fever, acute renal failure, microangiopathic hemolytic anemia (MAHA), and thrombocytopenia are suggestive of what disorder?**

Hemolytic Uremic Syndrome.

❏❏ **What malignancy is <u>most frequently</u> associated with MAHA?**

Gastric Adenocarcinoma.

❏❏ **What is the most common worldwide cause of hemolytic anemia?**

Malaria.

❏❏ **What are the components of whole blood that are used for transfusion?**

RBCs
Platelets
Plasma
Cryoprecipitate

❏❏ **By how much will the infusion of one unit of PRBCs raise the hemoglobin and hematocrit in a 70 kg patient?**

Hemoglobin: 1 g/dL.
Hematocrit: 3%.

❏❏ **What are the three conditions under which the transfusion of PRBCs should be considered?**

Acute hemorrhage (blood loss > 1,500 ml).
Surgical blood loss > 2 L.
Chronic anemia (Hgb < 7 - 8 g/dL, symptomatic, or with underlying cardiopulmonary disease).

❏❏ **What factors indicate the need for typing and cross-matching of blood in the ED?**

Evidence of shock from whatever cause.
Known blood loss > 1,000 ml.
Gross GI bleeding.
Hgb < 10; Hct < 30.
Potential of going to surgery with further significant blood loss.

❏❏ **What are the contents of cryoprecipitate?**

Factor VIII C.
von Willebrand Factor.
Fibrinogen.
Factor XIII.
Fibronectin.

❏❏ **What is the first step in treating all immediate transfusion reactions?**

Stop the transfusion.

❏❏ **What type of immediate transfusion reaction is not dose related and can often be completed following patient evaluation and treatment with diphenhydramine?**

Allergic transfusion reaction.

❑❑ **What infection carries the highest risk of transmission by blood transfusion?**

Hepatitis C (1: 3,300 units).

❑❑ **What is the currently approved emergency replacement therapy in the ED for massive hemorrhage?**

Type-specific, uncrossmatched blood (available in 10 - 15 min).
Type O negative, whereas immediately life saving in certain situations, carries the risk of life-threatening transfusion reactions.

❑❑ **In current practice, which blood components are routinely infused along with PRBCs in a patient receiving a massive transfusion?**

None (the practice of routinely using platelet transfusion and FFP is costly, dangerous and unwarranted).

❑❑ **What is the only crystalloid fluid compatible with PRBCs?**

Normal saline.

❑❑ **What condition would be suspected in a patient with multiple myeloma who presents to the ED with paraparesis, paraplegia and urinary incontinence?**

Acute spinal cord compression. Seen primarily with multiple myeloma and lymphoma, but also encountered with carcinomas of the lung, breast and prostate.

❑❑ **What are the two most common neoplasms causing pericardial effusion and tamponade?**

Carcinoma of the lung and breast.

❑❑ **A 48 y male, cigarette smoker presents to the ED complaining of headache, swelling of the face and arms, and a feeling of fullness in the face and neck. He is noted on PE to have JVD, and papilledema on funduscopic exam. What is the most likely diagnosis?**

Superior Vena Cava Syndrome.

❑❑ **What is the most common cause of hyperviscosity syndrome?**

Waldenstrom macroglobulinemia.

❑❑ **What diagnosis should be considered in a patient who presents to the ED with coma, anemia and rouleau formation in the peripheral blood smear?**

Hyperviscosity Syndrome.

❑❑ **What are the major causes of GI bleeding in cancer patients?**

Hemorrhagic gastritis.
Peptic ulcer disease.

❑❑ **Vitamin K dependent factors of the clotting cascade include:**

X, IX, VII and II. REMEMBER 1972.

❏❏ **An adult patient receives a major head injury. He also suffers from classic hemophilia, what treatment should be given?**

Give Factor VIII 50 U/kg.

❏❏ **What is von Willebrand's disease?**

It is an autosomal dominant disorder of platelet function.
It causes bleeding from mucous membranes, menorrhagia and increased bleeding from wounds.
Patients with vW disease have less (or dysfunctional) vW factor.
vW factor is a plasma protein secreted by endothelial cells. vW factor serves two functions - it is required for platelets to adhere to collagen at the site of vascular injury (initial step in forming a hemostatic plug) and it forms complexes in plasma with factor VIII which are required to maintain normal factor VIII levels.

❏❏ **What lab abnormalities does DIC cause?**

Increased PT, elevated fibrin split products, decreased fibrinogen and thrombocytopenia.

❏❏ **What is appropriate treatment for a life threatening level of hypercalcemia of 16 mg per deciliter?**

Start giving the patient 0.9 NS at 5 to 10 liters per day. In addition, administer furosemide. A typical dose of Lasix would be 80 mg IV every 1 to 2 h. Watch out for hypokalemia. Consider glucocorticoids if the patient is obtunded or comatose.

The admitting internist may also administer agents to counteract parathyroid hormone which include calcitonin and mithramycin.

❏❏ **What factors are deficient in Classic hemophilia, Christmas disease, and von Willebrand's disease, respectively?**

Classic hemophilia -   Factor VIII.
Christmas disease -   Factor IX.
Willebrand's disease -   Factor VIIIc + von Willebrand's cofactor.

❏❏ **Which pathway involves factors VIII and IX?**

Intrinsic pathway.

❏❏ **What effect does deficiency of factors VIII and IX have on PT and on PTT?**

Deficiency leads to increase in PTT.

❏❏ **What pathway does the PT measure and what factor is unique to this pathway?**

Extrinsic, factor VII.

❏❏ **How may hemophilia A be clinically distinguished from hemophilia B?**

Hemophilia A is not clinically distinguishable from Christmas disease (Hemophilia B).

❏❏ **Which blood product is given when the coagulation abnormality is unknown?**

FFP.

❏❏ **What agent can be used for treating mild hemophilia A and von Willebrand's disease type 1?**

D-Amino-8, D-arginine vasopressin (DDAVP) induces a rapid rise in factor VIII levels.

OB/GYN PEARLS

"A great part, I believe, of the Art is to be able to observe."

Hippocrates (460 - 370 B.C.)

❑❑ **What percentage of known pregnancies end in spontaneous abortion?**

About 15-20%.

❑❑ **Most spontaneous abortions occur before what gestational age?**

8-9 weeks.

❑❑ **Beyond what gestational age is a COMPLETE spontaneous abortion unlikely to occur?**

Seven weeks.

❑❑ **What is the incidence of coexistent ectopic and intra-uterine pregnancies?**

Traditionally quoted as 1/30,000-more recently estimated at 1/4000 in the general population and 1-8% after in vitro fertilization.

❑❑ **What is the minimal ß-hCG titer for which an experienced ultrasonographer should be able to visualize a viable intrauterine pregnancy?**

Transvaginal, > 2000 hCG mIU/ml. Transabdominal, 6500.

❑❑ **Who is eligible for methotrexate treatment of their ectopic pregnancy?**

Hemodynamically stable, unruptured gestations of less than 4 cm in diameter by ultrasound.

❑❑ **Transient pelvic pain frequently occurs 3-7 d after methotrexate therapy for ectopic pregnancy. What is your concern?**

Rupture may be difficult to differentiate from this pain presumed due to tubal abortion, typically lasting 4-12 h.

❑❑ **What is the most likely non-gynecologic condition presenting with lower abdominal pain?**

Appendicitis.

❑❑ **Virtually all severe cases of dysfunctional uterine bleeding (DUB) occur in what age group?**

Adolescent girls shortly after the onset of menstruation.

❑❑ **What is the number one cause of maternal mortality?**

Thromboembolism. The risk progressively increases throughout pregnancy, peaking at >5 times non-pregnant controls during the post-partum period.

Claire

(718)

281-0877

❑❑ **What is the most common medical complication in pregnancy?**

Urinary tract infections.

❑❑ **What is the indication for RhoGAM in the first trimester?**

An unsensitized Rh-negative woman with any vaginal bleeding.

❑❑ **Against how much fetomaternal hemorrhage (FMH) does the standard 300 microgram dose of RhoGAM protect?**

Approximately <30 ml whole blood. Following trauma, FMH should always be considered. In the setting of trauma, order a quantitative Kleihauer-Betke assay to determine the amount of FMH, then calculate the appropriate RhoGAM dose.

❑❑ **What is the most serious complication of gynecologic laparoscopy?**

Thermal injury. When initially unrecognized, this insidious necrosis presents 3-7 d post-operatively with peritonitis and/or viscous perforation. Bleeding and sharp dissection complications are usually recognized intra-operatively.

❑❑ **How much blood does a standard size pad absorb?**

20 - 30 ml blood.

❑❑ **How soon after implantation can ß-HCG be detected?**

2-3 d.

❑❑ **What percentage of pregnancies are ectopic?**

1.5%. Ectopic pregnancies are the leading cause of death in the first trimester.

❑❑ **What is the most common presentation of ectopic pregnancy?**

Amenorrhea followed by pain.

❑❑ **How does a spontaneous abortion most commonly present?**

Pain followed by bleeding.

❑❑ **What is the most common finding on pelvic exam in a patient with an ectopic pregnancy?**

Unilateral adnexal tenderness.

❑❑ **Does a negative culdocentesis rule out an ectopic pregnancy?**

No. It only rules out hemoperitoneum.

❑❑ **When can abdominal ultrasound find an intrauterine gestational sac?**

5th week. Fetal pole, 6th week. Embryonic mass with cardiac motion, 7th week.

❑❑ **A 3 mo pregnant patient presents with pelvic pain. On exam, a retroverted and retroflexed uterus is found. What diagnosis should come to mind?**

Incarceration of the uterus. Patients typically complain of rectal and pelvic pressure . Urinary retention may also be found. The knee-chest position or rectal pressure may correct the problem.

❏❏ **Which patients with PID should be admitted?**

Pregnant; temperature > 38 °C (100.4 °F); nausea and vomiting which prohibits po antibiotics; pyosalpinx or tubo-ovarian abscess; peritoneal signs; IUCD present; no response to oral antibiotics; and uncertain diagnosis.

❏❏ **What are the criteria for diagnosis of PID?**

All three of the following: adnexal tenderness, cervical and uterine tenderness, and abdominal tenderness. Also one of the following: T >38 °C, endocervix gram stain positive for gram negative intracellular diplococci, leukocytosis greater than 10,000/mm^3, inflammatory mass on US or pelvic, and WBC and bacteria in the peritoneal fluid.

❏❏ **What is the most common cause of toxic shock syndrome?**

The most common cause is S. aureus. Other causes which are clinically similar include group A Streptococci, Pseudomonas aeruginosa, and Streptococcus pneumoniae.

❏❏ **What criteria are necessary for the diagnosis of toxic shock syndrome?**

All of the following must be present: T > 38.9 °C (102 °F), rash, systolic BP < 90 and orthostasis, involvement of three organ systems (GI, renal, musculoskeletal, mucosal, hepatic, hematologic, or CNS), and negative serologic tests for such diseases as RMSF, hepatitis B, measles, leptospirosis, VDRL, etc.

❏❏ **What type of rash is seen with TSS?**

Blanching erythroderma which resolves in 3 d and is followed by a desquamation (full thickness). This typically occurs between the 6th and 14th d with peeling prominent on the hands and feet.

❏❏ **How should a patient with toxic shock syndrome be treated?**

FLUIDS, pressure support, FFP or transfusions, vaginal irrigation with iodine or saline, and antistaphylococcal penicillin or cephalosporin with anti-ß-lactamase activity (nafcillin or oxacillin). Rifampin should be considered to eliminate the carrier state.

❏❏ **What anticoagulant should be used in pregnant patients?**

Heparin does not cross the placenta.

❏❏ **What antiemetic should be used in pregnant patients?**

Prochlorperazine (Compazine) or trimethobenzamide (Tigan).

❏❏ **What dose of radiation to a fetus increases the risk of inhibiting fetal growth?**

10 rad. A typical abdominal or pelvic film delivers 100 to 350 mrad. A shielded chest x-ray should deliver < 10 mrad to the fetus. Necessary x-rays should not be withheld.

❏❏ **Define preeclampsia.**

HTN after 20 wk EGA with generalized edema or proteinuria.

❏❏ **Define eclampsia.**

Preeclampsia plus grand mal seizures or coma.

❏❏ **Should BP be lowered acutely in a preeclampsia patient?**

Dangerous HTN (>170/110) should be gradually lowered with hydralazine 10 mg IV followed by a drip. Definitive treatment for preeclampsia and eclampsia is delivery.

❏❏ **What level of serum glucose warrants admission in a patient with gestational diabetes?**

Hyperglycemia (>200 mg %) which is persistent requires admission.

❏❏ **Can iodinated radiodiagnostic agents be used in a pregnant patient?**

Use should be avoided as concentration in the fetal thyroid can cause permanent loss of thyroid function. Nuclear medicine scans, pulmonary angiography with pelvic shielding, and impedance plethysmography are preferred.

❏❏ **What viral or protozoal infections require extensive work-up during pregnancy?**

Herpes genitalis, rubella, cytomegalovirus, and Toxoplasma gondii. These patients require full work-ups and referral for genetic counseling.

❏❏ **What is the most common cause of vaginitis?**

Candida albicans.

❏❏ **A 26 y old female complains of dysuria and mild lower abdominal pain. On pelvic exam, punctate hemorrhages are noted on the cervix. Diagnosis?**

Trichomonas vaginitis. The cervix is called "strawberry cervix." The diagnosis can be confirmed by obtaining <u>vaginal vault secretions</u> using the "hanging drip" slide test. The sexual partner must be treated.

❏❏ **A wet prep of vaginal secretions reveals clue cells. Diagnosis?**

Gardnerella vaginitis. Male partners should be treated.
Sherlock Holmes looks for "clues" in the "Garden."

❏❏ **A pregnant patient presents in a coma. The husband indicates the patient has had been itching for a few days, seemed slightly yellow, and earlier in the day her daughter said "Mom was confused". Diagnosis?**

Acute fatty liver of pregnancy. Conjugated bilirubin and transaminase levels will be increased.

❏❏ **Is appendicitis more common during pregnancy?**

No (1/850). Outcome is worse. As pregnancy progresses, the appendix moves, at term it is near the right subcostal margin. The distal end is pointed toward the diaphragm. The WBC count usually does not increase beyond the normal value of 12-15,000. In a pregnant patient, pyuria with no bacteria suggest appendicitis. Pregnant patients may lack GI distress, fever may be absent or low grade.

❏❏ **3 d post-partum a patient presents with fever. On exam, a foul lochia and tender boggy uterus is present. Diagnosis?**

Endometritis typically occurs 1-3 d post-partum.

❏❏ **Why is Rh status important in a pregnant patient?**

Rh negative with Rh positive fetus can result in fetal anemia, hydrops, and fetal loss. Rh immunoglobulin should be given to all Rh negative patients. The usual amount of RhoGAM may be inadequate in the setting of trauma; a Kleihauer-Betke assay can quantitate fetomaternal hemorrhage.

❏❏ **What is the expected finding on culdocentesis in a patient with a ruptured ectopic pregnancy?**

Non-clotting blood.

❏❏ **When can transvaginal and abdominal ultrasound identify an intrauterine sac?**

Transvaginal, 31-32 days. Abdominal, 5 wk.

❏❏ **A 24 y old, 10 w pregnant patient presents with bleeding per vagina. She also complains of nausea, vomiting, and abdominal pain. Physical findings reveal a blood pressure of 150/100 and a uterus which is larger than dates. Lab studies reveal proteinuria. Diagnosis?**

Molar pregnancy. Uterus may be larger or smaller than expected dates.

❏❏ **An 8 mo pregnant patient presents to the ED with profuse bleeding. What must be ruled out with ultrasound before a pelvic exam is performed?**

Placenta previa.

❏❏ **Risk factors for placenta previa?**

Previous cesarean section, previous placenta previa, multiparity, multiple induced abortions, and multiple gestations.

❏❏ **Risk factors for abruptio placenta?**

Smoking, hypertension, multiparity, trauma, and previous abruptio placenta.

❏❏ **What effect does pregnancy have on: Cardiac output, BP, HR, coagulation, sed rate, leukocytes, blood volume, arterial blood gases, tidal volume, bladder, BUN/CR, and GI.**

Cardiac Output	Increases. Moving the uterus off the IVC increases CO 25%.
BP	Falls in second trimester. Returns to normal state in third trimester.
Heart Rate	Increases.
Coagulation	Factors 7, 8, 9, 10, and fibrinogen increase, the others remain unchanged.
Sed Rate	Elevated.
Leukocytes	Increase to as much as 18,000.
Blood volume	Increases, RBC unchanged, dilutional "anemia" is physiologic.
Tidal volume	Increases 40%.
Bladder	Displaced superiorly and anteriorly.
BUN/Cr	Decrease because of increased GFR and renal blood flow.
GI	Gastric emptying and GI motility decrease. Peritoneal signs such as rigidity and rebound are diminished or absent. Alkaline phosphatase is increased.

❏❏ **What are the presenting signs and symptoms of abruptio placentae?**

Placental separation before delivery is associated with vaginal bleeding (78%), abdominal pain (66%), as well as tetanic uterine contractions, uterine irritability, and fetal death.

❏❏ **What dose of oxytocin (Pitocin) should be administered following a postpartum hemorrhage?**

20 to 40 units of oxytocin added to 1000 ml normal saline or Ringer's lactate infused at 200 - 500 ml/h.

❏❏ **How can ruptured membranes be diagnosed?**

Nitrazine paper turns blue and a "ferning" pattern is seen under a microscope in the presence of amniotic fluid.

❏❏ **What are the indications for cardiotocographic monitoring in a trauma patient?**

All women past 20 w gestation with indirect or direct abdominal trauma require 4 h of monitoring. Loss of beat-to-beat variability, uterine contractions, or fetal brady- or tachycardia demands immediate obstetrical consultation.

❏❏ **Is life threatening hemorrhage due to trauma during pregnancy most often intra- or retroperitoneal?**

Retroperitoneal.

❏❏ **What type of incision should be used in a post-mortem cesarean section?**

Vertical (Classical) incision.

❏❏ **What is the normal fetal heart rate?**

120 to 160 beats per minute. If bradycardia is detected, position the mother on her left side, give oxygen and an IV fluid bolus.

❏❏ **A pregnant patient presents with fetal bradycardia and tetanic contractions. Delivery is not imminent. Treatment?**

Tocolytic agents to relax the uterus: magnesium sulfate 4 to 6 g IV over 20 min or terbutaline 0.25 mg subcutaneously.

❏❏ **What technique can be used to identify intravaginal semen?**

Semen will fluoresce with a Wood's Lamp.

❏❏ **How long after intercourse can acid phosphatase be detected?**

2-9 h.

❏❏ **How quickly must a patient be treated to provide pregnancy prevention after a being raped?**

72 h. Common treatment is Ovral, 2 tablets po and 2 tablets 12 hours later.

DERM PEARLS

"Adventure is worthwhile in itself."

Amelia Earhart

❏❏ **What type of reaction is erythema multiforme?**

Hypersensitivity.
Bullae are subepidermal, the dermis is edematous, and a lymphatic infiltrate may be present around the capillaries and venules. In children, infections are the most important cause and in adults, drugs and malignancies. EM is often seen during epidemics of adenovirus, atypical pneumonia, and histoplasmosis.

❏❏ **A patient presents with fever, myalgias, malaise, and arthralgias. On exam, findings include bullous lesions of the lips, eyes, and nose. The patient indicates eating is very painful. What should the family be told about the patient's prognosis?**

Stevens-Johnson syndrome has a mortality of 5 - 10% and may have significant complications including corneal ulceration, panophthalmitis, corneal opacities, anterior uveitis, blindness, hematuria, renal tubular necrosis, and progressive renal failure. Scarring of the foreskin and stenosis of the vagina can occur. Treatment in a burn unit is supportive; steroids may provide symptomatic relief but are not of proven value, and may be contraindicated.

❏❏ **What are the two distinct causes of toxic epidermal necrolysis (scalded skin syndrome)?**

Staphylococcal and drugs or chemicals. Both begin with appearance of patches of tender erythema followed by loosening of the skin and denuding to glistening bases.
Staphylococcal scalded skin syndrome is commonly found in children less than 5y and is due to toxin that cleaves <u>within the epidermis</u> under the stratum granulosum.

❏❏ **What area does Staphylococcal scalded skin syndrome usually affect?**

The face around nose and mouth, neck, axillae, and groin. Disease commonly occurs after upper respiratory tract infections or purulent conjunctivitis. Nikolsky's sign is present when lateral pressure on the skin results in epidermal separation from the dermis.

❏❏ **How can SSSS be distinguished from scalded skin syndrome caused by drugs or chemicals?**

Pull out your microscopes and call in the pathologists trivia fans, in drug or chemical etiologies the skin separates at the dermoepidermal junction. This drug induced TEN carries up to 50% mortality as a result of fluid loss and secondary infection.
On microscopic exam of SSSS intraepidermal cleavage occurs with a few acantholytic keratinocytes will be seen.
In non-staphylococcal type, cellular debris, inflammatory cells, and basal cell keratinocytes are present.

❏❏ **Treatment of SSSS?**

Oral or IV penicillinase-resistant penicillin, baths of potassium permanganate or dressings soaked in 0.5% silver nitrate, and fluids. Corticosteroids and silver sulfadine are contraindicated.

Great quote series:

"Hawaii has always been a very pivotal role in the Pacific. It is in the Pacific. It is a part of the United States that is an island that is right here."

Dan Quale during a speech in Hawaii, 1989

❏❏ What is the most common gram-negative anaerobe found in human feces?

Bacteroides fragilis. It is also the <u>most common</u> organism found in abscesses involving the perineal region. Its other claim to fame is being the only anaerobe resistant to penicillin.

❏❏ Where are cutaneous abscesses caused by Escherichia coli and Neisseria gonorrhoeae commonly found?

"Sorry about that chief," but they are <u>not</u> typically seen in cutaneous abscesses.

Staphylococcus aureus is the <u>most common</u> aerobe in cutaneous abscesses, two-thirds are found in the upper torso, 97% are resistant to penicillin G. It is most commonly isolated in axilla abscesses.

❏❏ What is the most common gram-negative aerobe found in the upper torso?

Proteus mirabilis, most commonly isolated in the axilla.

❏❏ What is the most common aerobe seen in stool and intra-abdominal abscesses?

Escherichia coli. The pus of E. coli is odorless. The "sweat succulent" smell of abscesses in the perirectal area is due to anaerobic bacteria.

❏❏ How may the Toxicodendron species be recognized?

Poison oak and ivy have leaves with 3 leaflets per leaf. They also have U- or V-shaped leaf scars. The milky sap becomes black when exposed to air.

❏❏ How quickly will people react to the Toxicodendron antigen?

Contact dermatitis typically develops within 2 d of exposure; cases have been reported in as quickly as 8 h to as long as 10d. Lesions appear in a linear arrangement of papulovesicles or erythema. Fluid from vesicles does not contain antigen and does not transmit the dermatitis.

❏❏ How should steroids be prescribed in a patient with poison ivy?

Prednisone 40 - 60 mg q d tapered over 2 to 3 wk. Short courses may result in rebound.

❏❏ What are the causes of exfoliative dermatitis?

Chemicals, drugs, and cutaneous or systemic diseases. Usually scaly erythematous dermatitis involves most or all of the surface skin. It can be recognized by erythroderma with epidermal flaking or scaling. Acute signs and symptoms may include low-grade fever, pruritus, chills, and skin tightness. The chronic condition may produce dystrophic nails, thinning of body hair, and patchy hyperpigmentation or hypopigmentation. Cutaneous vasodilation may result in increased cardiac output and high-output cardiac failure. Splenomegaly suggests leukemia or lymphoma.

❏❏ What is a furuncle?

Deeeeep-inflammatory nodule which grew out of superficial folliculitis.

❏❏ What is a carbuncle?

Deep abscess that interconnects and extends into the subcutaneous tissue. Commonly seen in patients with diabetes, folliculitis, steroid use, obesity, heavy perspiration, and areas of friction.

❏❏ What is a Bartholin's cyst?

Obstructed Bartholin's duct resulting in an abscess.

❑❑ **What is a pilonidal abscess?**

Abscess which occurs in the gluteal fold as a result of disruption of the epithelial surface. They do not originate from rectal crypts and bacteria are from the cutaneous surface.

❑❑ **Where does a perirectal abscess originate?**

Anal crypts and burrows through the ischiorectal space. They may be perianal, perirectal, supralevator, or ischiorectal.
Perianal abscesses which involve the supralevator muscle, ischiorectal space, or rectum require operative drainage.

❑❑ **What is hidradenitis suppurativa?**

Chronic suppurative abscesses found in the apocrine sweat glands of the groin and/or axilla. Proteus mirabilis overgrowth is common.

Great quote series:

"Hawaii is a unique state. It is a small state. It is a state that is by itself. It is a...it is different from the other 49 states. Well, all states are different, but it's got a particularly different situation."

Dan Quale

❑❑ **What is the cause of tetanus?**

Tetanospasmin, which is an exotoxin produced by a gram-positive anaerobic rod, Clostridium tetani.

❑❑ **What is the mechanism of action of tetanospasmin?**

Enters peripheral nerve endings and ascends the axons to reach the brain and spinal cord. At this point it binds four areas of the nervous system:

1. Anterior horn cells of the spinal cord - impairs inhibitory interneurons resulting in neuromuscular irritability and generalized spasms.
2. Sympathetic nervous system - resulting in sweating, labile blood pressure, tachycardia, and peripheral vasoconstriction.
3. Myoneural junction - inhibits release of acetylcholine.
4. Binds to cerebral gangliosides - thought to cause seizures.

❑❑ **What is the treatment of a tetanus prone wound?**

Surgical debridement, 3,000 to 10,000 units of human tetanus immune globulin [TIG (h), (Hyper-tet)] IM (Do Not Inject Into Wound), penicillin G or metronidazole.

❑❑ **What is the danger of giving tetanus toxoid boosters in a pleonastic fashion (e.g., with only a 9 mo interval)?**

Arthus-type hypersensitivity reaction, with onset about 4 - 6 h after injection. History of a severe hypersensitivity reaction or of a severe neurologic reaction are the only contraindications to tetanus toxoid.

❑❑ **What is the most common cause of gas gangrene?**

C. perfringens. The first symptom is a sensation of weight or heaviness in the muscle followed by severe pain. The DOC is penicillin G, an alternative is chloramphenicol.

❏❏ **A patient presents with a raised, red, small, and painful plaque on the face. On exam, a distinct, sharp advancing edge is noted. What is the cause?**

Erysipelas is caused by group A streptococci. When the face is involved, the patient should be admitted.

IMAGING PEARLS

"Decide promptly, but never give your reasons. Your decision may be right, but your reasons are sure to be wrong."

Lord Mansfield

❏❏ **What is the purpose of ultrasound gel?**

It serves to displace air and provide a medium for coupling the probe to the skin surface without impedance mismatching.

❏❏ **"Duplex" combines what two features?**

A high-resolution <u>image</u> and <u>doppler</u> capability.

❏❏ **What audible characteristics differentiate arterial from venous flow when using doppler?**

Arterial flow is characterized by sharp, brisk changes in pitch throughout the cardiac cycle (higher pitched during peak systole and lower pitched during diastole; also termed multiphasic) whereas venous signals are lower pitched and more consistent throughout the cardiac cycle (monophasic). Venous flow also varies with the respiratory cycle.

❏❏ **What is an ABI and what is its significance?**

ABI = ankle/brachial index. The ankle systolic pressure (numerator) is compared to the higher of the two brachial arterial pressures (denominator). It is used to determine if arterial obstruction is present.
Normal ABI = greater than or equal to 1
ABI 0.5-0.9 = obstructive disease of a single peripheral arterial segment e.g. claudication
ABI < 0.5 indicates multiple arterial segments are obstructed

❏❏ **What technical factors can effect the accuracy of the ABI?**

Probe pressure, probe placement (should be longitudinal to the vessel and 30-60 degree angle to the skin surface), too rapid deflation of the BP cuff, and arterial wall calcifications

❏❏ **What is the diagnostic test of choice for documenting DVT?**

Duplex ultrasound. Although it is highly operator dependent and not utilized in all centers, its sensitivity and specificity are virtually identical to venography. In addition, its benefits include being noninvasive and not utilizing contrast dye. The accuracy of physical examination for DVT is generally quoted to be approximately 50%.

❏❏ **List some of the advantages/disadvantages of CT, ultrasound and DPL for assessing trauma patients?**

	Advantages	*Disadvantages:*
DPL	low complication rate done at bedside	invasive, time consuming, can't ID retroperitoneal injury, significant false positive rate
CT	IDs location/extent injury including the retroperitoneum	cost, time consuming, interpretation expertise, patient monitoring not optimal, requires travel
US	cheap, noninvasive, done at bedside, good for hemoperitoneum, fast	operator dependent, not good for IDing specific organ injury

❑❑ **Surgical repair of abdominal aortic aneurysms is generally indicated for those measuring >**
_____.

5 cm. Ultrasound is extremely sensitive for detecting AAA but is not sensitive for the detection of ruptured AAA.

❑❑ **Name some ultrasonographic abnormalities seen in patients with acute cholecystitis.**

Wall thickening, gallstones, surrounding fluid, US Murphy's sign, air in the biliary tree.

❑❑ **An intrauterine gestational sac without a fetal pole, yolk sac or cardiac activity can be confused with what structure?**

The pseudosac of ectopic pregnancy (seen with 10-20% ectopics).

❑❑ **What is the most common site for ectopic implantation?**

The ampullae of the fallopian tube.

❑❑ **Name 6 risk factors for ectopic pregnancy.**

Advanced maternal age, PID, prior ectopic, history of pelvic surgery or tubal ligation, IUDs, in vitro fertilization.

❑❑ **What is the primary use of ultrasonography in females with a positive hCG who present with abdominal pain and/or vaginal bleeding?**

To verify the presence of an intrauterine pregnancy. The incidence of simultaneous intrauterine and extrauterine pregnancies is approx. 1 in 30,000. Ultrasound may not be able to definitively verify that an ectopic pregnancy exists.

❑❑ **What is the only true diagnostic sign of en ectopic pregnancy with ultrasound?**

A fetus with cardiac activity outside the uterus. Complex masses and fluid in the cul-de-sac can be seen in other conditions e.g. pelvic abscess, ruptured ovarian cyst.

❑❑ **In early pregnancy, what is the average doubling time of serum hCG?**

1.5-2 d.

❑❑ **What is the role of ultrasound in detecting placenta previa and abruption?**

Ultrasound is not sensitive for detecting placental abruption. However, in the patient with third trimester vaginal bleeding, ultrasound is used primarily to rule out placenta previa. An experienced ultrasonographer can detect a placenta previa. Uterine contraction, incorrect scanning techniques and an overfilled bladder can result in false positives.

❑❑ **What is the incidence of allergic reaction to IV contrast materials?**

Severe allergic reactions occur in approximately 1 in 14,000 patients, whereas fatal reactions occur about 1 in 40,000 cases.

❑❑ **What is the prevalence of adverse reactions to ionic and nonionic contrast materials?**

12.7 % with ionic and 3.1% with nonionic.

Nonionic contrast causes hypotension, bronchospasm, arrhythmia and angioneurotic edema, urticaria, flushing, nausea, vomiting, etc. less often than ionic contrast materials. Whether or not nonionic materials are less nephrotoxic is still controversial.

❏❏ **T/F: Oral contrast should be avoided in patients with marginal renal function.**

False. Little nephrotoxic iodine is absorbed with oral contrast administration. When barium is used, it is inert and not absorbed.

❏❏ **What are the contraindications to administration of oral iodine or barium contrast?**

Barium cannot be given when complete colon obstruction exists or intestinal perforation is suspected. Severe allergy to iodine is the only contraindication to the oral iodine-containing preparations.

❏❏ **T/F: IV contrast material is contraindicated in chronic renal failure.**

False. The contrast material can be dialyzed and the kidney is already maximally impaired.

❏❏ **Describe the typical shape and vessel origin of subdural hematomas (SDH) and epidural hematomas (EDH)?**

SDH are typically crescent-shaped and although can be arterial in origin are most often caused by the tearing of bridging veins. Acute SDH are hyperdense relative to the brain and become isodense to the brain (1-3 weeks). EDH are biconvex (lenticular) is shape and are usually arterial in origin. An EDH does not cross intact skull sutures but can cross the tentorium and the midline.

❏❏ **What percentage of SDH are bilateral?**

About 25%

❏❏ **Why does the performance of a DPL make the evaluation of a subsequent CT more difficult?**

Air and fluid are introduced during the DPL.

❏❏ **What is the test of choice for evaluating and staging renal trauma?**

IV contrast-enhanced CT has replaced IVP for this purpose. CT is more accurate as IVP is not sensitive for renal injuries.

❏❏ **The magnetic fields of an MRI can be detrimental to patients with_____.**

Ferrous metal in their body or electrical equipment whose function can be disrupted by strong magnetic fields. Examples include pacemakers, metal foreign bodies in the eye (welders, sheet metal workers, artists who work with metal, etc), ferromagnetic cerebral aneurysm clips (nonmagnetic steel clips are not dangerous), and cochlear implants. Relative contraindications for the MRI include: certain prosthetic heart valves, implantable defibrillators, bone growth and neurostimulators. One might also include patients who are claustrophobic.

❏❏ **Technetium 99m-labeled studies of the gallbladder are viewed every 10 minutes for 1 hour. If the gallbladder is not visualized at 1 hour, what does this signify?**

Either complete obstruction of the cystic duct due to inflammation and stones (acute cholecystitis) or partial obstruction with a slow filling rate (due to scarring). Delayed images up to 4 hours are obtained to rule out the latter possibility (chronic cholecystitis).

❏❏ **Although bone scans are useful for detecting subtle fractures missed on x-ray, why is it not always useful in the emergent setting for recent fractures?**

Skeletal uptake is dependent on blood flow and osteoblastic activity, thus a bone scan may not pick up the increased bone turnover until h or d after trauma. A positive scan demonstrates asymmetric skeletal uptake.

❑❑ **Radionuclide studies are most helpful in determining the bleeding site in upper or lower GI bleeds?**

Lower.

❑❑ **What 2 studies can detect testicular torsion and differentiate it from epididymitis, orchitis or torsion of the appendix testis?**

Technetium 99m nuclear studies and (in some centers) duplex ultrasound.

ECG 1

This tracing demonstrates a supraventricular tachycardia. It also displays a very tall R wave in the precordial V leads, in particular in V_2. This is consistent with a posterior wall myocardial infarction. Mild ST depression in leads V_2 and V_3 are the equivalent of ST elevation in AMI (ST elevation might be seen if the leads had been placed on the posterior thorax). The ST segment elevates in posterior wall infarction in V_2 because the posterior wall of the LV has infarcted (its "dead") and there is now unmasking of the normal anterior wall, anterior forces which have vectors directed primarily at V_2. Subendocardial infarction can also cause ST segment depression in the precordial leads.

ECG 2 (3 simultaneous rhythm tracings)

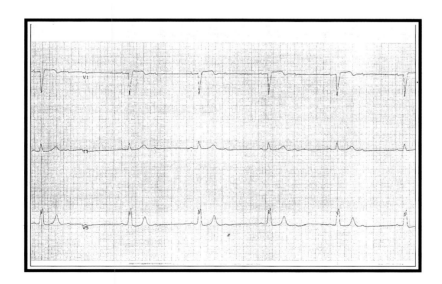

This tracing demonstrates three leads (V_1, II, V_5) recorded simultaneously. Both P waves and QRS complexes are seen. The P waves are not "related" to the QRS complexes (some are appearing after the QRS and several do not have a QRS complex which immediately follow the P wave). The QRS rate is very slow. Thus, the PR interval would be interpreted as variable. The QRS complexes are moderately widened. This patient is experiencing complete heart block with atrioventricular dissociation. The ventricles and atria are depolarizing in an independent fashion. This is an indication for immediate placement of a transcutaneous pacing device or transvenous pacemaker. This disturbance is associated with ischemia to the infranodal conduction pathways during an acute myocardial infarction. It may have been preceded by a Mobitz II AV block which has now progressed to complete heart block.

ECG 3a

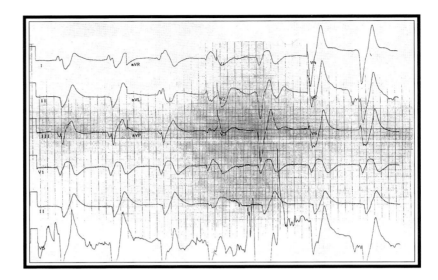

This tracing was recorded 19 minutes prior to ECG 3b from the same patient (see below). The first tracing demonstrates a very wide QRS complex in all leads depolarizing at a slow rate. The P waves are not visible and the T waves are tall. At very high serum potassium levels, e.g., above 7 mEq/L, impulses may be conducted from the SA node to the ventricles. However conduction may be very impaired through the AV node and result in an idioventricular rhythm. The tracing below occurred after initial treatment for the hyperkalemia.

ECG 3b

This tracing was recorded 19 minutes after ECG 3a from the same patient. It demonstrates loss of the P waves, some widening of the QRS complexes, sagging ST segments and narrow ("pinched waist"), peaked T waves. These findings are the primary electrocardiographic findings of hyperkalemia. Acute treatment might include various agents including parenteral calcium chloride (gluconate), bicarbonate, insulin and glucose (coadministered), ß-agonist inhalation, loop diuretics (lasix), and dialysis (hemodialysis or peritoneal dialysis). The cause of the hyperkalemia, e.g., postobstructive uropathy, digitalis toxicity, should be sought and corrected immediately, when possible. Oliguric renal failure is the most common cause of dangerous hyperkalemia. This tracing demonstrates the classic findings of hyperkalemia after improvement occurred from acute therapy for very severe hyperkalemia (ECG 3a).

ECG 4 (Rhythm strip)

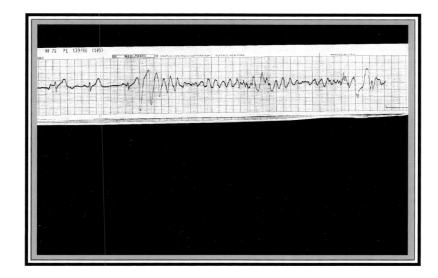

This tracing is a single lead (unspecified) rhythm tracing. It demonstrates three sinus beats with ST elevation followed by a wide complex tachyarrhythmia which has a gradually changing (rotating) QRS axis. This is consistent with Torsades de Pointes ("a twisting of the points"), a specfic type of atypical ventricular tachycardia which involves a single focus. It is associated with conditions that prolong the QT interval and results from a triggered arrhythmic mechanism after a period of prolonged, uneven ventricular repolarization. There are both acquired (administration of type Ia antiarrhythmic drugs [procainamide, disopyramide, quinidine], cyclic antidepressants, phenothiazines, electrolyte disturbances, hypothermia) and congenital (Jervell-Lange-Nielson syndrome, Romano-Ward syndrome) forms. Electrolyte disturbances especially hypomagnesemia, hypokalemia, and hypocalcemia should be considered and corrected. This rhythm may be seen in patients with any serious myocardial disease. Treatment with lidocaine is usually ineffective. Acceleration of the heart rate to shorten the QT interval using a pacemaker is the safest and most effective treatment. Intravenous bolus and infusion of magnesium sulfate is useful (especially with drug-induced torsades), but may be associated with recurrences during the infusion.

ECG 5

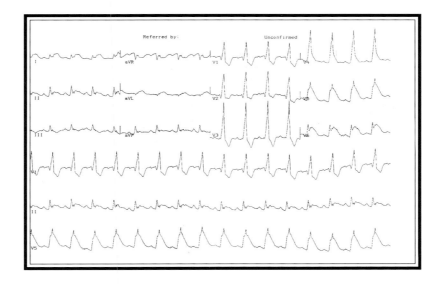

This tracing reveals a sinus rhythm with a wide complex QRS (180 msec) at approximately 100 beats per minute. The wide (and tall) QRS complexes in the right precordial leads may be consistent with right ventricular hypertrophy. The inferior lead (II, III, aVF) ST elevation, and lateral lead ST elevation (V5, V6, I, aVL), are consistent with inferior and anterolateral injury or acute infarction. Although no clinical information has been provided, keep in mind that any grouping of ECG findings can occur in the setting of acute pulmonary embolism. Poor cardiac output can contribute to myocardial hypoperfusion (with resulting left ventricular ischemia or injury) in the setting of right ventricular strain due to an obstructed pulmonary artery outflow tract.

This tracing reveals a bradycardia at 42 beats per minute with P waves and narrow QRS complexes visible. In the lead II rhythm strip the P waves are independent of the QRS complexes. This is most consistent with AV dissociation with an infranodal (His-Purkinje) pacemaker initiating ventricular depolarization (conduction is blocked through the AV node). Ventricular pacemaker sites always result in a wide QRS complex, so the pacemaker origin is eminating from a site higher in the conduction system. The inferior leads demonstrate ST elevation (reciprocal changes are seen in the anterolateral V leads); this is most consistent with inferior wall injury in the setting of acute myocardial infarction. Conduction through the AV node is impaired when the node is ischemic (as in the setting of inferior wall MI). The conduction block is usually transient in this situation and will spontaneously resolve or respond to atropine or pacing measures.

This tracing reveals a sinus rhythm at 91 beats per minute with normal P waves (look at lead II) and wide QRS complexes visible (QRS duration is 152 msec). The anterolateral V leads and leads I and aVL (lateral leads) demonstrate ST elevation consistent with acute anterolateral injury (infarction). Reciprocal ST-T wave changes (depressions) are seen in the inferior leads (II, III, aVF).

ECG 8

This tracing reveals a bradycardia at 45 beats per minute. An absence of P waves in the setting of a narrow QRS bradycardia is most consistent with a junctional rhythm. A junctional impulse is considered one that arises from the AV node or bundle of His proximal to the bifurcation of the main bundle branches. Atrial activation may not be seen if retrograde conduction is blocked or if atrial depolarization is occuring simultaneously with ventricular depolarization (P waves are obscured by the QRS complexes). AV junctional beats usually pace the ventricles at a rate of 40-60 beats per minute depending on the level of the pacemaker site. Junctional rhythms occur whenever there is a long enough delay in the impulses reaching the AV junction. This is seen in many conditions including congestive heart failure, hypokalemia, or digitalis toxicity. Myocarditis may also present with this rhythm disturbance. The primary treatment is to treat the underlying condition.

ECG 9

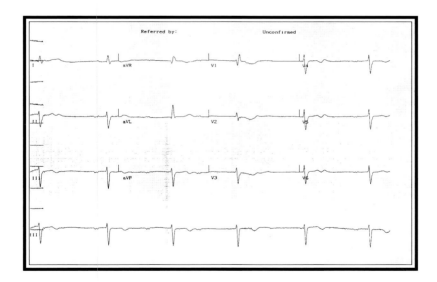

This tracing from a 78-year-old patient reveals a sinus rhythm with a prolonged PR interval of more than .2 msec (1° AV block), an rSR' configuration of V$_1$ (consistent with a right bundle branch block), and left axis deviation more negative than minus 45° (consistent with a left anterior superior fasicle block, i.e., the R wave in lead I is greater than the R waves in leads II and III, a qR wave is seen in lead aVL, and deep S waves are seen in leads II, III and aVF). The primary concern in the setting of a "trifasicular block" is the sudden development of complete heart block; most patients with this type of tracing have advanced organic heart disease. However, placement of a ventricular (demand) pacemaker is indicated only when symptoms are due to documented bradyarrhythmias (most still have a relatively low risk of sudden death from ventricular asystole in this setting).

ECG 10a

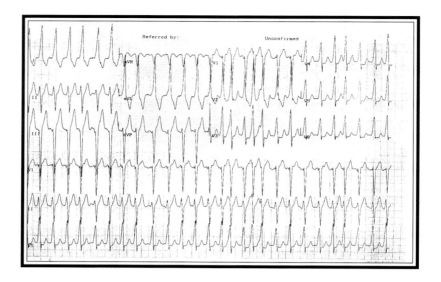

This tracing reveals a wide QRS complex tachyarrhythmia at approximately 163 beats per minute. Some irregularity in the rhythm is seen. Because it is irregular, one should suspect supraventricular arrhythmia with abberant conduction. Ventricular tachycardia is always considered initially as the most important diagnosis (in the setting of a rapid wide complex), but the irregularity in this case is a clue in favor of SVT with aberrancy, although P waves are not apparent. The same patient had a repeat ECG after an intervention (ECG 10b-see below) during the same visit to the emergency department. It reveals the diagnosis!

ECG 10b

This tracing reveals a sinus rhythm with a short PR interval and a delta wave (slurred upstroke of the QRS complex-look at leads I, V_1, V_5, V_6). These findings are consistent with a particular type of preexcitation syndrome, i.e., Wolff-Parkinson-White (WPW) syndrome. In this case it is WPW type B (there are three subtypes-A, B, and C). The short PR is due to a bypass tract originating in the atrium and inserting into the ventricular muscle (bypasses the normal His-Purkinje network). The bypass tract allows for rapid conduction which is more rapid than the conduction through the normal AV node (the AV node is responsible for the normal length of the PR interval—its relatively slower conduction allows time for the ventricles to fill). Now that the patient who was previously in a circus movement, wide-complex tachyarrhythmia (ECG 10a), has been converted to a sinus rhythm, the classic findings for Wolff-Parkinson-White syndrome are apparent.

Visual Pearl

This adult patient complained of a severe generalized headache and subsequently became severely obtunded. What is your diagnosis based on the appearance of this cranial CT obtained without radiographic contrast enhancement (C – CT)?

Answer

This study demonstrates a diffuse subarachnoid hemorrhage (the increased fuzzy density along the sulci and gyri) and bilateral ventricular enlargement. Blood in the subarachnoid space is causing a convexity (outflow) obstruction preventing the normal flow of cerebrospinal fluid from the arachnoid granulations into the venous sinuses. Expansion of the body of both lateral ventricles is evidence of a convexity block in this circumstance.

Visual Pearl

This adult patient complained of a severe headache which began on the right after an episode of syncope. He had vomited at the time of arrival to the hospital and had decorticate posturing. What is your interpretation of this cranial CT obtained without radiographic contrast enhancement?

Answer

There is a large irregular very hyperintense intracerebral hemorrhage with some increased intensity (acute hemorrhage) in the posterior horns of the lateral ventricles bilaterally. The left posterior horn demonstrates a meniscus which represents increased density in its most posterior aspect where blood has collected (dotted markers).

Visual Pearl

This adult patient was intoxicated with ethanol and quite confused. She suddenly became unresponsive in the emergency department. What is your diagnosis based on the appearance of this C – cranial CT?

Answer

There is a large epidural (lenticular shape) hematoma of the right parieto-occipital region with a shift of the intracranial structures to the left. The anterior horn of the right lateral ventricle is compressed. This is usually a high pressure hemorrhage due to arterial vessel injury. Occasionally, epidural hemorrhage is venous in origin since the location of the dural venous sinuses is between the periosteal (lateral) and meningeal (medial) layers of the dura. Dural venous sinus injury will therefore produce a lens shaped collection of blood on a CT image.

Visual Pearl

This adult male patient complained of a severe generalized headache and subsequently became severely obtunded. What is your diagnosis based on the appearance of this cranial CT obtained without radiographic contrast enhancement?

Answer

There is a large subdural (cresecent shape) hematoma compressing the entire right hemispheric region. The right lateral ventricle is completely compressed. This hemorrhage also extends along the falx cerebri (dotted markers) and is causing a shift of the intracranial structures to the left.

Visual Pearl

This 17-year-old male complained of a sore throat two days after playing football. He stated, "I had the wind knocked out of me during the game." On presentation, he was afebrile and appeared well. There were no findings on the initial physical examination. What is your diagnosis based on this chest film?

Answer

This film demonstrates a vertical linear lucency in the right paramediastinal region which travels cephalad into the neck. The diagnosis was pneumomediastinum (not a ruptured esophagus). The patient had an uneventful recovery.

Visual Pearl

This teenage female patient presented with general malaise, arthralgias and a few of these sparsely distributed, tender lesions on her extremities. What is the most likely diagnosis?

Answer

The finding is a small pustule on an erythematous base. The primary clinical consideration is disseminated gonococcemia. The lesions in meningococcemia are generally larger and hemorrhagic. The diagnosis of disseminated gonococcemia is problematic because only 20 to 50% of lesion, blood, or joint cultures become positive. Pharyngeal, cervical, and rectal smears are the most helpful in making a culture diagnosis.

Visual Pearl

This toddler was brought to the emergency department with this rash. There was no history of a previous similar rash. The child is afebrile and feeding well. There is no other significant finding on physical examination. What is your diagnosis based on this clinical information?

Answer

Hives (urticaria). Hives are due to local capillary vasodilation and result in an erythematous or white nonpitting plaques. They may be confused with many conditions including erythema multiforme. Up to 20% of the general population will experience one episode. Both acute and chronic forms exist. Therapy includes eliminating potential causes, and treatment using one or several agents including antihistamines, steroids, and epinephrine in severe cases.

Visual Pearl

This adult male complained blisters on his penis. He was mildly ill, with inguinal discomfort, but no adenopathy. What is your diagnosis based on this appearance?

Answer

Genital herpes (herpes simplex). This is a primary infection based on the patient's presntation. He denied any prior similar lesions. Acyclovir is an effective therapy. Recurrences are usually less painful. Frequency of recurrence varies in different patients.

Visual Pearl

This adult patient complained of a severe sore throat and dysphagia of several hours duration. He was febrile and appeared acutely ill, but was not initially in respiratory distress. What is your diagnosis based on this lateral neck film?

Answer

This film demonstrates a markedly swollen epiglottis with a dilated proximal airway, i.e., acute epiglottitis in an adult. The primary age for this infection is 2 to 7 years old, but it may occur at any age. It is most commonly due to *H. influenzae* type B, but may also be caused by *Streptococcus* or *Staphylococcus* species. After protection of the airway, the primary therapy includes the parenteral administration of a third generation cephalosporin. Adults with epiglottitis may be managed in an intensive care setting without intubation.

Visual Pearl

This adult female was toxic and febrile. She developed this facial rash with subsequent bulla formation, but rapidly improved with intravenous penicillin in twenty-four hours. What is your diagnosis? What is the causative organism?

Answer

The diagnosis is erysipelas–a superficial cellulitis with lymphatic involvement usually caused by group A *Streptococcus*. The physical findings are essentially diagnostic. The plaques are sharply demarcated, red, shiny, and painful. Local lymphadenopathy is common.

Visual Pearl

This ambulatory 12-year-old female complained of back pain after a motor vehicle accident. She was a rear-seat passenger and her vehicle was struck from the rear. She was restrained by a lap belt without a shoulder harness. What is your diagnosis?

Answer

There is a large horizontal-oblique fracture extending from the spinous process of L_1 anteriorly through the laminae and pedicles, to the posterior border of the vertebral body–a Chance fracture. This injury is seen with hyperflexion of the thoracolumbar (TL) region. Distraction of the posterior and middle column occurs with simultaneous impaction of the anterior column of the TL spine. The bony injury may be associated with a neurologic deficit. Up to 50% have an associated intraperitoneal injury, involving primarily the intestine.

Visual Pearl

This adult male patient presents with an itchy blistering rash which began 2 days after hiking through a wooded area. He now has several regions of involvement with a linear distribution on skin surfaces that were previously protected by clothing during the hike.

Answer

Toxicodendron (Rhus) dermatitis. Principle causes include poison ivy and poison oak in North America, but it may also occur after exposure to poison sumac. Scratching disseminates the antigen contained in sap under a person's fingernails. Blister fluid contains no antigen. Treatment may include oral steroid therapy.

Visual Pearl

This 27-year-old female complained of repetitive episodes of swelling of her lips, abdominal pain and this very itchy rash. This is the appearance of the rash. What is your diagnosis based on this clinical information?

Answer

Angioedema is a well demarcated localized edema of the deeper skin layers and subcutaneous tissue. Classifications of urticaria with angioedema include IgE-dependent, complement mediated, nonimmunologic (mast cell-releasing agents: antibiotics, opiates, radiocontrast media), and idiopathic. Most chronic cases are idiopathic. Elimination of the etiologic factor(s) is the best therapeutic approach. Topical steroids are of no benefit. H1 antihistamines and sympathomimetics provide symptomatic relief. Hydroxyzine, and a combination of H1 and H2 antihistamines may be even more effective.

Visual Pearl

This female patient complained of a mildly tender, weeping, red tender area of her right earlobe after wearing a new pair of earings. Her ears are not pierced. What is your diagnosis?

Answer

This is nickel-induced contact dermatitis (one of the most common causes of allergic contact dermatitis). The acute problem will resolve, but the patient should be advised that it will reoccur upon repeat contact with earings made of nickel. Some gold earings contain nickel. Stainless steel or plastic earings are clinically safe for nickel sensitive patients.

Visual Pearl

This male patient presented with a tender papule on his penis which ulcerated. Multiple lesions then developed; some of them coalesced. The patient complained of left inguinal pain, but had minimal constitutional symptoms and no skin rash. What is the most likely diagnosis and the treatment?

Answer

Chancroid is due to a pleomorphic gram-negative coccobacillus (*Haemophilus ducreyi*) that causes irregular-shaped, genital ulcers with red halo formation and lymphadenitis after the initial appearance of a painful, red papule. Ulcers are deeper than those in herpes and they spread laterally; autoinoculation produces multiple lesions. Painful inguinal adenopathy may be followed by bubo formation with spontaneous rupture. Diagnosis is made clinically, but syphilis should be considered. Azithromycin, ceftriaxone, or erythromycin base are all recommended treatments.

Visual Pearl

This known alcoholic adult patient was confused, severely dyspneic with a rectal temperature of 104°F and a productive cough. There is a foul odor to the breath. What are the primary findings on this chest film? What is the likely diagnosis?

Answer

There is a large, diffuse infiltrate in the left hemithorax with elevation of the left hemidiaphragm. There is a central lucency with a meniscus within the infiltrate. The most likely diagnosis is anaerobic lung abscess after an episode of emesis with aspiration.

Visual Pearl

This adult patient complained of a relatively sudden uniocular complete loss of vision. He denied any pain. He has a history of hypertension. What is the most likely diagnosis?

Answer

The diagnosis in this case is central retinal vein occlusion. Pressure from the retinal artery has collapsed the retinal vein preventing the outflow of blood out of the eye. The retina appears chaotic with blood-streaked areas. There is no immediate therapy the emergency physician can provide that will ameliorate the problem. The patient requires immediate ophthalmologic consultation.

Visual Pearl

This patient complained of a sudden choking spell. What is your diagnosis?

Answer

This film hilights a radiolucent foreign body in the esophagus anterior to the vertebral bodies of C$_{6-7}$ after water soluble contrast ingestion.

Visual Pearl

This diabetic was febrile with severe erythema, swelling, and a dusky appearance to the foot after minor trauma to the soft tissues of the volar surface several days ago. There is also blister formation on the dorsal skin. A lateral radiograph was obtained. What is your concern? What is the likely diagnosis?

Answer

There is a large amount of subcutanenous gas visible within the plantar and distal posterior soft tissues. This implies a gas-forming infection. The primary concern is gas gangrene due to *Clostridium perfringens* although other organsisms (synergistic infections) may produce this radiographic appearance. The patient requires tetanus prophylaxis, immediate surgical consultation, and broad spectrum, parenteral antibiotics. Hyperbaric oxygen therapy might be employed.

Visual Pearl

This female patient presents with a progressive area of granulation tissue which is elevated, red and painless. She has had the problem for "several months." The lesions began as a papule which ulcerated. What is the most likely diagnosis?

Answer

Granuloma inguinale (Donovanosis) is a mildly contagious, chronic, progressive, autoinocuable, ulcerative disease. It involves skin and lymphatics of perianal and genital areas. It is sexually transmitted and associated with the presence of an intracellular microorganism (the Donovan body) in affected tissues. Lesions appear within 30 days after sexual exposure. Lesions in women progress anteriorly over the genitalia in a V shape along the vulva. Extragenital lesions may occur. Erythromycin or trimethoprim-sulfamethoxazole are effective antimicrobial therapy.

Visual Pearl

What is your diagnosis based on the appearance of this rash? The rash evolved as per the listed sequence. The patient complained of burning pain in the areas of the lesions over the left hemithorax and left upper extremity for several days prior to the appearance of the rash.

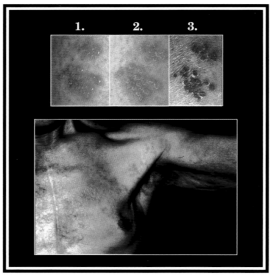

Answer

Varicella-zoster with thoracic neuralgia presents with multiple, small, erythematous, grouped vesicles which evolve into crusted ulcerations. Impaired immunity, elderly age, debilitation, or malnourishment may all contribute to activation of the virus. Diagnosis of neuralgia can be difficult if vesicles are not evident, but the patient has pain within a dermatome (zoster sine herpete). Acute thoracic radiculopathy may precede the rash by many days. Treatment may include systemic steroids (some studies show a decrease incidence of postherpetic neuralgia if given early), and oral (or intravenous) acyclovir.

Visual Pearl

This adult patient complained of a mild viral syndrome with a subsequent rash which began as a single lesion on the posterior thorax. Susequently, multiple small patches of skin became covered with a dry epidermis and then desquamated to form a collarette of scale at their periphery. What is the most likely diagnosis?

Answer

The first lesion of pityriasis rosea is a solitary erythematous or salmon-colored herald plaque. It is most often seen on the trunk and extremities, followed by the development of smaller maculopapular lesions similiar to the initial lesion. These latter lesions erupt over time in groupings and often appear in the pattern of a christmas tree following the lines of skin tension on the posterior thorax. This is probably a viral condition and may last 3-8 weeks. Care is only symptomatic. Lesions heal without sequelae. In general, a diagnosis of secondary syphilis should be ruled out.

Visual Pearl

This adult male was intoxicated, but complained of left chest pain after a motor vehicle accident. A chest tube was placed and immediately drained 250 mL of blood. The patient's vital signs improved after 1500 mL of crystalloid were administered. What are the key findings and primary diagnostic concern?

Answer

There is obvious widening of the upper mediastinum with bilateral apical capping. Widening of the superior mediastinum is significant if it is more than 8 cm on an upright PA CXR. Although this is a portable AP film, the findings strongly suggest traumatic rupture of the aorta (TRA), or mediastinal venous bleeding which is significant enough to warrant suspicion for TRA. The patient requires angiography to establish the nature of the injury and the need for urgent surgical repair.

Visual Pearl

This 7-year-old male child presented with multiple lesions of the left buttock and upper thigh. There is no history of injury to the area. The original lesion appeared as a red papule. This progressed over several days to multiple lesions with erythema, a rim of adherent golden crust, and central clearing. The child is not acutely ill. What is the diagnosis and the treatment?

Answer

The diagnosis is impetigo contagiosa. The causative organism is Group A ß-hemolytic streptococcus, but it may occasionally be due to staphylococcus. Effective therapy includes one of these: parenteral PCN, erythromycin, cephalexin, dicloxacillin, or mupurocin topically. Glomerulonephritis is associated with nephritogenic strains of streptococcus, and is not prevented by antibiotic therapy.

Visual Pearl

This adult male complained of blisters with this appearance on the hand. There is no history of burn or injury. On presentation, he was afebrile and appeared well. There are no other lesions on the skin surfaces. There is no regional lymphadenopathy. What is your diagnosis based on this appearance?

Answer

Bullous impetigo, is caused by an epidermolytic toxin which causes separation of the skin at the granular layer. The lesions usually are not contaminated by streptococci. Respiratory colonization predates colonization of normal skin (opposite sequence occurs in vesicular, i.e., streptococcal impetigo) by more than 10 days. The condition is most common in infants and children, especially on the face, and lesions may persist for months. Regional lymphadenitis is uncommon. Rarely, serious secondary infections (e.g., septic arthritis, pneumonia) develop.

Visual Pearl

This 3-year-old child presented with a temperature of 101.5 °F, a mild sore throat and a brassy cough. The parents became concerned when they heard a "noise" on inspiration. There was no drooling, and the child was taking po liquids without difficulty. He appeared moderately ill, but was not in obvious distress. What is your diagnosis based on this AP film?

Answer

"Steeple sign" seen in croup (laryngotracheal bronchitis). The noise was stridor (it typically begins abruptly at night). Croup mainly affects children less than 4 years old, and is usually caused by viruses (especially the parainfluenza group). Other etiologies include influenza virus, respiratory syncytial virus, and measles. Primary treatment includes oxygen and humidification. Corticosteriods are generally not utilized. Antibiotics are only indicated in the uncommon situation of secondary bacterial infection.

Visual Pearl

This patient was found unconscious after a "gang fight." What is the most likely diagnosis?

Answer

This is a coronal reformatted cranial CT. The finding is a penetrating injury to the skull with an irregularly shaped intracranial hematoma of high density (acute hemorrhage) and subcutaneous hematoma. Note the low density border around the hematoma which is representative of cerebral edema. There is some shift of the midline structures to the left. When an intracranial hematoma is irregular in shape, think of a traumatic injury. Spontaneous intracranial hemorrhage is more typically round in appearance.

Visual Pearl

This baby had an initial umbilical infection. Moderate dehydration was managed with intravenous fluids. The illness also required intravenous methicillin, but corticosteroids were specifically withheld. Healing occurred without scar formation. Cultures from intact bullae were negative. What is your diagnosis based on this information and clinical appearance?

Answer

Staphylococcal scalded skin syndrome (*Ritter's disease)* is a staphylococcal epidermolytic toxin-mediated syndrome that begins with a localized *S. aureus* infection. A diffuse erythema with tenderness evolves with bullae formation, wrinkling of the skin, and subsequent desquamation in large sheets. Minor pressure will induce skin separation (Nikolsky's sign).

Visual Pearl

This adult patient complained of painless "bumps" on his penis. He admits to a history of homosexual behavior. What is your diagnosis based on this clinical appearance?

Answer

This photograph demonstrates genital warts. The incidence is significantly increasing even exceeding that for genital herpes. There is a strong correlation between genital warts due to human papilloma virus, HPV (several types), and genital cancer. Warts may spread rapidly and may extend into the urethra, rectum, or, in the female, into the vagina. Visualization is enhanced after application of dilute acetic acid. Treatment includes podophyllum resin and may result in significant pain with local inflammation.

Visual Pearl

This adult female complained of pruritis and a migratory rash with tracks that changed position and shape on her skin. She had episodes of abdominal pain and diarrhea containing some mucus and blood. Her blood demonstrated eosinophilia. What is the diagnosis and treatment?

Answer

Creeping eruption (cutaneous larva migrans) is an infestation of migrating hookworm larva (most common is *Ancyclostoma braziliense*) after they penetrate the skin. The patient has usually been walking barefoot on soil. Moderate itching and eosinophilia occur. Loffler's syndrome is a transitory, patchy pulmonary infiltrate in patients with a severe cutaneous infestation. Parasites may be found in the sputum. Treatment includes topical thiabenda-zole or ivermectin. Oral antibiotics and topical steroids are used for secondary bacterial infection or eczematous inflammation. Oral thiabendazole induces nausea, vomiting and dizziness in a significant number of patients but may be indicated.

Visual Pearl

This adult male awoke in the morning with this problem on his left dorsal wrist. He had been drinking heavily and fell asleep in his barn. His temperature is 100.2°F. He complains of chills, nausea, and muscle aches. What is your diagnosis based upon this appearance and clinical information?

Answer

The initial bite of a brown recluse spider usually produces a minor burning or sudden sharp pain. Severe bites may demonstrate necrosis of the bite area within 4 hours and severe pain. Within 12 hours after the bite the victim may demonstrate systemic toxicity. The toxin may induce thrombocytopenia, generalized hemolysis, DIC, renal failure, or even death (severe reactions are more likely in children). Primary treatment includes bedrest, elevation, tetanus toxoid, antibiotics, dapsone, and pain management. Immediate surgical excision is avoided.

Visual Pearl

This child had been on vacation in Florida and developed a sudden pruritic dermatitis after swimming in the ocean. She had been wearing a bathing suit that covered her abdomen. This is the appearance of the rash after 3 days. She had associated headache and conjunctivitis. The dermatitis resolved after 10 days. She had no sequelae. What is the diagnosis?

Answer

Seabather's eruption is a pruritic dermatitis that primarily involves skin surfaces previously covered by a bathing suit after exposure to the larval form of the thimble jellyfish, *Linuche unguiculata*. Systemic complaints may occasionally occur and include general malaise, headache, conjunctivitis, and urethritis. Treatment is symptomatic. Swimmer's itch (due to parasitic flatworm schistosomes in fresh water–usually in the Great Lakes region of the United States) occurs on any exposed areas and may be associated with secondary infection. Treatment for this infestation may include cool compresses, calamine lotion, and antihistamines. Topical steroids are occasionally indicated.

Visual Pearl

This 22-year-old male complained of neck pain after being kicked in the back of the head with a boot. He was ambulatory and had an odor of ketones on his breath. There was no obvious neurologic deficit. What is your diagnosis based on this clinical information and the film?

Answer

This patient presents with bilateral interfacetal dislocation of C6 on C7. 50% or more override of one vertebral body anteriorly over the next body implies this injury. The mechanism is hyperflexion without rotation. This is an unstable injury and would likely present with, or develop, an acute neurologic deficit. The patient requires immediate C-spine immobilization, further diagnostic evaluation, and orthopedic and/or neurosurgical consultation.

Visual Pearl

This 37-year-old physician complained of severe pain in the left inguinal region. He presented with a chief complaint of left inguinal hernia. On physical examination no hernia was detectable. He had direct tenderness in the left lower abdomen with some tenderness on rectal examination. Genitourinary examination was normal. What is your diagnosis?

Answer

This patient has a diverticular abscess (phlegmon). Multiple tiny dark gas-filled pockets surround a hyperintense (white) thickened bowel wall on the patient's left side of the study. A fever would be expected although its absence does not rule out the diagnosis. The patient was treated with broad spectrum intravenous antibiotics and did not require surgery.

Visual Pearl

This male patient presented with acute loss of consciousness after complaining of a severe headache. Decerebrate posturing, hyperreflexia, and a positive Babinski reflex were present. His breathing pattern was irregular and rapid with pauses. He died shortly after this study was obtained. What is your diagnosis?

Answer

The diagnosis is acute subarachnoid hemorrhage seen as a hyperintense outlining of the brainstem in the center of the image. This is an axial cranial CT without contrast (C-). New hemorrhage greatly attenuates the x-ray fan beam on CT, and therefore, appears white. The findings in this patient indicated a moribund presentation with increased intracranial pressure.

Visual Pearl

This patient was confused and has a history of intravenous drug abuse. He is severely dyspneic with a rectal temperature of 104.2°F and a nonproductive cough. His posterior thorax also demonstrates skin lesions with this appearance (lower portion of image). What is the likely diagnosis? What do the skin lesions represent?

Answer

Bilateral alveolar and interstitial infiltrates on chest film in this patient were due to *Pneumocystis carinii* pneumonia. The skin lesions represent Kaposi's sarcoma. This patient had previously contracted the HIV virus.

Visual Pearl

This adult male complained of rash, low grade fever, swollen glands, and a general malaise. He had no known tick exposure. His GU exam is normal. Bilateral nontender inguinal lymphadenopathy is present. Small ulcerations are visible in the mouth. The musculoskeletal examination is normal. What is the most likely diagnosis?

Answer

This patient presents with a maculopapular rash with intraoral lesions all consistent with secondary syphillis. The rash may be maculopapular, papular, macular, annular, psoriasiform, or follicular. The intraoral lesions are hightly contagious as are the lesions of condylomata lata. The patient requires antibiotic therapy with parenteral benzathine penicillin G. A falling RPR after measurement of a baseline serum titer indicates successful therapy. Alternate antibiotics for PCN sensitive patients include tetracycline and doxycycline; spectinomycin is not effective.

Visual Pearl

This 65-year-old male fell from a ladder. He complained of sudden, severe, anterior chest pain and was profoundly hypotensive and anuric shortly after his arrival in the ED. A systolic murmur was heard over the posterior thorax. The initial CXR was normal. The following study was obtained just prior to the episode of hypotension. What is your diagnosis?

Answer

This CT demonstrates acute traumatic rupture of the ascending aorta with extension into the descending aorta. A portion of the calcified aortic wall is seen centrally in the descending aorta. Both true and false lumen are visible in the ascending and descending aorta. This is a surgical emergency. Untreated, the condition is lethal. Preoperative aortography is performed, when possible, to define anatomy and delineate the extent of injury. Pulse deficits and asymmetric bilateral blood pressure measurements may be present. Sudden anuria indicates obstruction of blood flow to the kidneys or severe hypotension with renal hypoperfusion.

Visual Pearl

This adult male presents with a chronic pruritic rash with flat topped closely spaced pink-purple papules. Fine white scale is visible on the surface of the lesions. Some have angular margins. He is otherwise well and afebrile. There is no known exposure to medication or toxins. What is your diagnosis?

Answer

Lichen planus is an inflammatory cutaneous reaction of unknown etiology. It may affect the mucous membranes. Drugs and toxins have been implicated; there is no known viral or bacterial etiology associated. 10% of patients have a positive family history primarily as adults. The lesions are pruritic, planar, polyangular, purple papules (the five P's). The fine lacy scale or lines on the surface are called Wickham's stria (areas of epidermal thickening). Treatment includes topical steroids for localized disease, intralesional steroids, and sometimes systemic steroids. Antihistamines effectively relieve itching.

Visual Pearl

This adult male presents with a lesion on his proximal penis. What is the likely diagnosis?

Answer

3 serotypes of *Chlamydia trachomatis* cause lymphogranuloma venereum. A small papule or herpetiform vesicle appears on the genitalia after an incubation period of 5-21 days. Rapid evolution leads to painless ulcer formation and healing occurs without scarring. Primary lesions are rare in women and the initial lesion may go unnoticed. Unilateral or bilateral inguinal lymphadenopathy develops 1-4 weeks after healing of the ulcer. This is accompanied by headache, fever, arthralgia, and migratory polymyalgia. Rupture of lymph nodes (buboes) and lymphatic obstruction with genital edema (the latter in females) are chronic sequelae. Diagnosis is made using microimmunofluorescent techniques or culture. Treatment is with tetracycline.

RANDOM PEARLS

Errors, like straws, upon the surface flow;
He who would search for pearls must dive below.

John Dryden 1631-1700, Prologues and Epilogues:
Prologue, All for Love.

❑❑ **Cricothyroidotomy is not recommended in children of less than what age?**

10 years.

❑❑ **Name, in order, the 5 Kübler-Ross stages.**

1.) Denial.
2.) Anger.
3.) Bargaining.
4.) Depression.
5.) Acceptance.

❑❑ **Use of an EOA is contraindicated in patients of less than _____ years of age.**

16.

❑❑ **Is succinylcholine a depolarizing or a non-depolarizing neuromuscular blocking agent?**

It is the only commonly used depolarizing agent.
It binds to post-synaptic acetylcholine receptors causing depolarization.
It is enzymatically degraded by pseudocholinesterase (serum cholinesterase).
Onset within 1 minute with duration of paralysis of 7-10 min.

❑❑ **What is the rationale for pre-treating a patient with a subpolarizing ("defasciculating") dose of a non-depolarizing agent prior to administration of succinylcholine?**

Attenuates fasciculations from succinylcholine induced depolarization - this may decrease subsequent muscle pain.
Blunts increased intragastric and intraocular pressure associated with succinylcholine.

❑❑ **What is the appropriate dose of midazolam (Versed) to cause loss of consciousness and amnesia during a rapid sequence induction?**

≈ 0.1 mg/kg.
5 mg seems to work for most people.

❑❑ **What is the appropriate dose of thiopental to induce anesthesia during a rapid sequence induction?**

≈4 mg/kg.

❑❑ **Onset of loss of consciousness with thiopental usually occurs within 15 s. What is the usual duration of action?**

2-30 min, depending on source. < 5 min commonly referenced.

❑❑ **What is the appropriate dose of vecuronium for "defasciculating" or "priming" dose?**

≈ 0.01 mg/kg.

❏❏ **What is the appropriate dose of vecuronium for paralysis (no "priming")?**

0.15 - 0.20 mg/kg.

❏❏ **What is the appropriate dose of pancuronium (Pavulon) for "defasciculating" or "priming" dose?**

0.015 mg/kg.
≈ 1 mg common adult dose.

❏❏ **Dermacentor andersoni (wood tick) is a pesky arthropod associated with <u>four</u> tick-borne illnesses! Name each and its cause.**

Rocky Mtn. Spotted Fever caused by Rickettsia rickettsii for which Dermacentor andersoni is a vector.

Tick paralysis caused by neurotoxin. Its ascending paralysis with decrease or loss of DTRs can be similar to symptoms of Guillain-Barré syndrome.

Q Fever caused by Coxiella burnetii (a rickettsiae).

Colorado Tick Fever from arbovirus.

❏❏ **What is the <u>most</u> <u>common</u> opportunistic infection of AIDS?**

PCP. It is the initial opportunistic infection in 60% of AIDS patients and eventually affects 80%.

❏❏ **What is appropriate initial treatment of PCP?**

TMP/SMX or pentamidine.

❏❏ **Describe "AIDS dementia" complex (aka HIV-I encephalopathy).**

A progressive disease caused directly by HIV-I present in 1/3 of AIDS patients characterized by impairment of recent memory, concentration deficit, increasing DTRs, seizures and frontal release signs.

❏❏ **What is the <u>most</u> <u>common</u> cause of *focal* encephalitis in AIDS patients?**

Toxoplasma gondii.

❏❏ **Ethylene glycol is <u>the</u> alcohol that may present with hypocalcemia (1/3 of cases). Where does the calcium go?**

Oxalic acid is one of the metabolites of ethylene glycol.
Calcium precipitates with oxalate and forms calcium oxalate crystals.
The + birefringent calcium oxalate dihydrate crystals are pathognomonic of this ingestion.

❏❏ **What is the LD$_{50}$ for falling in adults?**

48 feet.

❏❏ **A laryngeal fracture is suggested by finding the hyoid bone elevated above what cervical level on x-ray?**

C3.

❏❏ **Describe the action and side effects of diazoxide.**

Diazoxide is a direct arterial vasodilator. The onset of action is within one to two min and lasts up to 12 h. Side effects may include nausea, vomiting, fluid retention and hyperglycemia. Diazoxide is contraindicated in patients with aortic dissection or angina.

❏❏ **What species of plasmodium are resistant to chloroquine?**

Falciparum.

❏❏ **In children greater than one year of age, where are foreign bodies in the airway usually located?**

In the lower airway.

❏❏ **In a child with malrotation, what is the most likely age of presentation, what is a common complication, and what signs and symptoms are usually present?**

Malrotation usually occurs in children under 12 months of age.
Volvulus is a common complication.
Signs and symptoms usually include vomiting, blood streaked stools, and abdominal pain.

❏❏ **Name 2 causes of Toxic Epidermal Necrolysis (aka scalded skin syndrome).**

1.) Drug or Chemical. Usually in adults. Cleavage at dermo-epidermal junction.

2.) Staphylococcal. Usually in children < 5 y. SSSS results in intraepidermal cleavage beneath stratum granulosum.

❏❏ **Describe the presentation of SSSS.**

Disease begins after URI or purulent conjunctivitis. First lesions are tender, erythematous and scarlatiniform, usually found on face, neck, axillae and groin. Skin peels off in sheets with lateral pressure, a + Nikolsky's sign.

❏❏ **What is appropriate treatment for Toxic Epidermal Necrolysis?**

Regardless of cause, treat skin loss similarly to partial thickness burns. Do not use silver sulfadiazine. Adults can have large fluid loss. Admit patients with >10% BSA to burn unit.
For SSSS treat with IV penicillinase-resistant penicillin.

❏❏ **In bullous impetigo, which of the following drugs may not be effective: erythromycin, amoxicillin, cefaclor, or doxycycline?**

Amoxicillin.

❏❏ **Methanol intoxication causes early death by what cause?**

Respiratory arrest. Unknown pathophysiology.

❏❏ **Reiter's syndrome diagnostic triad:**

Conjunctivitis, polyarthritis, and non-gonococcal urethritis.

❏❏ **Nerve most commonly injured in glenohumeral dislocation?**

Axillary nerve, numb area over lateral deltoid.

❏❏ **Permanent pacemakers have a coding system of 5 letters. The first letter signifies the Chamber Paced. What does the second letter signify?**

Chamber Sensed.

❏❏ Describe and contrast regional enteritis and ulcerative colitis.

Category	Regional Enteritis	Ulcerative Colitis
Name	Crohn's disease Regional enteritis Terminal ileitis Granulomatous ileocolitis	Ulcerative colitis
Area	**Stem-to-stern** = social to anti- social (mouth to anus) **Segmental** (skip areas) <u>Most</u> <u>common</u> area is ileum	95% rectosigmoid **Contiguous** (no skip areas)
Demographics	15 - 22 y 55 - 60 y Common in Europeans Jews White > Black 10-15 % have family hx	10 - 20 y 20 - 30 y 15 x greater risk with 1st° relative

Bowel	**ALL LAYERS**
	Thick Bowel Wall
	Narrow lumen
	Creeping fat - mesenteric fat over
	  bowel wall
	
	"Cobblestone" mucosal appearance
	
	Fissures
	Fistulas
	Abscesses
		Mucosa and Submucosa
		Mucosal ulceration
		Epithelial necrosis
		
		Mild - Mucosa is fine, granular and
		  friable
		
		**Severe - Spongy, red, oozing
		ulcerations**
		
		Crypt abscesses
		Toxic Megacolon

❏❏ Describe the mechanism and cause of a boutonniere deformity.

Boutonniere deformity is secondary to rupture of the extensor apparatus of the PIP joint. The result of the injury is a PIP joint which is flexed and a DIP joint which is hyperextended. It is treated by splinting the PIP joint in full extension.

❏❏ A cyanotic patient has a low oxygen saturation measured on ABG. What flavor of cyanosis does this patient have?

Central.

❏❏ What is a peripheral cyanosis?

ABG reveals an oxygen saturation within normal; shunting or increased O_2 extraction is taking place.

❏❏ Name the two primary causes (groups) of peripheral cyanosis.

Cyanosis with a normal SaO_2 can be due to:
    Decreased cardiac output.
      Redistribution - may be 2° to shock, DIC, hypothermia, vascular obstruction.

❏❏ Name the causes of central cyanosis.

The causes of cyanosis with a decreased SaO_2 are:

Decreased PaO_2, or decreased O_2 diffusion.
Hypoventilation.

V-Q mismatch, pulmonary shunting.
Dysfunctional hemoglobin (includes sickle cell crisis, drug induced hemoglobinopathies).
NOTE: Hb-CO does not cause cyanosis (though the cherry red appearance of skin and mucous membranes could suggest a cyanosis).

❏❏ **A pulmonary embolism causes which flavor of cyanosis?**

Central cyanosis, although secondary shock and right-heart failure can lead to peripheral cyanosis.

❏❏ **What is a positive Chvostek's sign?**

Twitch in the corner of the mouth occurring when the examiner taps over the facial nerve in front of the ear.
It is present in approximately 10 to 30 percent of normal individuals. Eyelid muscle contraction with Chvostek's maneuver is generally considered to be diagnostic of hypocalcemia.

❏❏ **What is Trousseau's sign and when is it seen?**

Trousseau's sign is a carpal spasm induced when a blood pressure cuff on the upper arm maintains a pressure above systolic for approximately three minutes. Fingers become spastically extended at the interphalangeal joints and flexed at the metacarpophalangeal joints.
Trousseau's sign is generally a more reliable indicator of hypocalcemia than is Chvostek's sign.
Positive Trousseau's sign may also be found in hypomagnesemia, severe alkalosis, and strychnine poisoning.

❏❏ **Activated charcoal is <u>not</u> effective treatment for what substances?**

Alcohols, ions, and acids and bases.

❏❏ **Permanent pacemakers have a coding system of 5 letters. In this system the letter A refers to the Atrium and V to the Ventricle. What does the letter D refer to?**

D = Double, meaning both Atrium and Ventricle.

❏❏ **Describe a patient with Sjogren's syndrome.**

Sjogren's syndrome is usually seen in women more than 50 years of age. Symptoms often include diminished lacrimal and salivary gland secretions, salivary gland enlargement and arthritis. Sjogren's syndrome predisposes a patient to corneal irritation, ulceration and superimposed infection. It may complicate many rheumatic diseases or may occur independently. The likely cause of Sjogren's syndrome is lymphatic infiltration of the lacrimal and salivary glands, resulting in dry eyes and dry mouth.

❏❏ **Describe the DeBakey classification of regions of aortic dissection.**

(I) Ascending and descending aorta.
(II) Ascending aorta.
(III) Descending aorta distal to the left subclavian artery.

❏❏ **What is the <u>most common</u> conduction disturbance in acute myocardial infarction?**

First degree AV block.

❏❏ **What is the <u>most common</u> foot fracture?**

Calcaneus (60%). The talus is a distant second most common.

❏❏ **Where does the <u>most common</u> metatarsal fracture occur?**

At the base of the fifth metatarsal, a Jones fracture.

❏❏ **Which tendons are involved in de Quervain's tenosynovitis?**

The abductor pollicis and the extensor pollicis brevis tendons.
Diagnosis is confirmed with positive Finkelstein's test.

❏❏ **Describe Dupuytren's (Guillaume, 1777-1835) contracture.**

Contraction of the longitudinal bands of the palmar aponeurosis.

❏❏ **What is the <u>most</u> <u>common</u> form of anorectal abscess?**

Perianal abscess. Anorectal abscesses are usually mixed infections, both gram negative and anaerobic organisms. Fistula formation is a frequent complication.

❏❏ **What is the <u>most</u> <u>common</u> rhythm disturbance in a pediatric arrest?**

Bradycardia.

❏❏ **How long does it take to prepare type-specific saline cross-matched blood?**

Ten minutes.

❏❏ **Describe the common features of a slipped femoral capital epiphysis.**

Injury usually occurs in adolescence. The rupture typically presents with an insidious development of knee or thigh pain, and a painful limp. Frequently hip motion is limited, particularly that of internal rotation. Evaluation is aided by anteroposterior and frogleg lateral films of both hips.

❏❏ **A core temperature of less than 32 °C (90 °F) is commonly associated with:**

Poor prognosis, complications including arrhythmias resistant to treatment, and loss of the shivering reflex.

❏❏ **What is the treatment for torsade de pointes?**

Treatment includes techniques to accelerate the heart rate, shortening the duration of ventricular repolarization. This may be accomplished with isoproterenol, temporary pacing, or with magnesium sulfate.

Drugs which increase or prolong repolarization, and therefore exacerbate torsade de pointes, include: Class IA antiarrhythmics (quinidine, procainamide, disopyramide), tricyclic antidepressants and phenothiazines.

❏❏ **Dobutamine in moderate doses causes what cardiovascular effects?**

Decreased peripheral resistance and pulmonary occlusive pressure, and inotropic stimulation of the heart.

❏❏ **Permanent pacemakers have a coding system of 5 letters. The first letter refers to chamber Paced, the second to chamber Sensed. What does the third letter refer to?**

Mode or Response. It comes in several flavors including I = Inhibited, T = Triggered, D = Double, R = Reverse and O = nOne.

❏❏ **What are the two most common causes of fatal anaphylaxis?**

#1 = Drug reactions, 95% to penicillin. Parenteral most dangerous. 300 people/y.
#2 = Hymenoptera stings. 100 people/y.

❏❏ **Which type of hypersensitivity reaction is responsible for anaphylaxis?**

Type I, (IgE mediated).

Hypersensitivity Reaction	Mediator	Example
Type 1 - Immediate	IgE binds allergen, includes mast cells and basophils	Food allergy. **Asthma in children.**
Type 2 - Cytotoxic	IgG & IgM antibody reactions to antigen on cell surface activates complement and killers	Blood transfusion rxn. ITP, hemolytic anemia, ITP.
Type 3 - Immune complex, Arthrus	Complexes activate complement	Tetanus toxoid in sensitized persons. **Poststreptococcal glomeru-lonephritis.**
Type 4 - Cell mediated, delayed hypersensitivity	Activated T-lymphocytes	Skin tests

❏❏ **What are the common concerns with anterior dislocation of the shoulder?**

Axillary nerve injury, axillary artery injury (elderly patients), compression fracture of the humeral head (Hillsack's deformity), a rotator cuff tear, fractures of the anterior glenoid lip, and fractures of the greater tuberosity.

❏❏ **Describe a Monteggia fracture/dislocation.**

A fracture of the proximal ulna with dislocation of the radial head.

Treatment usually requires open reduction and internal fixation. When a Monteggia fracture is suspected, x-rays should include the forearm, elbow and wrist.

<u>M</u>ichigan <u>U</u>niversity <u>P</u>olice <u>D</u>epartment = <u>MUPD</u>

<u>MUPD</u> = <u>M</u>onteggia, <u>U</u>lnar fracture, <u>P</u>roximal <u>D</u>islocation.

❏❏ **Describe a Galeazzi's fracture/dislocation.**

A radial shaft fracture with dislocation of the distal radioulnar joint.

<u>G</u>reat <u>R</u>ays <u>D</u>own <u>D</u>eep! = GRDD

<u>GRDD</u> = <u>G</u>aleazzi, <u>R</u>adius fracture, <u>D</u>istal <u>D</u>islocation

This is a little-known but true story. Galeazzi's fracture/dislocation is named for the famous orthopod who suffered this injury in a fatal diving accident. Dr. Galeazzi, it seemed, was following a large ray off the coast of Cozumel when he smashed his arm into an unseen coral outcropping. The pain caused him to hyperventilate and head up. His last words as he made the surface (before his dysbaric air embolism) were "Great Rays Down Deep!"

❏❏ **Describe the clinical characteristics of carboxyhemoglobin concentrations, specifically for ranges of near 10%, 20%, 30%, 40%, 50%, 60% and 70%.**

10%-	Frontal headache.
20%-	Headache and dyspnea.
30%-	Nausea, dizziness, visual disturbance, fatigue, and impaired judgment.
40%-	Syncope and confusion.
50%-	Coma and seizures.
60%-	Respiratory failure and hypotension.
70%-	May be lethal.

❑❑ **What is the appropriate treatment for cyanide poisoning?**

Amyl nitrite, sodium nitrite IV, followed by sodium thiosulfate IV.

❑❑ **Organisms which produce focal nervous system pathology via an exotoxin include:**

C. diphtheria.
C. botulinum.
C. tetani.
Wood and dog tick (Dermacentor A&B).
Staph aureus.

❑❑ **Signs and symptoms of diphtheria infection include:**

Infection is heralded by acute onset of exudative pharyngitis, high <u>fever</u> and malaise. A pseudomembrane may form in the oropharynx with possible respiratory compromise. Powerful exotoxin has direct effects on the heart, kidneys and nervous system. Diphtheria infection may lead to paralysis of the intrinsic and extrinsic eye muscles.
You will never see such paralysis in your practice, but you may need to differentiate it from bulbar palsy caused by C. botulinum on an exam. Botulism does not cause fever.

❑❑ **Describe botulism intoxication.**

Botulism exotoxin is elaborated by C. botulinum. It affects the myoneural junction and prevents the release of acetylcholine. In the United States, it is caused principally by ingestion of foods that have been inadequately prepared.
The most common neurologic complaints are related to the bulbar musculature. Neurologic symptoms usually occur within 24 to 48 hours of ingestion of contaminated foods.
Muscle paralysis and weakness usually spread rapidly to involve all muscles of the trunk and extremities. It is important to distinguish between botulism poisoning and myasthenia gravis. This distinction can be made by using the edrophonium (Tensilon) test, usually performed by a neurologist.

❑❑ **What are some of the key features of Guillain-Barré syndrome?**

Guillain-Barré syndrome is a lower motor neuron disease which commonly affects persons in their 30's and 40's. It presents as an ascending weakness involving the legs more than the arms. A sensory component may be present.
Bulbar muscles are usually involved late in the course of the disease. Reflexes are affected early. Paralysis can progress rapidly and recovery is usually slow, but almost always complete.

Lower motor neuron.
Ascending.
Bulbar late.
Reflexes early.

❑❑ **What formula should be used to calculate fluid requirements for resuscitation of a burn victim?**

2-4 ml/kg / %TBSA / day.
One-half of this is given in the first 8 hours.

❑❑ **Poor prognostic signs <u>on admission</u> of a patient with pancreatitis include:**

Age over 55 years.
Glucose level greater than 200 mg/dl.
LDH level greater than 700 IU/l.
WBC count greater than 16,000.
SGOT level greater than 250 U/l.

NOTICE - <u>NO</u> <u>AMYLASE</u> INVOLVEMENT!

❏❏ **Poor prognostic signs <u>at 48° after admission</u> of a patient with pancreatitis include:**

Hematocrit fallen more than 10% with a rise in BUN more that 5 mg/dl, declining calcium level to less than 8 mg/dl, PaO_2 less than 60 mm Hg, large fluid accumulation and base deficit greater than 4 mEq/L. NOTICE - <u>NO AMYLASE</u> INVOLVEMENT!

Great quotes series:

"That's just something for your trivia basket."

Professor John "Jack" Nolte, formerly of University of Colorado Health Sciences Center which could not retain this outstanding teacher and author of <u>The Human Brain - An introduction to its functional anatomy</u>.

"My trivia basket is full." Medical student response.

❏❏ **What test is considered to be the gold standard in establishing the diagnosis of acute cholecystitis?**

Radionuclide scan of the biliary tree.

❏❏ **What pain medicine is theoretically contraindicated in the treatment of pain from acute diverticulitis?**

Codeine and morphine are contraindicated, as their use may increase intraluminal colonic pressure. Meperidine (Demerol) is a good substitute as it inhibits segmental contraction of the colon.

❏❏ **What test is best to confirm the diagnosis of Boerhaave's syndrome?**

An esophagram using a water soluble contrast medium should be used in place of barium to confirm the diagnosis.

❏❏ **What pseudonyms are associated with regional enteritis (4)?**

Crohn's disease.
Terminal ileitis.
Regional enteritis.
Granulomatous ileocolitis.

❏❏ **What are the other terms used to refer to ulcerative colitis?**

NONE. If any other pseudonym is used it refers to that other similar disease.

❏❏ **A patient presents with Mallory-Weiss syndrome, and a Sengstaken-Blakemore tube is being considered to control hemorrhage. What problem could a patient have by history that would prevent its use?**

Hiatal hernia, since proper placement of the balloon, as well as proper traction, cannot be applied in such persons.

❏❏ **What are the signs and symptoms of a patient with Boerhaave's syndrome?**

Substernal and left sided chest pain with a history of forceful vomiting leading to spontaneous esophageal rupture.

❏❏ **What is the <u>most common</u> cause of intestinal obstruction?**

Adynamic ileus is the <u>most common</u> cause of intestinal obstruction.

❏❏ **What is the <u>most</u> <u>common</u> cause of small bowel obstruction?**

<u>Adhesions</u> (#1) and hernias are the <u>most</u> <u>common</u> causes of small bowel obstruction.

❏❏ **What is the <u>most</u> <u>common</u> cause of large bowel obstruction?**

<u>Carcinoma</u> (#1), volvulus and sigmoid diverticulitis are the most common causes of large bowel obstruction.

❏❏ **What is the single <u>most</u> <u>common</u> cause of upper GI tract hemorrhage?**

Duodenal ulcers.

❏❏ **Which layers of the bowel wall and mesentery are affected by regional enteritis (Crohn's disease, granulomatous ileocolitis)?**

Inflammatory reaction of regional enteritis involves all layers of the bowel wall.

REGIONAL enteritis involves ALL layers, of course!

❏❏ **What is the <u>most</u> <u>common</u> hernia in women?**

<u>Inguinal hernia</u>, as it is in men.
Though not as common overall, femoral hernias are more common in women than in men.

❏❏ **What are Kanavel's four cardinal signs of infectious digital flexor tenosynovitis?**

Tenderness along the tendon sheath,
finger held in flexion,
pain on passive extension of the finger,
finger swelling.

❏❏ **What symptoms are associated with presentation of regional enteritis (Crohn's disease, granulomatous ileocolitis)?**

Patients with regional enteritis may present with fever, abdominal pain, weight loss and diarrhea.
Fistulas, fissures and abscesses may be noted.
Ulcerative colitis, on the other hand, usually presents with bloody diarrhea.

❏❏ **The <u>most</u> <u>common</u> cause of subacute infectious endocarditis is:**

S. viridans.

❏❏ **Subacute bacterial endocarditis <u>most</u> <u>frequently</u> affects which valve?**

SBE usually involves the left side of the heart, specifically the <u>mitral</u> valve.
The aortic valve is the second most commonly involved valve. Rheumatic fever is the most likely cause of valvular damage associated with SBE. Mitral stenosis is a very common predisposing factor in SBE. Drug addicts tend to develop right-sided SBE, usually involving the tricuspid valve.

❏❏ **The <u>most</u> <u>common</u> cause of acute infectious endocarditis is:**

S. aureus.

❏❏ **A good initial antibiotic choice for empiric treatment of acute infectious endocarditis is:**

Gentamycin (1.0 - 1.5 mg/kg q 8° for normal adults) and oxacillin (12 gm/d).

❏❏ **A patient presents to your emergency department after being bitten by a wild raccoon. What treatment would you provide?**

Wound care, tetanus prophylaxis, RIG 20 IU/kg (1/2 at bite site and 1/2 IM), and HDCV 1 cc IM.

❏❏ **Describe the skin lesions found in a patient with disseminated gonococcemia.**

Umbilicated pustule with a red halo.

❏❏ **Describe the skin lesions associated with Pseudomonas aeruginosa infection.**

Pseudomonas aeruginosa bacteremia typically produces pale, erythematous skin lesions that are approximately 1 cm in size with an ulcerated necrotic center (ecthyma gangrenosum for you Zebe-hunters).

❏❏ **Defect of sickle cell disease?**

Valine is substituted for glutamic acid in the 6th amino acid of the ß-chain.

❏❏ **Describe the intracorporeal travel of the rabies virus.**

The virus is spread centripetally up peripheral nerve into the CNS. The incubation period for rabies is usually 30 to 60 d with a range of 10 d up to one yr. Transmission is usually by infected secretions, saliva or infected tissue. Stages include the upper respiratory tract infection symptomatology followed by encephalitis, and the final stage involving the brainstem.

❏❏ **What animals are the <u>most</u> <u>common</u> vectors of rabies a.) in the world, b.) in the U.S.?**

Worldwide, the dog is the most common carrier of rabies.
In the United States, the skUnk has become the <u>most</u> <u>common</u> source of disease. Bats, raccoons, cows, dogs, foxes and cats (descending order) are also sources.

Recall, parenthetically, that your rodents (Rocky (the flying squirrel), Dale (the chipmunk), Micky and Ratfink) and your lagomorphs (wild wangy wabbits) , are <u>NOT</u> carriers of rabies.

❏❏ **A septic appearing adult has multiple 1 cm diameter skin lesions with a necrotic, ulcerated center and an erythematous surrounding region. What is the likely pathogen?**

Pseudomonas aeruginosa.

❏❏ **What is the IM treatment for adult streptococcal pharyngitis?**

1.2 million units of benzathine penicillin G.
0.6 million units of benzathine penicillin G for kids under 27 kg.

Mercedes "Benz" last a long time.

❏❏ **What is the <u>most</u> <u>common</u> initial symptom in botulism poisoning?**

Visual disturbance.
Visual difficulties have been reported in up to 90 percent of cases. Abducent nerve (CN VI) palsy is common and severe cases may show third cranial nerve involvement with dilated and fixed pupils. Other common initial symptoms include headache, dizziness, weakness, malaise and a dry mouth. Nausea and vomiting is found in about 35% of cases. Symptoms usually appear within the first 24 to 72 hours after exposure.

❏❏ **Describe the signs and symptoms of spinal shock.**

Spinal shock represents complete loss of spinal cord function below the level of injury. Patients have flaccid paralysis, complete sensory loss, areflexia and loss of autonomic function.

Such patients are usually bradycardic, hypotensive, hypothermic and vasodilated.

❏❏ **Active adduction of the thumb tests which nerve?**

Ulnar nerve.

Great quote series:

The life so short, the craft so long to learn.

Hippocrates, c. 460-357 B.C.

❏❏ **Describe the rash found in exanthem subitum (roseola).**

The rash is usually found on the trunk and neck, and is maculopapular.

❏❏ **What is the <u>most</u> <u>common</u> cause of death among children between 1 and 12 months of age?**

SIDS.

❏❏ **Alkali causes what type of necrosis?**

Liquefactive necrosis.

❏❏ **What is the antibiotic of choice in the treatment of Rocky Mountain spotted fever in a patient allergic to tetracycline?**

Chloramphenicol.

❏❏ **Describe the chest x-ray of Mycoplasma pneumonia.**

Patchy densities involving the entire lobe are most common. Pneumatoceles, cavities, abscesses and pleural effusions can occur, but are uncommon. Erythromycin.

❏❏ **What type of bacterial pneumonia is commonly seen with viral illness?**

Staphylococcal infection.

❏❏ **What two types of pneumonia are often seen in the summer months?**

Staph pneumonia and Legionella.

❏❏ **Describe the chest x-ray findings in Legionella pneumonia.**

Dense consolidation and bulging fissures. Expect elevated liver enzymes and hypophosphatemia. Relative bradycardia on physical exam.

❏❏ **What are the classic signs and symptoms of TB?**

Night sweats, fever, weight loss, malaise, cough, and a green/yellow sputum most commonly seen in the mornings.

❏❏ **What are the chest x-ray findings in tuberculosis?**

Right upper lobe cavitation is classic.
Lower lung infiltrates, hilar adenopathy, atelectasis, and pleural effusion are common.

❏❏ **Where is the most likely location of a Boerhaave's tear?**

Left posterolateral region of the mid-thoracic esophagus.

❏❏ **How does a coin in the trachea appear on AP view?**

On its side.

❏❏ **How does a coin in the esophagus appear on AP?**

Like a solid circle.

❏❏ **Is GI bleeding common with a perforated ulcer?**

No.

❏❏ **During which trimester is acute appendicitis most common?**

Second.

❏❏ **What is the <u>most</u> <u>common</u> cause of paralytic ileus?**

Surgery.

❏❏ **What is the second most common cause of small bowel obstruction?**

Incarcerated hernia. The <u>most</u> <u>common</u> cause is adhesions.

❏❏ **An elderly female patient presents with the complaint of pain in the knee and also the medial aspect of the thigh. What GI diagnosis might you entertain?**

An obturator hernia may produce pain in the knee and thigh.

❏❏ **What is the second most common cause of colonic obstruction?**

Diverticulitis. Cancer of the sigmoid is the <u>most</u> <u>common</u> cause. Volvulus is the third most common cause.

❏❏ **What is the <u>most</u> <u>common</u> site of volvulus?**

Sigmoid colon.

❏❏ **Describe the location of an indirect inguinal hernia.**

Found <u>lateral to the epigastric vessels</u>, protrudes through the inguinal canal.

❏❏ **Describe a femoral hernia.**

Through the femoral canal and below the inguinal ligament.

❏❏ **Describe the location of a Spigelian hernia.**

Located 3-5 cm above the inguinal ligament.

❏❏ **What is a Pantaloon hernia?**

A hernia with both direct and indirect inguinal hernia components.

❏❏ **What is a sliding hernia?**

A hernia in which one wall of the hernia sac includes viscus.

❏❏ **Describe a Richter's hernia.**

An incarceration which contains only one wall of viscus.

❏❏ **What is the single <u>most</u> <u>common</u> hernia in children?**

An indirect hernia. Direct inguinal hernia is more common in the elderly.

❏❏ **When do umbilical hernias typically close?**

Age two.

❏❏ **List three other names for regional ileitis.**

Crohn's disease, terminal ileitis, and granulomatous ileocolitis.

❏❏ **What are other names for ulcerative colitis?**

None.

❏❏ **What is the most common site of Crohn's disease?.**

The ileum. It can actually involve any part of the GI tract from the social end to the antisocial end. It is segmental, often involving granuloma formation along with inflammatory reactions. Crohn's disease has two incidence peaks, one in the 15-22 y old age group and a second in the 55-60 y old age group.

❏❏ **How many layers of the bowel does Crohn's disease involve?**

All layers. Associated with *fissures, abscesses and fistulas.*

❏❏ **What are the signs and symptoms of Crohn's disease?**

Fever, diarrhea, right lower quadrant pain with mass possible, *fistulas,* rectal prolapse, perianal *fissures,* and *abscesses.* Associated with arthritis, uveitis, and liver disease.

❏❏ **What is the <u>most</u> <u>common</u> <u>complication</u> of Crohn's disease?**

Perianal abscess.
Also ischiorectal *abscess, fissures,* rectovaginal *fistulas,* rectal prolapse, and strictures.

❏❏ **Is toxic megacolon commonly associated with Crohn's disease?**

No. Toxic megacolon <u>is</u> a complication of ulcerative colitis.
Cancer is also an uncommon complication of Crohn's disease.

❏❏ **Systemic diseases associated with Crohn's disease?**

Pyoderma gangrenosum, uveitis, episclerosis, scleritis, arthritis, erythema nodosum, and nephrolithiasis.

❏❏ **Patient's with inflammatory bowel disease have ankylosing spondylitis what percentage of the time?**

20%.

❏❏ **What are the expected contrast x-ray findings with Crohn's disease?**

Segmental involvement in the colon with abnormal mucosal pattern and fistulas, often without involvement of the rectum. May see small intestinal narrowing.

❏❏ **What is the chief clinical feature of ulcerative colitis?**

Bloody diarrhea and involvement of the colon and rectum.
Peak incidence is in 20-30 y olds. The most common site is the rectosigmoid colon. Ulcerative colitis typically involves only the submucosal and mucosal layers. May see crypt abscesses and ulcerations present. Pseudopolyps are associated with ulcerative colitis.

❏❏ **What are the principal signs and symptoms of ulcerative colitis?**

Fever, weight loss, tachycardia, pancolitis, and six bloody bowel movements per day.

❏❏ **Is toxic megacolon more commonly seen in ulcerative colitis or Crohn's disease?**

Toxic megacolon is a very common, serious complication of ulcerative colitis.

❏❏ **What medications may be used in the treatment of Crohn's disease that are absolutely contraindicated in the treatment of ulcerative colitis?**

Antidiarrheal agents may be used in Crohn's disease, they should not be used to treat ulcerative colitis.

❏❏ **Is ulcerative colitis or Crohn's more commonly associated with perirectal fistulas and abscesses?**

Crohn's.

❏❏ **Is cancer more commonly seen in ulcerative colitis or Crohn's disease?**

Ulcerative colitis.
Remember, with ulcerative colitis, think of toxic megacolon and cancer. Avoid antidiarrheal agents.

❏❏ **What are the two <u>most common</u> causes of acute diarrhea?**

Rotavirus and Norwalk.

❏❏ **What is the <u>most common</u> cause of diarrhea in a child less than one year old?**

Rotavirus.

❏❏ **What type of diarrhea is most commonly associated with seizures?**

Shigella.

❏❏ **What type of diarrhea is associated with rose spots and watery diarrhea, as well as high fever and relative bradycardia?**

Salmonella. Particularly common in IV drug abusers with new pet turtles! Salmonella typhi may not have much diarrhea.

❏❏ **Treatment for Salmonella?**

Supportive care without antibiotics.
Severe fever may require antibiotic therapy.

❏❏ **What bacteria is associated with mesenteric adenitis and pseudoappendicitis?**

Yersinia.

❏❏ **What is the <u>most common</u> food born pathogen?**

Staphylococcus which presents 6-12 h post ingestion with diarrhea and vomiting. Enterotoxin.

❏❏ What gastroenteritis with diarrhea is associated with oysters, clams, crabs, and seafood?

Vibrio parahaemolyticus. Symptomatic treatment usually.

❏❏ What type of diarrhea is associated with perfuse, bloody diarrhea and no vomiting?

Entamoeba histolytica.
Diarrhea that is not necessarily bloody and that is associated with contaminated meat could be due to Clostridium perfringens.

❏❏ What is the most common parasite in the United States?

Giardia. Presents with foul smelling floating stools, abdominal pain, and perfuse diarrhea. It may be diagnosed with a positive string test, or duodenal aspiration for trophozoites.

❏❏ What type of diarrhea is commonly seen in AIDS patients?

Cryptosporidiosis. Diagnosed with a positive acid fast stain. Presents with profuse, watery diarrhea, no blood.

❏❏ What is the incubation period for Hepatitis A?

30 days. It is caused by an RNA virus.

❏❏ How is hepatitis A transmitted?

Oral fecal route. No carrier state exists.

❏❏ What does an elevated IgM anti-HBc mean?

Exposure to hepatitis B with antibody to the core antigen. High titers associated with contagious disease, low titers with chronic hepatitis B. M = might have the disease.

❏❏ What type of hepatitis is caused by a DNA virus?

Hepatitis B. Incubation period is 90 days.

❏❏ What does anti-HBs mean?

Suggests prior infection and immunity. Pt. has antibodies to the surface antigen just waiting for a chance...S = stopped.

❏❏ What type of defects cause left to right shunt murmurs?

ASD, VSD, and PDA.

❏❏ What type of defect produces diminished pulses in the lower extremities of a pediatric patient?

Coarctation of the aorta.

❏❏ What are two fairly common conditions in pediatrics which produce cardiac syncope?

Aortic stenosis, which is not cyanotic and tetralogy of Fallot, which is cyanotic.

❏❏ What are two unique clinical findings of tetralogy of Fallot?

A boot shaped heart on x-ray and exercise intolerance which is relieved by squatting. TOF is treated by placing the patient in the knee chest position and giving morphine.

❏❏ What would be the signs and symptoms of aortic stenosis in a child?

Exercise intolerance, chest pain, and a systolic ejection click with a crescendo, decrescendo murmur, radiating to the neck with a suprasternal thrill. No cyanosis!

❏❏ **What are the signs of left sided heart failure in an infant?**

Increased respiratory rate, shortness of breath, and sweating during feeding.

❏❏ **What is the single most common cause of CHF in the second week of life?**

Coarctation of the aorta.

❏❏ **What is the most common cause of otitis media?**

Strep pneumonia.

❏❏ **What is the most common cause of impetigo?**

Group A ß-hemolytic streptococcus.

❏❏ **What is the most common cause of bullous impetigo?**

Staph aureus.

❏❏ **What is the most common cause of sinusitis?**

Streptococcus pneumoniae.

❏❏ **What is the most common cause of orbital infections?**

Staph aureus. Periorbital infections are most commonly caused by H flu.

❏❏ **What is the most common cause of pediatric bacteremia?**

Strep pneumonia.

❏❏ **A patient presents with a staccato cough and a history of conjunctivitis in the first few weeks after birth, what type of pneumonia does this patient have?**

Chlamydia.

❏❏ **Most common cause of viral pneumonia in the pediatric patient?**

RSV.

❏❏ **What is the most common type of asthma in children?**

Extrinsic asthma which is a type I, immediate hypersensitivity reaction mediated by IgE. Common causes are molds and pet dander.

❏❏ **How do steroids function in the treatment of asthma?**

They increase cAMP, decrease inflammation, and help restore the function of ß-adrenergic responsiveness to adrenergic drugs.

❏❏ **What two viral illnesses are prodromes for Reye's syndrome?**

Varicella (chicken pox) and influenzae B.

❏❏ **Signs and symptoms of Reye's syndrome:**

Irritable, combative, and lethargic, right upper quadrant tenderness, history of influenzae B or recent chicken pox, papilledema, hypoglycemia, and seizures.
Lab findings would include hypoglycemia, and an elevated ammonia level greater than 20 times normal. Bilirubin level is NORMAL.

❑❑ **Describe stage I and stage II of Reye's syndrome.**

Stage I - vomiting, lethargy and liver dysfunction.
Stage II - disorientation, combativeness, delirium, hyperventilation, increased deep tendon reflexes, liver dysfunction, hyperexcitable, tachypnea, fever, tachycardia, sweating and pupillary dilatation.

❑❑ **Describe Stages III, IV, and V of Reye's syndrome.**

Stage III - coma, decorticate rigidity, increased respiratory rate, mortality rate of 50%.
Stage IV - coma, decerebrate posturing, no ocular reflexes, loss of corneal reflexes, and liver damage.
Stage V - loss of deep tendon reflexes, seizures, flaccid, respiratory arrest, 95% mortality.

❑❑ **What are the first, second, and third drugs of choice for treatment of seizures in children?**

The first is phenobarbital, second is phenytoin, and third is carbamazepine.

❑❑ **What is the drug of choice to treat a febrile seizure?**

Phenobarbital.

❑❑ **Use of diazepam (Valium) is avoided in neonatal seizures. Is part of the reason for this because it may cause hyperbilirubinemia by uncoupling the bilirubin-albumin complex?**

Yes.

❑❑ **Serious complication of valproic acid?**

Hepatic failure.

❑❑ **Complications of phenytoin use?**

Folate deficiency, osteomalacia, neutropenia, neuropathies, lupus and myasthenia.

❑❑ **What is the <u>most common</u> viral gastroenteritis in children?**

Rotavirus.

❑❑ **What is the most common cause of bacterial gastroenteritis in the world?**

E. coli.

❑❑ **What is the most common cause of diarrhea in infants and young children in day care centers?**

Giardia.

❑❑ **What bacterium is associated with mesenteric adenitis or appendicitis?**

Yersinia.

❑❑ **What enteritis causing bacterium produces watery diarrhea, encephalopathies, and convulsions.**

Shigella = seizures.

❏❏ **A child presents with vomiting and a moderate amount of blood in the stool. What is the diagnosis?**

Malrotation of the mid-gut.

❏❏ **What is the most common cause of painless lower GI bleeding in an infant or child?**

Meckel's diverticulum.

❏❏ **A 16 mo old presents with bilious vomiting, a distended abdomen, and blood in the stool. Diagnosis?**

Malrotation of the mid-gut.

❏❏ **A child presents with abdominal cramps which come and go, current jelly stools, and a sausage like tumor mass in the right lower quadrant. Contrast x-ray shows a coil spring sign. Diagnosis?**

Intussusception.

❏❏ **A child presents with a history of drug ingestion; she now has convulsions, coma, and cardiac collapse. What drug might have caused this?**

Salicylate with secondary hypoglycemia.

❏❏ **What side effect of propranolol may be concerning for a diabetic patient?**

Hypoglycemia.

❏❏ **What are some possible complications of sodium bicarbonate therapy?**

Hypokalemia, paradoxical CSF acidosis, impaired O_2 dissociation, and sodium overload.

❏❏ **Differentiate between non-ketotic hyperosmolar coma and DKA.**

In non-ketotic hyperosmolar coma, glucose is very high, often > 800. The serum osmolality is also very high, with average about 380. Nitroprusside test is negative.
In DKA, glucose is more often in the range of 600, the serum osmolality is approximately 350, nitroprusside test is positive.

❏❏ **What focal signs may be present in a patient with non-ketotic hyperosmolar coma?**

These patients may have hemisensory deficits or perhaps hemiparesis. 10-15% of these patients have a seizure.

❏❏ **What is the most common cause of hyperthyroidism?**

Grave's disease (toxic diffuse goiter).

❏❏ **What is the most common precipitating cause of thyroid storm?**

Pulmonary infection.

❏❏ **What is another name for life threatening hypothyroidism?**

Myxedema coma. Commonly seen in elderly women in the winter months and is stimulated by infection and stress.

❏❏ **What is the <u>most</u> <u>common</u> cause of hypothyroidism?**

Overtreatment of Grave's disease with iodine or subtotal thyroidectomy.

❏❏ **What is the second most common cause of hypothyroidism?**

Autoimmune Hashimoto's thyroiditis.

❏❏ **How may primary hypothyroidism be distinguished from secondary?**

In primary hypothyroidism the TSH levels are high, patients often have a history of thyroid surgery and may have a goiter; in secondary the TSH levels are low or normal, no hx of surgery and no goiter.

❏❏ **What drugs may make myxedema worse?**

Propranolol and phenothiazines.

❏❏ **What is a common "surgical problem" in myxedema that should be treated conservatively?**

Acquired megacolon.

❏❏ **What is primary adrenal insufficiency?**

Addison's disease, that is, failure of the adrenal cortex.

❏❏ **What hormones are produced by the adrenal cortex?**

Mineralocorticoids, glucocorticoids and androgenic steroids.
Salt, sugar, sex.

❏❏ **What is the major mineralocorticoid?**

Aldosterone. Aldosterone is regulated by the renin angiotensin system. Aldosterone increases sodium reabsorption and increased K^+ excretion.

❏❏ **What is the major glucocorticoid?**

Cortisol.

❏❏ **What does the medulla of the adrenal gland produce?**

Epinephrine and norepinephrine.

❏❏ **A patient presents two weeks after suffering a myocardial infarction. The patient takes warfarin and has sudden onset of hypotension, right flank pain, right CVA pain, epigastric pain, fever, nausea, and vomiting. Diagnosis?**

Adrenal gland hemorrhage - adrenal apoplexy.

❏❏ **What is Waterhouse-Fredrickson syndrome?**

Septicemia secondary to meningococcemia with associated bilateral adrenal gland hemorrhage. The patient will have a petechial rash, purpura, shaking chills, and severe headache.

❏❏ **What effect does Addison's disease have on cortisol and aldosterone levels?**

Cortisol and aldosterone levels are low.
Low cortisol levels mean nausea, vomiting, anorexia, lethargy, hypoglycemia, water intoxication, and inability to withstand even minor stress without shock.
Low aldosterone levels means sodium depletion, dehydration, hypotension, and syncope.

❏❏ **What are the signs and symptoms of Addison's disease?**

Hyperpigmentation, hyperkalemia, alopecia, and ascending paralysis secondary to hyperkalemia. Lab findings in Addison's disease include hypoglycemia, hyponatremia, hyperkalemia, and azotemia.

❏❏ **What ECG findings are expected in Addison's disease?**

Because of the hyperkalemia, expect peaked T-waves.

❏❏ **What are the principal signs and symptoms in adrenal crisis?**

Abdominal pain, hypotension and shock. The common cause is withdrawal of steroids. Treatment of adrenal crisis is hydrocortisone (Solu-Cortef), 100 mg IV bolus and 100 mg added to a the first liter of D_5 0.9 NS.

❏❏ **Does cyanide cause cyanosis?**

No, except secondarily when bradycardia and apnea precede asystolic arrest. Consider cyanide in an acidotic comatose patient without cyanosis and no hypoxia on ABG.

❏❏ **What key lab findings are expected in SIADH?**

Serum sodium would be low and urine sodium would be high, greater than 30.

❏❏ **What is the typical anatomic source of an epidural hematoma?**

The middle meningeal artery.

❏❏ **What is the most common anatomic source of a subdural hematoma?**

Bridging veins.

❏❏ **What is the most common source of a subarachnoid bleed?**

A saccular aneurysm.

❏❏ **If the lesion is in the right hemisphere, which way will the eyes deviate?**

Eyes will deviate toward the lesion.

❏❏ **If there is a lesion in the brain stem, which way will the eyes deviate?**

They will deviate away from the lesion in the brain stem.

❏❏ **What is the single most common intraparenchymal site of intracranial bleeding?**

The putamen.

❏❏ **In the pediatric esophagus, what is the most common site of a foreign body?**

Cricopharyngeal narrowing.

❏❏ **Most common hernia in population?**

Inguinal.

❏❏ **Do household pets transmit Yersinia?**

Yes.

❏❏ **What is the most common cause of conjunctivitis in the newborn?**

Chlamydia.

❏❏ **Most common cause of urinary tract infection in a female child?**

E. coli.

❏❏ **First line of treatment of a seizure in a five year old?**

Phenobarbital.

❏❏ **What is the most common cause of intrinsic renal failure?**

Acute tubular necrosis.

❏❏ **What is the most common cause of cardiac arrest in an uremic patient?**

Hyperkalemia.

❏❏ **A "blue dot" sign suggests:**

Torsion of the epididymis or appendix testis.

❏❏ **What is the first cardiac finding in cyclic antidepressant overdose?**

Sinus tachycardia.

❏❏ **What is the most common cause of right sided endocarditis in IV drug addicts?**

Staph aureus.

❏❏ **What is the most common valve affected in IV drug addicts?**

Tricuspid.

❏❏ **What is the most common cause of osteomyelitis or septic arthritis in an IV drug addict?**

Serratia marcescens.

❏❏ **What is the most common cause of <u>chronic</u> heavy metal poisoning?**

Lead. Arsenic is most common acute.

❏❏ **What is the most commonly injured area of the mandible?**

Angle.

❏❏ **Most common cause of Erysipelas:**

Group A streptococci.

❏❏ **Are steroids effective in treatment of toxic epidermal necrolysis?**

No.

❏❏ **Erythema nodosa is associated with which type of gastroenteritis?**

Yersinia.
I've a particular <u>YEN</u> for this answer!!

❏❏ **Thyrotoxicosis may be treated with:**

Support and hydration, IV propylthiouracil 1 gram, sodium iodine IV 1 g q 12 h or IV propanolol 1 mg/min up to 10 mg.

❏❏ **What is the most reliable method of diagnosing a posterior shoulder dislocation?**

Physical exam. Order a "Y-view" x-ray - it may be helpful.

❏❏ **The mortise view of the ankle is important in the diagnosis of:**

Medial (deltoid) ligament disruption of the ankle.

❏❏ **A fracture of the proximal fibular shaft is commonly associated with:**

Medial ankle fracture or sprain.
This is a Maisonneuve fx, it may be present with a widened mortise and no fx seen in the ankle.

❏❏ **What is the best x-ray view for diagnosing lunate and perilunate dislocations?**

Lateral x-ray views of the wrist.

❏❏ **What is the formula for calculating the serum osmolarity?**

$$CalculatedOsmol(mOsm \, / \, l) = 2(Na) + \frac{glucose}{18} + \frac{BUN}{2.8}$$

❏❏ **What is a good way to remember the signs and symptoms of anticholinergic toxicity?**

Think of atropine, as most of the signs and symptoms of atropine use are similar.
Tachycardia, hyperthermia, mydriasis, Ø sweat, dry mucosa, blurred vision for near objects (poor accommodation), decreased GI activity, urinary retention, aberration of mentation including delirium, lethargy and hallucinations, seizure and coma.

Dry as a bone,
Red as a beet,
Mad as a hatter,
Hot as a stone,
(Blind as a bat).

❏❏ **What are common anticholinergic compounds?**

Atropine, tricyclic antidepressants, antihistamines, phenothiazines, antiparkinsonian drugs, belladonna alkaloids, and some Solanaceae plants (e.g. deadly nightshade , jimson weed).

❏❏ **For how long should a patient with TCA overdose demonstrating tachycardia and conduction disturbances be monitored?**

24 h.

❏❏ **A baby is brought to the emergency department with persistent crying for two hours and vomiting. On exam, a testicle is tender and enlarged. What is the most common cause?**

Testicular torsion.

❏❏ **A child is seen with bluish discoloration of the gingiva. What diagnosis do you suspect?**

Chronic lead poisoning. You would also expect erythrocyte protoporphyrin level to be elevated in chronic Pb poisoning.

❏❏ **What is the anatomical weakness of the esophagus?**

Lack of a serosa.

❏❏ **In a humeral shaft fracture, what nerve is most commonly injured?**

Radial nerve.

❏❏ **What is the most common hip dislocation?**

Posterior.

❏❏ **What disorder is most likely to be confused with erythema nodosum?**

Cellulitis.

❏❏ **What is erythema nodosum?**

An inflammatory disease of skin and subcutaneous tissue characterized by tender red nodules. Nodules are most commonly found in the pretibial area.
Most commonly affects young adults.
Most common cause in children - UTI, especially with streptococci.
Most common cause in adults - Streptococcal infections and sarcoidosis.
Other causes - leprosy, TB, psittacosis, ulcerative colitis, drug reaction.

❏❏ **Galeazzi's fracture implies:**

Fracture of the shaft of the radius with dislocation of the distal radioulnar joint.
"GREAT RAYS DOWN DEEP!"

❏❏ **What is the <u>most</u> <u>common</u> dysrhythmia in a child?**

Paroxysmal atrial tachycardia.

❏❏ **On an upright chest x-ray, what is the earliest radiographic sign of left ventricular failure?**

Apical redistribution of the pulmonary vasculature.

❏❏ **What is the <u>most</u> <u>common</u> cause of hyponatremia?**

Dilution.

❏❏ **Of the following, which is <u>not</u> a common cause of <u>large</u> <u>bowel</u> obstruction: diverticulitis, adhesions, sigmoid volvulus or neoplasms?**

Adhesions.

❏❏ **A fracture of the acetabulum may be associated with damage to what nerve?**

The sciatic nerve.

❏❏ **What are some <u>common</u> causes of increased anion gap?**

Aspirin, methanol, uremia, diabetes, idiopathic (lactic), ethylene glycol and alcohol are reasonably common.

Numerous etiologies may produce the entity above listed demurely as "lactic." Lactic acidosis may be the result of shock, seizures, acute hypoxemia, INH, cyanide, ritodrine, inhaled acetylene, carbon monoxide and ethanol. Sodium nitroprusside, povidone-iodine ointment, sorbitol and xylitol can cause an anion gap acidosis.

Other causes of anion gap acidosis include toluene intoxication, iron intoxication, sulfuric acidosis, short bowel syndrome (D-lactic acidosis), formaldehyde, nalidixic acid, methanamine and rhubarb (oxalic acid). Inborn errors of metabolism such as methylmalonic acidemia and isovaleric acidemia may also cause a gap acidosis.

Recall some pearls for sorting out the differential diagnosis:

Methanol- visual disturbances and headache common. Can produce quite wide gaps as each 2.6 mg/dl of methanol contributes 1 mOsm/L to gap. Compare this with alcohol, each 4.3 mg/dl adds 1 mOsm/L to gap.

Uremia- is quite advanced before it causes an anion gap.

Diabetic Ketoacidosis- usually has both hyperglycemia and glucosuria; alcoholic ketoacidosis (AKA) often has a lower blood sugar and mild or absent glucosuria.

Salicylates- high levels contribute to gap.

Lactic Acidosis- can check serum level. Itself has broad differential as above.

Ethylene glycol- causes calcium oxalate or hippurate crystals in urine. Each 5.0 mg/dl contributes 1 mOsm/L to gap.

A reasonably comprehensive mnemonic device for recalling causes of anion gap acidosis is A MUDPILE CAT.

A MUDPILE CAT

A   = alcohol,

M = methanol,
U   = uremia,
D   = DKA,
P   = paraldehyde,
I   = iron and isoniazid,
L   = lactic acidosis,
E   = ethylene glycol,

C   = carbon monoxide,
A   = ASA (aspirin),
T   = toluene.

❏❏ What are the causes of <u>normal</u> anion gap metabolic acidosis?

Causes include diarrhea, ammonium chloride, renal tubular acidosis, renal interstitial disease, hypoadrenalism, ureterosigmoidostomy, and acetazolamide.

❏❏ What are some common causes of respiratory alkalosis?

Respiratory alkalosis is defined as a pH above 7.45 and a pCO_2 less than 35. Common causes of respiratory alkalosis include any process that may cause hyperventilation including shock, sepsis, trauma, asthma, PE, anemia, hepatic failure, heat stroke and exhaustion, emotion, salicylate poisoning, hypoxemia, pregnancy and inappropriate mechanical ventilation. Alkalosis shifts the O_2 disassociation curve to the left. It also causes cerebrovascular constriction. Kidneys compensate for respiratory alkalosis by excreting HCO_3^-.

❏❏ Causes of right shift of O_2 disassociation curve:

"CADET! Right face!!"

Right = Release to tissues.

Hyper	Carbia,
	Acidemia,
2,3	DPG,
	Exercise,
and increased	Temperature.

❏❏ **How should a patient with hypertrophic cardiomyopathy be treated who presents with chest pain and normal vital signs except for a heart rate of 140?**

ß-antagonists are the primary treatment for hypertrophic cardiomyopathy. ß-antagonists are first-line treatment for any symptomatic patient even without tachycardia present. Calcium channel blocking drugs are second-line therapeutics.

❏❏ **What is the adult dose of epinephrine in acute anaphylactic shock?**

0.3 - 0.5 mg of 1:10,000 IV.

❏❏ **How should neurogenic shock be best managed?**

Neurogenic shock is treated with replacement of volume deficit followed by vasopressors.

❏❏ **What is the most appropriate medication to treat a hypertensive patient with an acute aortic dissection?**

Trimethaphan.
Trimethaphan reduces hydraulic stress on the aortic wall and as a consequence, minimizes further dissection. The mechanism of action is via decreasing myocardial contractility. Trimethaphan also functions as a vasodilator and therefore reduces intra-aortic pressure and concomitant total peripheral resistance. Esmolol, a new titratable short acting ß-blocker, may also be a valuable alternative.

❏❏ **An elderly male presents to your emergency department with ataxia, confusion, amnesia and ocular paralysis. The patient is apathetic to his situation and has an otherwise normal neurologic exam. What is the likely cause of the patient's problem?**

Vitamin B deficiency associated with Wernicke-Korsakoff's syndrome.

❏❏ **How is SVR calculated?**

$$\frac{(MAP - CVP) \times 80}{CO} \quad Nl = 800 - 1400 \ dyn \cdot s^{-1} \cdot cm^{-5}$$

❏❏ **What is the <u>most</u> <u>common</u> dysrhythmia associated with excess digitalis?**

PVC's.

❏❏ **What is the order of appearance of CHF on chest x-ray?**

Initially cephalization and redistribution of blood flow is seen, followed by interstitial edema with evident Kerley B lines, as well as a perihilar haze. This is followed by alveolar infiltrates in the typical butterfly appearance. Finally, flagrant pulmonary edema and effusions are present.

❏❏ **The most common cause of sporadic encephalitis?**

Herpes simplex virus.

❏❏ **What are the classic EKG findings of a patient with a posterior MI.**

A large R-wave and ST depression in V1 and V2.

❏❏ **What is the classic EKG finding in Wolff-Parkinson-White syndrome?**

A change in the upstroke of QRS, the delta wave.

❏❏ **The most common cause of endemic encephalitis?**

Arbovirus.

❏❏ **What is the best treatment for an unstable patient with Wolff-Parkinson-White syndrome presenting with rapid atrial fibrillation?**

Shock.

❏❏ **What is the <u>most</u> <u>common</u> dysrhythmia seen with digitalis?**

PVC's are the <u>most</u> <u>common</u>.
AV block and PSVT with block are second most common.
V-tach and junctional tachycardia are the least common arrhythmias associated with digitalis.

❏❏ **The <u>most</u> <u>common</u> cause of pelvic pain in adolescent females?**

Ovarian cyst.

❏❏ **What is the <u>most</u> <u>common</u> cause of valvular induced syncope in the elderly?**

Aortic stenosis is the most common valvular cause of syncope in the elderly.
Vasovagal mechanisms are the most common mechanism overall.

❏❏ **Describe the signs, symptoms and ECG finding associated with lithium toxicity.**

Tremor, weakness, and flattening of the T-waves.

❏❏ **How many days after a measles vaccine might a fever and a rash be expected to develop?**

Seven to ten days.

❏❏ **The most common complication of acute otitis media?**

Tympanic membrane perforation. Other complications include mastoiditis, cholesteatoma, as well as intracranial infections.

❏❏ **Compare and contrast the rashes and associated symptoms and signs of roseola and rubella.**

With roseola, a child usually develops a fever up to 40 °C (104 °F) which lasts for three to five days. The child does not look particularly ill during the symptoms, although adenopathy may be noted. As the fever falls, the child may develop a maculopapular rash which usually appears within 48 hours after the fever disappears and may last from a few hours to a few days.

Rubella (measles) usually begins with a prodrome of three to four days of fever, conjunctivitis and upper respiratory tract symptoms. The characteristic rash is also maculopapular, confluent, but distinctively begins on the face and moves down the body. Koplik's spots are diagnostic.

❏❏ **What is appropriate treatment for a non-immunized individual exposed to hepatitis B?**

Treat with immune globulin, specifically HBIG. Consider vaccination.

❑❑ **What is the most common cause of sigmoid volvulus in the elderly?**

Constipation.

❑❑ **The most common complications of Varicella infections in adults:**

Encephalitis, pneumonia, Staph and Strep cellulitis.

❑❑ **The anterior drawer test of the ankle is used to test what ligament?**

The anterior talofibular ligament.

❑❑ **A patient presents with a shortened, internally rotated right leg after an accident. What injury is suspected?**

Posterior hip dislocation.

❑❑ **Describe a mallet finger deformity.**

Mallet finger deformity is produced by forced flexion of the DIP joint when the finger is in full extension. The deformity is a result of either rupture of the distal extensor tendon, or an avulsion fraction of the tendon insertion on the distal phalanx with a dorsal plate avulsion.

❑❑ **The most common cause of laryngotracheitis?**

Parainfluenza virus type I.
Staph aureus is the most common bacterial pathogen.

❑❑ **A patient has a fracture of the proximal 1/3 ulna; what associated injury should be ruled out?**

Dislocation of the radial head. This is also known as a Monteggia fracture. Anterior dislocation is most common.

<u>M</u>ichigan <u>U</u>niversity <u>P</u>olice <u>D</u>epartment = <u>MUPD</u>

<u>MUPD</u> = <u>M</u>onteggia, <u>U</u>lnar fracture, <u>P</u>roximal <u>D</u>islocation.

Little known fact, this fracture/dislocation is named after the now world-famous quarterback, Joe Monteggia who suffered this injury during a scuffle with the Michigan University PD.

❑❑ **A patient has an orbital floor fracture; what symptoms and signs might be seen?**

The most common symptom would be diplopia due to entrapment of the inferior rectus and inferior oblique muscles, and resultant paralysis of upward gaze. In addition, one would worry that the inferior orbital nerve could be damaged with paresthesia resulting to the lower lid, infraorbital area and side of the nose.

❑❑ **What gynecological infection presents with a malodorous, itchy, white to grayish sometimes frothy vaginal discharge?**

Trichomoniasis.

❑❑ **What are the signs of an upper motor neuron lesion?**

Upper motor neuron lesion involves the corticospinal tract. The lesion usually gives paralysis with:
1. initial loss of muscle tone and then increased tone, resulting in spasticity;
2. Babinski sign;
3. loss of superficial reflexes;
4. increased deep tendon reflexes.

A lower motor neuron lesion is associated with the anterior horn cells' axons. The lesion gives paralysis with decreased muscle tone and prompt atrophy.

❏❏ What condition commonly presents with ocular bulbar deficits?

Botulism poisoning.
Patients with myasthenia gravis may present similarly.
Diphtheria toxin may rarely produce similar deficits.

❏❏ Describe the symptoms and signs of myasthenia gravis.

Weakness and fatigability with ptosis, diplopia and blurred vision are the initial symptoms in 40 to 70 percent of patients. Bulbar muscle weakness is also common with dysarthria and dysphagia.

❏❏ Describe the presenting symptoms of botulism poisoning.

Botulism poisoning often presents with ocular bulbar deficits. Symmetrical descending weakness, usually with no sensory abnormalities, classically develops. Common associated symptoms include dysphagia, dry mouth, diplopia, dysarthria. Deep tendon reflexes may be decreased or absent.

❏❏ Describe the signs and symptoms of Guillain-Barré disease.

Guillain-Barré disease classically presents with symmetric weakness in the leg which ascends to include the arms or trunk. Distal weakness is usually greater than proximal. Onset rarely involves the cranial nerves.

❏❏ Which nerve provides sensation to both dorsum and volar aspects of hand?

Ulnar. Radial is primarily dorsum, and median is primarily volar.

❏❏ Describe the key features of Ménière's disease, also known as endolymphatic hydrops.

Vertigo, hearing loss and tinnitus are the hallmarks of Ménière's disease.
Ménière's disease typically presents with rapid onset of vertigo, often with associated nausea and vomiting that lasts for hours to one day. Nystagmus may be spontaneous during the critical stage. Tinnitus may be present and is louder during the attacks. Sensorineural hearing loss may be present. There may also be an aura with a sensation of fullness in the ear during the attack. Symptoms are unilateral in over 90 percent of patients, and recurring attacks are typical.

❏❏ Describe the key features of benign positional vertigo.

Violent positional vertigo is usually provoked by certain head positions or movement. Nystagmus is also always positional, of brief duration with fatigability.

❏❏ What are the key features of viral labyrinthitis or vestibular neuritis?

Vertigo is severe, usually lasting three to five days, with nausea and vomiting. Symptoms usually regress over three to six weeks. Nystagmus may be spontaneous during the severe stage.

❏❏ What is a major concern in a patient that presents with unilateral Parkinsonian features?

Intracranial tumor.

❏❏ Describe the key features of acoustic neuroma.

Symptoms and signs may include unilateral high tone sensorineural hearing loss and tinnitus. Other signs and symptoms include decreased corneal sensitivity, diplopia, headache, facial weakness and positive radiographic findings. Vertigo usually appears late, more often presenting as a progressive feeling of imbalance. Vertigo may be provoked by changes in head movement. Nystagmus is frequently present and is usually spontaneous. The CSF may have elevated protein.

❑❑ **Describe the key features of vertebrobasilar insufficiency.**

Vertigo is nearly always positional, provoked by certain head positions. Nystagmus usually accompanies the vertigo. Other signs of arteriosclerosis may be found.
Vertebrobasilar insufficiency is usually seen in older persons and may occur with other symptoms of brainstem ischemia, visual symptoms being the most common.

❑❑ **What's that little bone seen behind the tympanic membrane?**

The malleus.

❑❑ **What disease would you expect in a patient with a two week history of lower limb weakness?**

Guillain-Barré is usually an ascending weakness which begins in the lower extremity.
With botulism poisoning, the weakness is descending.
Cranial nerves are typically affected first with myasthenia gravis.

❑❑ **What is the mortality rate of Wernicke's encephalopathy?**

10-20%. Treat with thiamine IV. Symptoms include ocular palsies, nystagmus, confusion, and ataxia.

❑❑ **Deep tendon reflexes are usually maintained in which of the following diseases: Myasthenia gravis, Guillain-Barré or Eaton-Lambert syndrome?**

Myasthenia gravis.
Reflexes are usually depressed in Eaton-Lambert syndrome and absent in Guillain-Barré.

❑❑ **On IVP, what is most indicative of severe urinary tract obstruction?**

A hyperdense nephrogram. Delayed filling may also be an indicator of obstruction.

❑❑ **How might a patient present with a hydatidiform mole?**

Hydatidiform mole presents with a larger than expected uterus and a positive pregnancy test.

❑❑ **Of the major tranquilizers, which one displays the most hypotensive tendency?**

Thorazine.

❑❑ **What is the most common cause for pain of odontogenic origin?**

Dental caries.

❑❑ **What factors and substances are known to decrease theophylline metabolism and increase theophylline levels?**

Age greater than 50, prematurity, liver and renal disease, pulmonary edema, CHF, pneumonia, obesity and viral illness in children. Drugs which increase theophylline levels include cimetidine, erythromycin, allopurinol, troleandomycin, BCP's, and quinolone antibiotics.

In smokers, however, theophylline half-life is decreased, causing decreased levels of serum theophylline. In addition to smoking, phenobarbital, phenytoin, rifampin, carbamazepine, marijuana smoking and exposure to environmental pollutants can decrease serum theophylline levels. Eating charcoal broiled foods may cause lowered theophylline levels.

❑❑ **What therapy should be used for a patient with hemophilia A who suffers a head injury?**

Treat this patient with cryoprecipitate. Keep total volume as low as possible. Cryoprecipitate has an increased concentration of factor VIII complex and has less volume than fresh frozen plasma.

❏❏ **What is the most serious complication of abscessed anterior maxillary teeth?**

Septic cavernous sinus thrombosis. Results from extension of infection into the canine space and facial venous system.

❏❏ **What is the first therapy to initiate for a bleeding patient on warfarin with a high PT?**

D/C warfarin. Then administer a water soluble form of vitamin K. Give IM, consider test dose. If the bleeding is severe, or in a dangerous location (e.g. brain), fresh frozen plasma should be given containing active factors X, IX, VII and II (REMEMBER 1972).

❏❏ **What is a common electrolyte abnormality associated with transfusion of packed red blood cells?**

Hypocalcemia secondary to citrate toxicity. Citrate, when rapidly infused, binds ionized calcium and therefore decreases the calcium level. Hyperkalemia may also develop with rapid packed red blood cell transfusion, especially if the patient is in renal failure or if the blood products are old.

❏❏ **What invasive measurement should be performed to evaluate a patient with swelling of the face, neck and arms?**

CVP. Swelling of the face, neck and arms is suggestive of superior vena cava syndrome. To confirm superior vena cava syndrome, increased CVP pressure in the upper body and normal pressure in the lower extremities must be documented. Chest x-ray will detect only about 10 percent of the masses causing superior vena cava syndrome.

❏❏ **Describe Leriche's syndrome.**

Leriche's syndrome is characterized by buttock, calf, and back pain with impotence. It is usually seen with aortoiliac disease.

❏❏ **What diagnosis should be suspected for a patient who has suffered loss of vision and whose fundus is pale?**

Central retinal artery occlusion usually presents with acute, painless loss of vision.

❏❏ **Describe a patient with sigmoid volvulus.**

Patients with sigmoid volvulus are typically either psychiatric patients or elderly who suffer from severe chronic constipation. Symptoms include intermittent cramping, lower abdominal pain and progressive abdominal distention.

❏❏ **Describe a typical patient with intussusception.**

Intussusception typically occurs in children of ages 3 months to 2 years. The majority are in the 5 to 10 mo age group. It is more common in boys. The area of the ileocecal valve is usually the source of the problem.

❏❏ **What are the common symptoms and signs of hyperthyroidism?**

Symptoms include weight loss, palpitations, dyspnea, edema, chest pain, nervousness, weakness, tremor, psychosis, diarrhea, hyperdefecation, abdominal pain, myalgias and disorientation.
Signs include fever, tachycardia, wide pulse pressure, CHF, shock, thyromegaly, tremor, weakness, liver tenderness, jaundice, stare, and hyperkinesis. Mental status changes include somnolence, obtundation, coma, or psychosis. Pretibial myxedema may be found (a true misnomer!)

❏❏ **A patient suffers a rotational knee injury and hears a pop. Within 90 minutes hemarthrosis develops. What is the suspected location of the injury?**

The anterior cruciate.

❑❑ **What are radiological and laboratory findings of duodenal injury?**

Retroperitoneal air and increased serum amylase.

❑❑ **A patient has a fracture of the radial shaft. What associated injury should be ruled out?**

Distal radius-ulna joint dislocation, also known as a Galeazzi's fracture/dislocation.
Great Rays Down Deep! = GRDD

GRDD = Galeazzi, Radius fracture, Distal Dislocation

❑❑ **G-6-PD is the first enzyme in the hexose monophosphate shunt pathway that generates NADPH. NADPH helps maintain reduced glutathione. In G-6-PD deficiency, which affects 11% of black American males, this enzyme deteriorates with age. So?**

Glutathione serves to protect hemoglobin from injury due to oxidants. If such injury occurs, denatured Hb or hemolysis may follow.

❑❑ **What drugs should be avoided in G-6-PD deficiency?**

ASA, phenacetin; primaquine, quinine and quinacrine; nitrofurans; sulfamethoxazole and sulfacetamide; and methylene blue are all associated with hemolysis. These are all oxidants.

❑❑ **What is the current therapeutic regimen for treatment of meningitis in a neonate?**

Initially, ampicillin and aminoglycoside were favored for treating the neonate with meningitis. However, today recommendations include ampicillin and cefotaxime.
A combination used in infants up to 2 months of age will cover coliform, Group B streptococci, Listeria, and enterococcus. Over 2 months of age up to 6 years, cefotaxime alone is indicated.

❑❑ **What is the formula for calculating a change in potassium with changes in pH?**

For each pH increase of 0.1, expect the potassium to drop by 0.5 mmol/l.

❑❑ **A patient has alcoholic ketoacidosis (aka AKA); what is appropriate treatment?**

Alcoholic ketoacidosis usually presents with nausea, vomiting and abdominal pain occurring 24 to 72 h after cessation of drinking. No specific physical findings are typically evident, though abdominal pain is a common complaint/finding.
AKA is thought to be secondary to increased mobilization of free fatty acids with lipolysis to acetoacetate and ß-hydroxybutyrate.

Treatment usually includes normal saline and glucose. As acidosis is corrected, K^+ may drop. Sodium bicarbonate should not be given unless pH drops below 7.1.

❑❑ **A patient presents to the emergency department and is very sick. Your diagnosis is alcoholic ketoacidosis. Urine dip is _trace_ positive for ketones. Now what do you think?**

God, I LOVE biochemistry!! I expect urine ketones to be few to none in some patients with AKA, as the nitroprusside test (Acetest®) is the common method used to test for ketones. I recall that this test measures positive for Acetoacetate and is less reactive to Acetone and is not affected by ß-hydroxybutyrate. _I know that ß-hydroxybutyrate is preferentially produced in AKA,_ thus it is both possible and likely to obtain a negative or weakly positive test for serum ketones in the presence of clinically significant AKA.

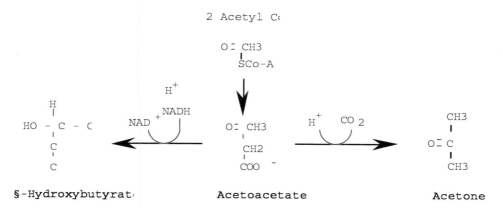

§-Hydroxybutyrate   Acetoacetate   Acetone

❑❑ **Describe the symptoms of optic neuritis.**

The patient suffers a variable loss of central visual acuity with a central scotoma and change in color perception. The patient also has eye pain. The disk margins are blurred from hemorrhage and the blind spot is increased.

❑❑ **Compare and contrast primary and secondary myxedema.**

Primary:	Secondary :
Source: Thyroid	Pituitary
Frequency: Common, 95%	Ø common, 5%
+ Coarse voice	Ø Coarse voice
+ Goiter	Ø Goiter
Heart Big	heart small
+ Pubic hair	Ø Pubic hair
TSH elevated	TSH low
Iodine <2µg/dl	Iodine >2µg/dl

❑❑ **Which renal calculi are radiolucent and which renal calculi are radiopaque?**

U̲r̲ic acid stones and blood clots are radiolU̲cent ureteral obstructions. 90 percent of all stones are radiopaque, composed of calcium oxalate, cysteine, calcium phosphate, or magnesium ammonium phosphate.

❑❑ **Antidote for arsenic?**

British Anti-Lewisite (BAL) 5 mg/kg IM.

❑❑ **Antidote for clonidine?**

Naloxone may help. Care is primarily supportive.

❑❑ **Cyanide's harmful effects are due to its propensity to bind to metals and to disrupt the function of metal containing enzymes. Which is the most important of these?**

Cytochrome A_3, aka cytochrome oxidase, necessary for aerobic metabolism.

❑❑ **Antidote for cyanide?**

Amyl nitrite followed by sodium nitrite followed by sodium thiosulfate.

❑❑ **Why give nitrites for cyanide?**

Theory says nitrites form methemoglobin and methemoglobin strongly binds cyanide, decreasing binding to cytochrome A_3.

❏❏ **Why give sodium thiosulfate for cyanide?**

Rhodanase, an intrinsic enzyme, transfers cyanide from its attachment to methemoglobin to sulfur, forming thiocyanate. Thiocyanate is excreted. Sodium thiosulfate acts as a sulfur donor for this process.

❏❏ **Antidote for ethylene glycol?**

Ethanol and dialysis.

❏❏ **Antidote for gold?**

BAL.

❏❏ **Antidote for iron?**

Deferoxamine.

❏❏ **Antidote for lead?**

Dimercaptosuccinic acid (DMSA) or calcium EDTA.

❏❏ **Antidote for mercury?**

BAL.

❏❏ **Antidote for methanol?**

Ethanol and dialysis.

❏❏ **Antidote for nitrites?**

Methylene blue 1% 0.2 ml/kg IV over 5 minutes.
Severe methemoglobinemia requires exchange transfusion.

❏❏ **Antidote for organophosphates?**

Atropine with 2-PAM as indicated.

Great quotes series:

"Fools take to themselves the respect that is given to their office." Aesop

❏❏ **What are the common features of organic brain syndrome?**

Onset may be at any age.
Symptoms include visual hallucinations and perception of the unfamiliar as familiar.
Signs include mental status changes such as disorientation, clouded sensorium, asterixis or mild clonus and focal neurologic signs. Vital signs are most often within normal limits.

❏❏ **Describe the features of functional syndromes.**

Onset is usually at age less than 40.
Symptoms include auditory hallucination and perception of the familiar as unfamiliar.

Patients are usually oriented, cognitive function is usually normal and the sensorium is usually clear. Asterixis or myoclonus is not a feature of functional disease. Vital signs are usually normal without focal neurologic deficit.

❑❑ **Is the stomach more commonly injured with penetrating trauma or blunt trauma?**

The stomach is more commonly injured with penetrating trauma.

❑❑ **What is the most common body area affected in trauma that results in death?**

The head.

❑❑ **What is the most common cause of airway obstruction in trauma?**

CNS depression.

❑❑ **What is the most common wound associated with pericardial tamponade?**

Right ventricular injury.

❑❑ **What are the signs and symptoms of acute pericardial tamponade?**

Triad of hypotension, elevated CVP, and tachycardia is usually indicative of either acute pericardial tamponade or a tension pneumothorax in a traumatized patient. Muffled heart tones may be auscultated.

❑❑ **What EKG finding is pathognomonic of pericardial tamponade?**

Total electrical alternans. Pulsus paradoxus is nonspecific. Muffled heart tones are subjective findings and are difficult to appreciate.

❑❑ **What is the formula for correct infusion of peritoneal lavage fluid in a child?**

10 cc/kg of lactated Ringer's solution should be infused to allow accurate interpretation of cell counts.

❑❑ **Name 2 retroperitoneal organs which may be injured without producing a positive DPL.**

Pancreas and duodenum.

❑❑ **Name 2 organs that do not tend to bleed enough to produce a positive DPL when injured.**

Bladder and small bowel.

❑❑ **What RBC count is considered positive in peritoneal lavage fluid analysis of a patient with blunt abdominal trauma?**

RBC counts of more than 100,000 per mm^3 are considered positive for both penetrating and blunt trauma to the abdomen.

5,000 RBCs per mm^3 is considered positive in a patient with low chest or high abdominal penetrating trauma where diaphragmatic perforation is a possibility.

❑❑ **Define sensitivity and specificity.**

Sensitivity is true positives divided by true positives plus false negatives. It represents how well a test identifies people who have a condition from among all the people who have the condition.

Specificity is true negatives divided by true negatives plus false positives. It is the percentage of people who do not have the disease correctly classified as negative by the test.

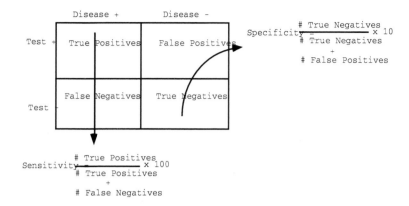

❑❑ Describe the zones of the neck and the appropriate treatment for injuries to each zone.

Zone 1 -- below the cricoid cartilage,
Zone 2 -- between the angle of the mandible and the cricoid cartilage,
Zone 3 -- above the angle of the mandible.

Treatment and evaluation:
Zones 1 and 3, angiography to evaluate major vessels.
Zone 2 requires surgical evaluation. ("2 surgery!!")

❑❑ What is the cause of death secondary to untreated tension pneumothorax?

Decreased cardiac output. The vena cava is compressed resulting in decreased right heart blood return and concomitant severe compromise in stroke volume, blood pressure and cardiac output.
[Editorial comment - 2° arrhythmias can also occur. V-tach in a young apparently healthy person is 2° to a tension pneumothorax until proven otherwise. JNA]

❑❑ How does a chronic pericardial effusion appear on chest x-ray?

Gradual pericardial sac distention results in a "water bottle" appearance of the heart.

❑❑ What are the symptoms and signs of adrenal insufficiency?

Fatigue, nausea, anorexia, abdominal pain, change in bowel habits and syncope are frequently reported symptoms.
Hyperpigmentation, hypertension, vitiligo and weight loss may be noted.
Laboratory abnormalities can include hypoglycemia, hyperkalemia, hyponatremia and azotemia.

❑❑ Treatment for myxedema coma may include:

IV thyroid replacement with thyroxine, IV glucose, hydrocortisone and consideration of water restriction.

❑❑ What are the symptoms and signs of thyrotoxicosis?

Weight loss and weakness may be reported.
Tachycardia and fever are common abnormal vital signs with hypotension and shock occurring less frequently. Mental status changes of decreased consciousness or psychosis may be present. Signs of CHF, thyromegaly, tremor, eye signs including lid lag and proptosis should also be sought.

❑❑ How do patients present with central retinal artery occlusion?

Patients present with a sudden, painless loss of vision in one eye.

❏❏ Describe a patient with acute narrow angle closure glaucoma.

Symptoms include nausea, vomiting and abdominal pain. Visual acuity is markedly diminished. The pupil is semi-dilated and nonreactive. There is usually a glassy haze over the cornea and the eye is red and very painful. Intraocular pressure may be as high as 50 or 60 mmHg.

❏❏ Describe the treatment of acute narrow angle glaucoma.

Mannitol to decrease intraocular pressure.
Miotics, such as pilocarpine, to open the angle.
Carbonic anhydrase inhibitor to minimize aqueous humor production. Iridectomy is eventually performed to provide aqueous outflow.

❏❏ What is the appropriate treatment for a hyphema?

Elevate the head.
Other treatment is controversial, however, most ophthalmologists believe patients should be hospitalized. Treatment <u>may</u> include double eye patch, topical cortisone and cycloplegics. Visual acuity is often decreased.

❏❏ Describe the classic symptoms and signs of retinal detachment.

The patient is typically myopic and will complain of seeing a curtain coming down across his or her eye. This is usually accompanied by flashes of light but no discomfort. The patient may also see flashing lights, black dots, or sudden change in vision.
On funduscopic exam, the detached areas will appear gray in comparison to the normal pink retina. Treatment includes bilateral eye patch, strict bed rest and consultation with an ophthalmologist for laser photocoagulation of the retinal detachment.

❏❏ What type of streptococci cause acute post-streptococcal glomerulonephritis?

Group A ß-hemolytic streptococci.
Physical exam may reveal facial edema and decreased urinary output that are the most common presenting findings. Urine may be dark. Laboratory findings include normochromic anemia due to hemodilution, increased sedimentation rate, numerous RBCs and WBCs in the urine with casts, and hyperkalemia. Hospitalization is advised.

❏❏ Name the five major modified Jones criteria.

Dr. Jones, the <u>EM</u> Physician, is <u>SN</u>oring, she <u>C</u>an't <u>C</u>ome.

Dr. Jones, the <u>EM</u>	<u>E</u>rythema <u>M</u>arginatum
<u>P</u>hysician,	<u>P</u>olyarthritis
is <u>SN</u>oring,	<u>S</u>ubcutaneous <u>N</u>odules
she <u>C</u>an't	<u>C</u>arditis
<u>C</u>ome.	<u>C</u>horea

Other criteria include rheumatic fever or rheumatic heart disease, arthralgias, fever, prolonged PR interval on EKG, C reactive protein, elevated sedimentation rate, or antistreptolysin O titer.

❏❏ What disorder is present when the five major modified Jones criteria are met?

Rheumatic fever.

❏❏ Describe the symptoms and signs of varicella (chickenpox).

Varicella rash onset is one to two days after prodromal symptoms of slight malaise, anorexia and fever. The rash begins on the trunk and scalp. It first appears as faint macules, later becoming vesicles.

❑❑ **Describe the signs of roseola infantum.**

Roseola infantum usually affects children ages 6 months to 3 years. It is characterized by high fever that begins abruptly and lasts 3 to 5 days, possibly precipitating febrile seizures. A rash appears as the temperature drops to normal.

❑❑ **Describe the symptoms and signs of rubella (German measles).**

Rubella begins after a mild 1 - 5 day prodrome of upper respiratory infection symptoms. A rash begins on the face and spreads quickly. Suboccipital and posterior auricular adenopathy are associated findings.

❑❑ **What is the standard dose of atropine in a child?**

0.02 mg/kg is the standard atropine dose.

❑❑ **What is the <u>most</u> <u>common</u> cause of bacterial meningitis in a child more than one month of age?**

Hemophilus influenzae.
S. pneumoniae is second most common.
N. meningitis is third most common.
This is treated with ampicillin and chloramphenicol. Single agent treatment with a third generation cephalosporin may also be used.

❑❑ **What is the initial dose of sodium bicarbonate in children during a cardiopulmonary arrest?**

1 mEq/kg.

❑❑ **How is the expected normal systolic blood pressure for a pediatric patient (toddlers and up) calculated?**

Multiply the age by 2 and add 90 to the result to determine expected systolic BP.

<u>Average</u> SBP (mm Hg) = (Age x 2) + 90

<u>Low normal limit</u> SBP (mm Hg) = (Age x 2) + 70.

SBP for a term newborn is about 60 mm Hg.

❑❑ **How does sickle cell disease usually present in a patient older than 12 months?**

Initial symptoms are often pain in the joints, bones and abdomen. The child may have abdominal tenderness and even rigidity. Mild icterus and anemia may be present.

❑❑ **How does a child present with erythema infectiosum (fifth disease or slapcheek syndrome)?**

Fifth disease typically does not infect infants or adults. There are no prodromal symptoms. The illness usually begins with sudden appearance of erythema of the cheeks followed by a maculopapular rash on the trunk and extremities that evolve into a lacy pattern.

❑❑ **What is the correct dose of epinephrine and atropine during a pediatric code?**

Epinephrine 0.01 mg/kg/dose.
Atropine 0.02 mg/kg/dose.

❑❑ **What are the signs and symptoms of Kawasaki's disease?**

Kawasaki's initial presentation is with a high spiking fever, conjunctivitis, morbilliform rash, strawberry tongue, and erythema of the distal extremities with cervical adenopathy. It is a disease of the mucocutaneous lymph nodes. Patients should be hospitalized to rule out myocarditis, pericarditis and coronary aneurysms. Aspirin is therapeutic.

❏❏ **What is the initial antibiotic treatment for a child with epiglottitis?**

The most likely cause is H. influenzae; the child should be treated with a second or third generation cephalosporin.

❏❏ **What are the characteristics of a posterior hip dislocation?**

Posterior hip dislocations are typically caused by posteriorly directed force applied to the flexed knee. The extremity is shortened, internally rotated and adducted. Acetabular fractures are associated with this injury. 90% of hip dislocations are posterior.

❏❏ **Describe the key features of central cord syndrome.**

Central cord syndrome typically occurs with hyperextension injuries in older patients with spondylosis, degenerative changes or stenosis in the cervical spine. Symptoms include weakness that is more pronounced in the arms than the legs.

❏❏ **Key features of anterior spinal cord syndrome?**

The anterior cord syndrome involves compression of the anterior cord causing complete motor paralysis and loss of pain and temperature sensation distal to the lesion. Posterior columns are spared - light touch and proprioception are preserved.

❏❏ **What is the typical organism of a paronychia?**

Staphylococcus.

❏❏ **How does myasthenia gravis typically present?**

Weakness of voluntary muscles, usually the extraocular muscles.
Diagnostic confirmation relies on the edrophonium (Tensilon) test that we don't do.
Treatment includes neurologic consultation, anticholinesterases, steroids and thymectomy.

❏❏ **What visual deficit is typically associated with lesions at the optic chiasm?**

Optic chiasm lesions typically produce bitemporal hemianopsia.

❏❏ **On CT scan of the brain of an immunocompromised patient, a ring lesion is noted. The patient also has lymphadenopathy, fever, headache and confusion. What diagnosis is suspected?**

Toxoplasmosis secondary to Toxoplasma gondii cyst. The disease is typically treated with pyrimethamine and sulfadiazine.

❏❏ **What are the signs and symptoms of posterior inferior cerebellar artery syndrome?**

Cerebellar dysfunction such as vertigo, ataxia and dizziness.

❏❏ **Describe the signs and symptoms of neuroleptic malignant syndrome.**

Patients present with muscle rigidity, autonomic disturbances and acute organic brain syndrome.
Blood pressure and pulse fluctuate wildly and temperature may reach as high as 42 °C (108 °F).
Muscle necrosis may occur with resultant myoglobinuria.
Mortality ranges as high as 20%.

❏❏ **Describe the presentation of placenta previa.**

Placenta previa typically presents with painless bright red vaginal bleeding.

❑❑ **Describe the presentation of abruptio placentae.**

Dark red, painful, vaginal bleeding.

❑❑ **What is the <u>most</u> <u>common</u> growth plate (Salter class) injury?**

Salter II fracture.

❑❑ **Where is the most common site for esophageal foreign bodies to lodge?**

The cricopharyngeus muscle.

❑❑ **What is the <u>most</u> <u>common</u> organism causing a septic joint in a child?**

S. aureus.

❑❑ **What is the <u>most</u> <u>common</u> organism to cause a septic joint in an adolescent?**

Neisseria gonorrhoeae.

❑❑ **Signs of tension pneumothorax on physical exam include:**

Tachypnea, unilateral absent breath sounds, tachycardia, pallor, diaphoresis, cyanosis, tracheal deviation, hypotension and neck vein distention.

❑❑ **What is the most common cause of bacterial pneumonia, except for the first week of life?**

Streptococcus pneumoniae.

❑❑ **What is the most common cause of abdominal pain in children?**

Constipation.

❑❑ **What is the <u>most</u> <u>common</u> cause of an intestinal obstruction in a child under 2 years of age?**

Intussusception.

❑❑ **What is the most frequent carpal fracture.**

Navicular fracture.

❑❑ **What is the most frequently dislocated bone in the wrist?**

Lunate.
It is also the second most common fractured bone in the wrist.

❑❑ **What medications should be used to treat preeclampsia and eclampsia?**

Magnesium and hydralazine.

❑❑ **Do local anesthetics freely cross the blood brain barrier?**

Yes.
Most systemic toxic reactions to local anesthetics involve the CNS or cardiovascular system.

❑❑ **What is the <u>most</u> <u>common</u> cause of hemoptysis in the United States?**

Bronchitis and bronchiectasis.

❑❑ **What is the most common site of thrombophlebitis?**

The deep muscles of the calves, particularly the soleus muscle.

❑❑ **What is the <u>most</u> <u>common</u> cause of acute aortic regurgitation?**

Infectious endocarditis.

❑❑ **What are the most common causes of aortic stenosis (2)?**

Rheumatic fever and congenital bicuspid valve disease.

❑❑ **What is the <u>most</u> <u>common</u> cause of acute mitral regurgitation?**

Inferior wall infarcts.

❑❑ **What are the most common causes of pulsus paradoxus (2)?**

COPD and asthma.

❑❑ **What does Beck's triad consist of?**

Hypotension, elevated CVP (distended neck veins) and distant heart sounds.

❑❑ **What's it good for (Beck's triad that is)?**

A cute pericardial tamponade.

❑❑ **What is the <u>worst</u> way to confirm the diagnosis of a delayed pericardial injury after blunt trauma?**

Autopsy.

❑❑ **What is the <u>most</u> <u>common</u> conduction disturbance in acute myocardial infarction?**

First degree AV block.

❑❑ **How much fluid is needed in the pericardial sac to increase the cardiac silhouette on chest x-ray?**

About 250 ml.

❑❑ **What is the most common site of rupture in abdominal aortic aneurysms?**

Posterior lateral aorta.

❑❑ **What is the most common symptom in abdominal aortic aneurysm?**

Pain.

❑❑ **What is the most common dysrhythmia associated with Wolff-Parkinson-White syndrome?**

Paroxysmal atrial tachycardia.

❑❑ **What are the symptoms and signs of aortic stenosis?**

Exertional dyspnea, angina and syncope.
Narrowed pulse pressure with decreased SBP.

Slow carotid upstroke.
Prominent S_4.

❏❏ **What drugs are commonly associated with torsade de pointes?**

Type I-A antiarrhythmics - quinidine and procainamide.

These drugs lengthen the Q-T interval.

❏❏ **What common metabolic disorder is associated with hypercalcemia?**

Hypokalemia.

❏❏ **What does the urine dipstick show from a patient with myoglobinuria?**

The dipstick is "heme-positive" with few or no RBCs.

❏❏ **What is the <u>most</u> <u>common</u> cause of hepatitis transmitted through blood transfusions?**

Hepatitis C.

❏❏ **Are males or females more likely to get symptomatic gallstones?**

Females.

❏❏ **What is the <u>most</u> <u>common</u> type of ulcers?**

Duodenal ulcers are more commonly seen than gastric ulcers.

❏❏ **What is the differential diagnosis of a red eye with decreased visual acuity?**

Iritis, glaucoma and central corneal lesions.

❏❏ **A patient has a non-red, painful eye with decreased visual acuity. What diagnosis do you suspect?**

Optic neuritis.

❏❏ **What disease is associated with retrobulbar optic neuritis?**

MS.

❏❏ **How could mydriasis caused by third cranial nerve compression be distinguished from mydriasis caused by anticholinergic drugs or mydriatics?**

Mydriasis caused by third cranial nerve compression is reversible with pilocarpine, other causes are not.

❏❏ **What is the best method to open an airway while maintaining C-spine precautions?**

Jaw thrust.

❏❏ **What is the absolute contraindication to MAST?**

Pulmonary edema.

❏❏ **T/F: Increased blood pressure in hypovolemic patients associated with MAST application is primarily due to autotransfusion.**

NOT!
The primary mechanism of MAST appears to be due to increased peripheral vascular resistance. Autotransfusion of a few hundred ml of blood may occur but is not of great significance.

❏❏ **What is the <u>most</u> <u>common</u> complication of using an EOA?**

Tracheal intubation, 10%.

❏❏ **At what child's age is a cuffed ET tube preferred?**

6 y.

❏❏ **What is the formula for appropriate ET tube size in children greater than 1 y old?**

ET size = (Age + 16) / 4.

❏❏ **What is the correct ET tube size for a 1 - 2 y old?**

4.0 - 4.5 mm.

❏❏ **What is the correct ET tube size for a 6 mo old?**

3.5 - 4.5 mm. Hey, we didn't *make up* these answers!...

❏❏ **What is the correct ET tube size for a newborn?**

3.0 - 3.5 mm.
Premature - 2.5 - 3.0 mm.

❏❏ **What is the distance from the mouth to 2 cm above the carina in men and women?**

Men 23 cm; women 21 cm.

❏❏ **What is the treatment of hyperkalemia?**

Diurese with loop diuretic, e.g.., furosemide or ethacrynic acid.

Sodium polystyrene sulfonate ion exchange resin (Kayexalate) enema (associated Na load can cause failure). Hours before effect is seen.

1 ampule of D_{50}, insulin 5 to 10 units IV for redistribution (follow by 50 g glucose and 20 U insulin over 1 h). About 30 minutes for effect.

Sodium bicarbonate 50 - 100 mEq IV over 10 - 20 minutes. Five to ten minutes for effect.

Calcium. Calcium chloride has more Ca per ampule (13.4 mEq) than gluconate (4.6 mEq) and is faster acting. Give one ampule (10 ml of 10% solution) over 10 - 20 minutes. WATCH OUT if giving to a patient on digitalis, it will potentiate toxicity. Very rapid onset.

3% sodium chloride IV may serve as a temporary antagonist.

Peritoneal or hemodialysis.

Digoxin specific Fab (Digibind) if 2° to digitalis overdose.

❏❏ **How should hypercalcemia be treated?**

Furosemide and normal saline. Mithramycin may be used, especially in hypercalcemia secondary to bone cancer. Other treatments include calcitonin, hydrocortisone, and indomethacin.

❏❏ **What is the <u>most</u> <u>common</u> cause of multifocal atrial tachycardia?**

COPD.

❑❑ **What is the treatment for multifocal atrial tachycardia?**

Treat underlying disorder.

Magnesium sulfate 2 grams over 60 seconds (with supplemental potassium to maintain serum K^+ above 4 mEq/l).
A second treatment is verapamil 10 mg IV.

❑❑ **What is the treatment of ectopic SVT due to digitalis toxicity?**

Stop digitalis, correct hypokalemia, consider digoxin specific Fab, magnesium IV, lidocaine IV or phenytoin IV.

❑❑ **What is the treatment of ectopic SVT not due to digitalis toxicity?**

Digitalis, verapamil or ß-blocker to slow rate.
Quinidine, procainamide or magnesium to decrease ectopy.

❑❑ **What is the treatment for verapamil-induced hypotension?**

Calcium gluconate 1 gram IV over several minutes.

❑❑ **What drugs are contraindicated for treatment of le torsade de pointes?**

A drug which prolongs repolarization (QT interval). For example, class Ia antiarrhythmics (quinidine, procainamide).
Other drugs that share this effect include TCAs, disopyramide, and phenothiazines.

❑❑ **What is the treatment of le torsade de pointes?**

Pacemaker cranked to 90 - 120 bpm to "overdrive" pace.
Isoproterenol.
Magnesium sulfate 2 grams IV.
The goal is to accelerate the heart rate and shorten ventricular repolarization. (If it's me, start with the mag, SHP & JNA).

❑❑ **Discuss the treatment of digitalis toxicity.**

Charcoal.
Phenytoin (Dilantin) for ventricular arrhythmias (it increases AV node conduction) or lidocaine.
Atropine or pace for bradyarrthymias.
Digoxin specific Fab (Digibind).

❑❑ **What hypos can lower the seizure threshold?**

Hypoglycemia, hyponatremia, and hypocarbia.

❑❑ **What are symptoms and signs of a vertebrobasilar artery lesion?**

Vertebral system supplies cerebellum and brain stem.
Vertigo, nausea, vomiting, ipsilateral 7th nerve deficit, contralateral hemiplegia.

Basilar artery occlusion leads to quadriplegia, coma or locked-in syndrome.

❑❑ **What motor function is spared in locked-in syndrome?**

Upward gaze.

❑❑ **What are signs and symptoms of a middle cerebral artery lesion?**

Hemiplegia or hemiparesthesias, homonymous hemianopsia and speech disturbance.

❏❏ **What is the most common cause of cerebral artery occlusion, embolic or thrombotic?**

Embolic.

❏❏ **What effects are likely to be present with an anterior cerebral artery lesion?**

Paralysis of contralateral leg with sensory loss in leg only and incontinence. No aphasia.

❏❏ **What deficits can result from ocular motor nerve paralysis?**

Ptosis as a result of levator palpebrae superioris/cranial nerve III injury. Lateral nerve gaze is controlled by cranial nerve VI, corneal reflex by cranial nerve V. The superior oblique muscle moves gaze downward and laterally; it is controlled by CN IV.

$$(LR_6 SO_4)_3$$

❏❏ **Describe the symptoms and signs of pressure on the first sacral root (S1).**

Symptoms of S1 injury include pain radiating to the mid-gluteal region, posterior thigh, posterior calf and down to the heel and sole of the foot.
Sensory signs are localized to the lateral toes. S1 root compression would typically involve the plantar flexor muscles of the foot and toes. The ankle reflex is decreased or absent.

❏❏ **In an infant, what is the most narrow segment of the airway?**

The cricoid cartilage ring. The glottic aperture is the most narrow part of the airway in the adult.

❏❏ **What is the ET tube size recommended for a term newborn infant?**

3 - 3.5 mm.
Premature infant requires a 2.5 mm tube.

❏❏ **What drug would you use to treat a patient in cardiac arrest secondary to hyperkalemia?**

Calcium chloride IV acts fastest.
Also provide $NaHCO_3$.

❏❏ **What are the potential complications of excess sodium bicarbonate?**

Cerebral acidosis, hypokalemia, hyperosmolality, and increased hemoglobin binding of oxygen.

❏❏ **What are the effects of dopamine at various doses?**

At 1 to 10 µg/kg, dopamine causes renal, mesenteric, coronary and cerebral vasodilation.
At 10 to 20 µg/kg, both α- and ß-adrenergic effects are present.
At 20 µg/kg, effects are primarily α-adrenergic.

❏❏ **What is the drug of choice for digitalis toxicity resulting in a ventricular arrhythmia?**

Phenytoin and digoxin specific Fab (Dilantin and Digibind).

❏❏ **What is the treatment for acute angle closure glaucoma?**

2% Pilocarpine drops every 15 minutes initially, acetazolamide (Diamox) 250 mg IV or 500 mg po, and po glycerol 1 g/kg with juice, or IV mannitol.

❏❏ **For each 100 increase in glucose, what is the effect on serum sodium?**

Each 100 increase in glucose decreases the serum sodium by 1.7 mEq/l.

❏❏ **What are common entities in the differential diagnosis of pinpoint pupils?**

Narcotic overdose, clonidine overdose, sedative hypnotic overdose including alcohol, cerebellar pontine angle infarct, and subarachnoid hemorrhage.

❏❏ **In a patient with tachycardia from cocaine abuse, what medications are appropriate?**

Sedation with benzodiazepines may calm the patient and decrease tachycardia. Nitroprusside may be used to treat hypertension.
Caution must be used with ß-adrenergic antagonist agents alone as they may leave α-adrenergic stimulation unopposed, increasing the patient's risk for intracranial hemorrhage or aortic dissection.

❏❏ **What traditional anti-arrhythmic agents may be used to treat digitalis induced ventricular arrhythmias in addition to phenytoin?**

Lidocaine and bretylium. Procainamide and quinidine are contraindicated in digitalis toxicity.

❏❏ **In a trauma patient receiving multiple units of transfused blood, when should the blood products be supplemented with fresh frozen plasma?**

For each five units of transfused blood, fresh frozen plasma is usually given.

❏❏ **What is a complication due to citrate present in stored blood?**

Citrate may bind calcium and result in hypocalcemia.

❏❏ **What is an anaphylactoid reaction?**

Anaphylactoid reactions are very similar to anaphylaxis, however, they do not require prior exposure to the reaction product. Cases may result from radiopaque contrast media or medications such as NSAIDs.

❏❏ **A child has a mild anaphylactic reaction. What is the correct route and dose of epinephrine?**

The correct dose is 0.01 ml/kg of a 1:1,000 solution, up to 0.3 ml, SQ.

❏❏ **What is universal donor blood?**

Type Rh negative blood with anti-A and anti-B titers of less than 1:200 in saline.

❏❏ **When would orthostatic hypotension typically develop in a 70 kg adult?**

Loss of over 1000 cc of blood would probably result in orthostatic hypotension.
Class II hemorrhage (loss of 750-1500 ml) presents with tachycardia, normal BP and narrow pulse pressure.
Class III hemorrhage (loss of 1500 to 2000 ml) presents with tachycardia > 120, hypotension and decreased urine output.

❏❏ **What are the common presentations of a transfusion reaction?**

Myalgia, dyspnea, fever associated with hypocalcemia, hemolysis, allergic reactions, hyperkalemia, citrate toxicity, hypothermia, coagulopathies and altered hemoglobin function.

❏❏ **What are the signs of the Cushing reflex?**

Increased systolic blood pressure and bradycardia.

❏❏ **In the Glasgow Coma Scale a dead person gets a 3. What number of points are possible measuring eye-opening response?**

4.
(I've an eye 4 U).

❏❏ **What number of points is the best verbal response worth in the Glasgow Coma Scale?**

5.

❏❏ **What number of points is the best motor response worth in the Glasgow Coma Scale?**

6.

❏❏ **What are normal findings in the oculocephalic reflex?**

Conjugate eye movement is opposite to the direction of head rotation.

❏❏ **In testing a patient's oculovestibular reflex, what is the direction of nystagmus anticipated in response to cold-water irrigation; toward or away from the irrigated ear?**

Recall that nystagmus is defined as the direction of the fast component of saccadic eye movement. Emergency physicians will commonly perform a crude but secure test of the oculovestibular reflex using ice water. After irrigation, nystagmus should be away from the irrigated ear.
Try the mnemonic COWS - Cold Opposite, Warm Same.

❏❏ **Signs and symptoms of an uncal herniation include:**

Ipsilateral pupillary dilation and either ipsilateral or contralateral hemiparesis. Blunting of corneal reflex may occur.
Oculovestibular response may be lost.

❏❏ **Tonic eye movement toward irrigated ear in response to caloric testing in a comatose patient signifies:**

Life.

❏❏ **What effect do ß-blockers have on Prinzmetal's variant angina?**

ß-blockers typically worsen the syndrome by allowing unopposed α-adrenergic stimulation of the coronary arteries.

❏❏ **What are the symptoms and signs of an ophthalmoplegic migraine?**

Typical duration is 3 to 5 days. Patient may complain of diplopia.
Mydriasis and exotropia may be noted.
Palsies of the muscles served by cranial nerves III, IV and VI may occur.

❏❏ **Define strabismus.**

A lack of parallelism of the visual axis of the eyes.
Esotropia = medially deviated,
Exotropia = laterally deviated.

❏❏ **What common drugs cause bradycardia?**

Agents such as ß-blockers, cardiac glycosides, pilocarpine and cholinesterase inhibitors such as organophosphates are responsible for bradycardia.

Sympathomimetics such as amphetamines and cocaine, and anticholinergics, such as atropine and cyclic antidepressants, commonly cause tachycardia.

❏❏ **What drug commonly causes both horizontal and vertical nystagmus?**

Phencyclidine (PCP).

❏❏ **What life-threatening mnemonic may help you recall the signs of cholinergic poisoning?**

DUELS. These fighters are wet.

D = diaphoresis,
U = urination,
E = eye changes (miosis),
L = lacrimation,
S = salivation.

❏❏ **What is the antidote for organophosphates?**

Atropine and pralidoxime (PAM).

❏❏ **How is an overdose of nitroprusside treated?**

Nitroprusside may induce methemoglobinemia. This is treated with 1% methylene blue solution.

❏❏ **For how long should sutures remain in the face, scalp or trunk, extremities and joints?**

Facial sutures	-3 to 5 days,
Scalp or Trunk	-7 to 10 days,
Extremities	-10 to 14 days,
Joints	-14 days.

❏❏ **What are the signs and symptoms of uncal herniation?**

Uncal herniation typically compresses the ipsilateral third cranial nerve resulting in ipsilateral pupil dilation. Contralateral weakness occurs because the pyramidal track decussates below this level. Occasionally, shift will be great enough to cause compression of both sides leading to a combination of ipsilateral or contralateral pupillary dilatation and weakness.

❏❏ **What is a common finding on sinus x-ray suggesting basilar skull fracture?**

Blood in the sphenoid sinus.

❏❏ **What bleeding sites are causes of subdural hemorrhages?**

Torn bridging veins.
Delayed hemorrhage from damaged parenchyma may also result in subdural hemorrhage.

❏❏ **In ordering x-rays of the face, what view gives the best view of the zygomatic arch?**

Modified basal view.
This is also called jug-handle, submentaloccipital or submental-vertical view.

❏❏ **What x-ray view should be ordered to evaluate the maxilla, maxillary sinus, orbital floor, inferior orbital rim or zygomatic bones?**

The Water's view.

❏❏ **How long can an extracted tooth survive?**

One percentage point of likely survivability is lost for each minute the tooth is out.
A tooth may survive 4 to 6 h longer in a commercial solution.
If no commercial solution is available place in milk or under patient's tongue.

❏❏ **Name five drugs or conditions that cause hypertension.**

Sympathomimetics
Withdrawal
Anticholinergics
MAO Inhibitors
Phencyclidine (PCP).   Mnemonic for this is SWAMP.

❏❏ **Name five drugs or conditions that cause tachycardia.**

Sympathomimetics
Withdrawal
Anticholinergics
MAO Inhibitors
Phencyclidine (PCP). SWAMP mnemonic.

❏❏ **Name six common drugs that can cause hyperthermia.**

Salicylates
Anticholinergics
Neuroleptics
Dinitrophenols
Sympathomimetics and PCP.

A psychotic friend of mine (on Stelazine) with bad allergies was on the beach smoking some Jimson weed laced with PCP. She took some antihistamine for the allergies and ASA for the sunburn. She was then stung by a beach-bee and required epi, but right about then the drugs were kicking in and it took 12 beach security guards to hold her down for her shot. Boy was she HOT!
The mnemonic is SANDS-PCP.

❏❏ **What drugs/environmental exposures can induce bullous lesion formation?**

Sedative hypnotics, carbon monoxide, snake bite, spider bite, caustic agents, and hydrocarbons.

❏❏ **What drugs cause an odor of acetone on the breath?**

Ethanol, isopropanol and salicylates.
Ketosis often has the same odor.

❏❏ **What substances induce an odor of almonds on the breath?**

Cyanide, Laetrile, and apricot pits (latter two contain amygdalin).

❏❏ **What drugs induce an odor of garlic on the breath?**

DMSO, organophosphates, phosphorus, arsenic, arsine gas and thallium.

❏❏ **What drug induces an odor of peanuts on the breath?**

Vacor (RH-787).

❏❏ **What drugs induce a pear-like odor on the breath?**

Chloral hydrate and paraldehyde.

❏❏ **What compounds induce an odor of rotten eggs on the breath?**

Hydrogen sulfide, mercaptans and sewer-gas.

❏❏ **What is the mnemonic for remembering what drugs or conditions commonly cause seizures?**

SHAKE WITH eL SPOC!

S	= salicylates,
H	= hypoxia,
A	= anticholinergics,
K	= Karbon Monoxide (KO),
E	= EtOH withdrawal,
W	= withdrawal,
I	= isoniazid,
T	= theophylline and tricyclics,
H	= hypoglycemia,
eL	= lead, lithium and local anesthetics,
S	= strychnine and sympathomimetics,
P	= PCP, phenothiazines and propoxyphene,
O	= organophosphates,
C	= camphor, cholinergics, carbon monoxide and cyanide.

❏❏ **What is a mnemonic for remembering the drugs that cause nystagmus?**

MALES TIP

M	= methanol,
A	= alcohol,
L	= lithium,
E	= ethylene glycol,
S	= sedative hypnotics and solvents,
T	= thiamine depletion and Tegretol (carbamazepine),
I	= isopropanol and
P	= PCP and phenytoin.

❏❏ **What is a mnemonic for remembering drugs that are radiopaque?**

BAT CHIPS!

B	= barium
A	= antihistamines,
T	= tricyclic antidepressants,
C	= chloral hydrate, calcium, cocaine condoms,
H	= heavy metals,
I	= iodine,
P	= phenothiazines, potassium,
S	= slow-release (enteric coated).

❑❑ **What is the antidote for Mercury, Arsenic and Gold (MAG) poisoning?**

BAL & Dimercaptosuccinic acid (DMSA).

Play BAL with a DMSAl named MAG!

❑❑ **What is the antidote for ß-blockers?**

Glucagon.

❑❑ **What is the antidote for ethylene glycol?**

Ethyl alcohol. Dialysis.

❑❑ **What three toxicologic emergencies require immediate dialysis?**

Ethylene glycol, methyl alcohol and Amanita phalloides.

❑❑ **What is the antidote for iron?**

Deferoxamine.

❑❑ **What is the antidote for isoniazid?**

Pyridoxine.

❑❑ **Antidote for reversing benzodiazepine overdose?**

Flumazenil.

❑❑ **What is the antidote for lead?**

EDTA. EDTA is ONLY used for treating lead poisoning.
Penicillamine.
BAL.

❑❑ **What is the antidote for mercury?**

Penicillamine and BAL.

What is the antidote for organophosphates?

Atropine and PAM.

❑❑ **What is the antidote for chronic bromide intoxication (bromism)?**

NaCl.

❑❑ **What is the antidote for tricyclic antidepressant overdose?**

Alkalinization.

❑❑ **Name some side effects of alkalization of the urine.**

Hypernatremia and hyperosmolality.

❑❑ **What drugs are commonly excreted using alkaline diuresis?**

BLIST

B = barbiturates (long-acting),
L = lithium (not so common),
I = INH,
T = TCAs,
S = salicylates.

❏❏ **What drugs require immediate dialysis?**

Ethylene glycol and methyl alcohol.
Come on, you know it...yup, Amanita phalloides does too.

❏❏ **Can theophylline be dialyzed?**

Yes.

❏❏ **For what drugs may hemoperfusion be indicated?**

Salicylates, theophylline and long-acting barbiturates.

❏❏ **For what drugs may dialysis be indicated?**

Salicylates, theophylline and long-acting barbiturates.
Also - Methyl alcohol, ethylene glycol, amphetamine, lithium and thiocyanate.

❏❏ **What are the four mechanisms by which tricyclics induce toxicity?**

(1) Anticholinergic atropine-like effects 2° to competitive antagonism of acetylcholine.
(2) Block the reuptake of norepinephrine.
(3) A quinidine-like action on the myocardium.
(4) Alpha blocking action.

❏❏ **What are the symptoms and signs of anticholinergic effects?**

Peripheral effects include tachycardia, hyperpyrexia, mydriasis, vasodilatation, urinary retention, decreased GI motility, decreased secretions. Central effects include anxiety, disorientation, hallucinations, hyperactivity, delirium, seizures, coma and death. These patients are dry. In fact,
Dry as a bone,
Red as a beet,
Mad as a hatter,
Hot as a stone,
(Blind as a bat).

❏❏ **What are the four stages of acetaminophen toxicity?**

I (within h)   - anorexia, nausea, vomiting and diaphoresis.

II (24 - 48 h)   - liver function test abnormalities and right upper quadrant pain.

III (72-96 h)   - jaundice, return of GI symptoms, peak of liver function abnormalities,   coagulation defects.

IV (4 d - 2 wk)   - Get better or die.

❏❏ **When does acetaminophen become toxic?**

When there is no glutathione to detoxify its toxic intermediate.

❏❏ **How does N-acetylcysteine act to interrupt acetaminophen toxicity?**

Exact mechanism unknown, however, likely that NAC enters cells, and is metabolized to cysteine which is a precursor for glutathione. Thus it may increase glutathione stores.

❏❏ **Would you like to have FOUR <u>ACE</u>s.**

Of course! So check <u>ACE</u>taminophen level FOUR h after ingestion.

❏❏ **What is the early acid base disturbance seen in salicylate overdose?**

Respiratory alkalosis. Approximately 12 hours later, one might see an anion gap metabolic acidosis or mixed acid base picture.

❏❏ **In salicylate overdose, is hyperglycemia or hypoglycemia expected?**

This may present with either hyperglycemia or hypoglycemia.

❏❏ **What are common symptoms and signs of chronic salicylism?**

Fever, tachypnea, CNS alterations, acid base abnormalities, electrolyte abnormalities, chronic pain, ketonuria, and noncardiogenic pulmonary edema.

❏❏ **A patient presents with an acute salicylate ingestion. What symptoms are expected with a mild, a moderate and a severe overdose?**

Mild - Lethargy, vomiting, hyperventilation and hyperthermia.

Moderate - Severe hyperventilation and compensated metabolic acidosis.

Severe - Coma, seizures and uncompensated metabolic acidosis.

❏❏ **What is the treatment of salicylate overdose?**

Decontaminate, lavage and charcoal, fluid replacement, potassium supplementation, alkalize the urine with use of bicarbonate, cooling for hyperthermia, glucose for hypoglycemia, oxygen and PEEP for pulmonary edema, multiple dose activated charcoal, and dialysis.

❏❏ **A patient presents with vomiting, hematemesis, diarrhea, lethargy, coma and shock. What cause is suspected?**

Iron intoxication. Order a flat plate of the abdomen to look for concretions.

❏❏ **What iron level is considered toxic?**

Moderate overdose is considered to be 350 µg/dl, best measured 4 h after ingestion.
The amount of <u>elemental</u> iron ingested is used in calculations. 20-40 mg elemental iron/kg is toxic.
Symptomatic patients receive treatment without waiting for lab tests.

❏❏ **Discuss the 4 stinking stages of iron toxicity.**

I (h) - Abdominal pain, vomiting, diarrhea, possible GI bleeding and 2° lethargy and metabolic acidosis. Due to direct corrosive effect of iron.

II (3-12 h) - GI symptoms resolve, M.D. falsely reassured.

III (>12 h) - Iron makes it into cells, blocks oxidative phosphorylation, catalyzes formation of free radicals. Cellular and organ disruption ensue with edema and venous pooling. Hepatic dysfunction, renal and cardiac failure can occur. Stage III occurs earlier in severe poisoning.

IV (days-wk) - Small bowel and gastric outlet obstruction.

❏❏ **What is the treatment of iron ingestion?**

If patient has Ø symptoms ever for 6 h and is completely normal on exam, go home.

If patient has minimal symptoms and appears fine and has iron level close to maximum normal level (150 µg/dl) measured 4 h after ingestion, go home.

Cathartics for patients without diarrhea (controversial).
Hydration and treat GI hemorrhage.

Deferoxamine if:
    Moderate or severely symptomatic,
    Serum iron level > TIBC,
    Serum iron level > 350 µg/dl.

Deferoxamine is a specific agent for iron and will not chelate other metals. The IV dose of deferoxamine is 10 to 15 µg/kg/h.

❏❏ **What are the symptoms and signs of cyanide overdose?**

Dryness and burning in the throat, air hunger, and hyperventilation. If not removed from the toxic environment loss of consciousness, seizures, bradycardia and apnea follow prior to asystole.

❏❏ **What is the treatment for cyanide overdose?**

(0) Oxygen, CPR prn.
(1) Amyl nitrite perle inhaled.
(2) Sodium nitrite 10 cc of 3% solution in an adult which is 300 mg, or 0.2 - 0.33 ml/kg.
(3) Sodium thiosulfate 12.5 mg, in an adult which is 50 cc of a 25% solution or 1.0 - 1.5 ml/kg in a child (five times the volume of sodium nitrite).

Excess nitrites may require treatment with methylene blue for very, very rare case of dangerous methemoglobinemia.

❏❏ **What are the classic signs of PCP overdose?**

Hypertension, agitation, confusion, ataxia, vertical nystagmus, miosis, muscle rigidity, and catatonia.

❏❏ **What drugs can cause methemoglobinemia?**

Nitrites, local anesthetics, silver nitrate, amyl nitrite and nitrites, benzocaine, commercial marking crayons, aniline dyes, sulfonamides and phenacetin.

❏❏ **Atropine is used to treat:**

Organophosphate and carbamate overdose.

❏❏ **Pralidoxime (2-PAM) is used to treat:**

Organophosphate overdose.

❏❏ **Sodium chloride is used to treat:**

Chronic bromism.

❏❏ **Vitamin K is used to treat:**

Warfarin overdose.

❏❏ **Methylene blue is used to treat:**

Methemoglobinemia.

❏❏ **Pyridoxine is used to treat:**

Isoniazid and Gyromitra mushroom poisoning.

❏❏ **Name two selective cardioselective ß-blockers.**

Just remember the main cardioselective ß-blockers <u>M</u>etoprolol and <u>A</u>tenolol from the mnemonic "Look <u>Ma</u>!, I'm cardioselective!"

❏❏ **Overdose of ß-blockers may result in:**

Nausea, vomiting, bradycardia, hypotension, respiratory depression, seizure, CHF, bronchospasm, hypoglycemia and hyperkalemia.

❏❏ **Evaluating a pediatric cervical spine film, what are the normal values?**

Predental space < 5 mm or < 3 mm in an adult.
The posterior cervical line attaching the base of the spinous process of C1 to C3 should be considered. If the base of C2 spinous process lies greater than 2 mm behind the posterior cervical line, a hangman's fracture should be suspected.
Anterior border of C2 to the posterior wall of the fornix distance < 7 mm.
Finally, anterior border of C6 to the posterior wall of the trachea distance would be 14 mm in children younger than 15 years of age, and less than 22 mm in an adult.

❏❏ **Describe a hangman's fracture.**

C2 bilateral pedicle fracture.

❏❏ **What are key features of a vertical compression fracture?**

Cervical and lumbar regions. Usually stable.

A Jefferson fracture of C1 may occur and is extremely unstable, although it is also very rare in occurrence.

❏❏ **Injury to what cervical area results in Horner's syndrome (ptosis, miosis, and anhidrosis)?**

Disruption of the cervical sympathetic chain at C7 to T2.

❏❏ **What spinal level corresponds with dermatomal innervation of:**

a. Perianal region,
b. Nipple line
c. Index finger
d. Knee
e. Lateral foot.

a.	Perianal region	S2-S4
b.	Nipple line	T4
c.	Index finger	C7
d.	Knee	L4
e.	Lateral foot	S1

❏❏ **Describe a patient with a central cord syndrome.**

Injury to the ligamentum flavum and to the cord causing upper extremity neurologic deficit greater than lower extremity deficit.

❏❏ Describe a patient with Brown-Séquard syndrome.

Ipsilateral motor paralysis.
Ipsilateral loss of proprioception and vibratory sensation.
Contralateral loss of pain and temperature sensation.

❏❏ Describe a patient with anterior cord syndrome.

Complete motor paralysis and loss of pain and temperature sensation distal to the lesion.
Posterior column sparing results in intact proprioception and vibration sense.
Cause - occlusion of the anterior spinal artery or protrusion of fracture fragments into the anterior canal.

❏❏ Under water conditions, oops. Under what conditions does trench foot or immersion foot develop?

Trench foot occurs with exposure to wet or cold for days where the temperature is above freezing. The extremity develops superficial damage resembling partial thickness burns.

❏❏ What is pernio (chilblain)?

Chilblain refers to exposure of an extremity for a prolonged period of time to <u>dry</u> cold at temperatures above freezing. Patients develop superficial, small, painful ulcerations over chronically exposed areas. Sensitivity of the surrounding skin, erythema and pruritus may develop.

❏❏ What is frost nip?

Frost nip is the name for the condition preceding frostbite in which the skin becomes numb and blanched followed by cessation of discomfort. Sudden loss of cold sensation at the location of injury is a reliable sign of precipitant frostbite. Frost nip will proceed to frostbite if treatment is not initiated.

❏❏ How is frostnip treated?

Frostnip is the only form of frostbite which can be treated at the scene. It is treated by warming by hand, by breathing on the skin or by placing the frostnipped fingers or toes in the armpit (FUN!).
The affected part should not be rubbed. This may cause skin breakage, increases chances of infection, and does not thaw the tissues completely.

❏❏ What is appropriate treatment for frostbite?

The extremity in question should be rapidly rewarmed. Immerse in 42 °C circulating water for 20 min or until flushing is observed. <u>Dry heat should not be used</u>. Refreezing thawed tissue greatly increases damage. Remember tetanus prophylaxis.
Débride white or clear blisters as they contain toxic mediators (prostaglandin and thromboxanes).
Hemorrhagic blisters should be left intact. Topical antibiotics such as silver sulfadiazine may be used.
After admission, whirlpool treatments in warm antibiotic solution should be used twice per day.

Great quotes series:

"But facts are facts and flinch not."

Robert Browning 1812-1889.

❏❏ What are some common complications of frostbite?

Rhabdomyolysis, permanent depigmentation of the extremity, and increased likelihood of subsequent cold injury.
X-ray approximately three to six months following frostbite injury reveals irregular, fine, punched out lytic lesions that may appear on the MTP, PIP and DIP joints, likely due to chronic subperiosteal inflammation.

❑❑ **Where do endoscopic perforations of the esophagus typically occur?**

They usually occur near the distal esophagus or at the site of pre-existing disease, such as a caustic burn.

❑❑ **What are the three most common sites of foreign body perforation of the esophagus?**

The levels of the cricopharyngeus muscle, the left mainstem bronchus, and the gastroesophageal junction.

❑❑ **What laboratory abnormalities may be anticipated in acute cyanide poisoning?**

An elevated anion gap - frequently 25 to 30 mEq/l, with lactic acidosis and decreased bicarbonate levels.

Venous PO_2 may be greater than 40 mm Hg due to decreased tissue oxygen extraction.

❑❑ **What is the most common site of penetrating ureteral injuries?**

Penetrating ureteral injuries typically occur in the upper one-third of the ureter.

In pelvic fractures the most common site of injury is where the ureter crosses the pelvic brim.

❑❑ **The most common cause of a coagulopathy in patients that require massive transfusions:**

Thrombocytopenia.

❑❑ **What percentage of ureteral injuries present without hematuria?**

One-third of ureteral injuries present without hematuria.

❑❑ **How may a posterior urethral tear be diagnosed in a male?**

High riding, boggy prostate suggests this injury.

❑❑ **Describe the mechanism of injury and signs & symptoms associated with an anterior urethral tear?**

Straddle or crush injury mechanism.
Severe perineal pain with blood usually found at the meatus.
Good urinary stream is maintained.

❑❑ **The best method of transporting an avulsed tooth?**

Under the patient's tongue. If unable, transport in milk, saline or a wet handkerchief.

❑❑ **What is the mechanism of a posterior urethral tear?**

Associated with pelvic fracture.
Urethral stricture, impotence and incontinence.

❑❑ **A patient has a pelvic fracture with suspected bladder or ureteral injury. What test should be performed first, a cystogram or an IVP?**

When a pelvic fracture is present or suspected, the cystogram is usually performed first so that distal ureteral dye from the IVP will not mimic extravasation from the bladder.

❑❑ **About what is the half-life of carboxyhemoglobin?**

6.0 h in 21% F_IO_2,
1.5 h in 100% F_IO_2 and
0.5 h in 3 atmospheres of hyperbaric 100% F_IO_2.

❑❑ **The most common cause of Ludwig's angina is:**

Odontogenic abscess of a lower molar. Most common pathogen is hemolytic strep.

❑❑ **The most common adverse effect of AZT:**

Granulocytopenia and anemia. Less commonly a myopathy.

❑❑ **Isopropyl alcohol, glycerol, or polyethylene glycol mixture is useful for treatment of what chemical burn?**

Phenol (carbolic acid).

❑❑ **The best means of transporting an amputated extremity:**

Wrapped in sterile gauze moistened with saline, placed in waterproof plastic bag, immersed in ice water.

❑❑ **What is the antidote for phosphorus poisoning?**

Copper sulfate 1% solution. Remove within 30 minutes.
Phosphorus may be identified by formation of insoluble black precipitate when swabbing with copper sulfate.

❑❑ **What is the dose of SQ/intradermal 10% calcium gluconate used to treat hydrofluoric acid skin burn.**

0.5 cc per cm^2 burned.

❑❑ **Explain the significant features of each "axis" in the DSM-III official diagnostic criteria and nomenclature for psychiatric illnesses.**

Axis I   - organic brain syndromes caused by intoxication or physical illness, and major psychiatric disorders including psychosis, affective disorders and disorders of substance use.
Axis II   - personality disorders including antisocial, schizoid and histrionic types.
Axis III   - medical problems such as heart disease and infections.
Axis IV   - life events that contribute to the patient's problems.
Axis V   - patient adaptation to these problems.

❑❑ **Which test is most reliable in predicting the severity of radiation exposure 48 h post exposure?**

Absolute lymphocyte count. Presence or absence of GI symptoms following near-lethal doses is a good indicator of mortality.

❑❑ **What local anesthetics may cause anaphylaxis?**

The ester derivatives containing para-aminobenzoic acid (PABA) are known to stimulate IgE antibody formation and cause anaphylaxis.

These include procaine and tetracaine.

❑❑ **What neighboring structures may be injured with a supracondylar distal humeral fracture?**

The anterior interosseous nerve (which is a branch of the median nerve) and the brachial artery.

❑❑ **Which test best discriminates between functional and organic blindness?**

Optokinetic nystagmus.

❑❑ **What is the <u>most</u> <u>common</u> carpal fracture?**

Scaphoid (navicular); the more proximal the fracture, the more likely to develop avascular necrosis.

❏❏ **How may a lunate dislocation be diagnosed?**

Lateral view x-ray - the lunate appears dorsal or volar to its usual position within the radial fossa.

❏❏ **The most common ligament injured after an inversion ankle sprain?**

Anterior talo-fibular ligament.

❏❏ **How may a perilunate dislocation be diagnosed?**

AP and lateral x-ray - the lunate remains in alignment with the radial fossa and the other carpal bones appear displaced.

❏❏ **What is the cause of lymphogranuloma venereum?**

Chlamydia trachomatis.
Painful unilateral suppurative nodes may present with sinus tract.

Sx: Transient <u>ULCER</u> <u>IS</u> <u>PAINLESS.</u>
Dx: Compliment fixation.
Rx: Tetracycline, erythromycin, doxycycline.

❏❏ **What is the cause of granuloma inguinale?**

The bacterium Donovania granulomatis, recently renamed Calymmatobacterium granulomatis.

Dx: Bright, beefy-red, granulomatous lesions. Confirm diagnosis with finding of intracytoplasmic bacilli in macrophages (Donovan bodies).
Rx: Streptomycin, tetracycline, erythromycin, chloramphenicol, TMP/SMX.

❏❏ **The best diluent in solid lye ingestion is:**

Milk.

❏❏ **What is the cause of condylomata acuminata?**

Papova virus.

❏❏ **What is the mechanism of injury responsible for the greatest portion of injuries in the elderly?**

Falls. Most falls are caused by tripping but other medical causes underlying the initial fall should always be sought.

❏❏ **The organ most severely affected in a blast injury:**

The lungs.

❏❏ **The organ most commonly affected in a blast injury:**

The ears.

❏❏ **A patient has previous focal deficits from CVA's. Is it true that such a patient may present with confusion when having suffered a new focal lesion.**

Yes. The presentation of a new focal lesion may be with generalized or non-focal symptoms in the context of previous insults.

❏❏ **A patient with a dementia gets a wound infection. Is it true that such a patient may present with a severe decrease in mental status.**

Yes. Normally minor insults may cause drastic changes in neurologic functioning in those with pre-existing deficits.

❏❏ **The most common cause of extrauterine surgical emergencies in pregnancy:**

Appendicitis.

❏❏ **A patient had right arm and hand paralysis from a previous CVA. That deficit is mostly compensated with only residual weakness remaining. Should that patient subsequently have an episode of hyponatremia, can the presentation be with a right arm and hand paralysis?**

Sure. Formerly compensated deficits may return in response to a generalized neurological insult.

❏❏ **Red blood cell basophilic stippling is seen in what two disorders?**

Thalassemia and lead poisoning.

Zebe alert!

❏❏ **What triad is associated with Reiter's syndrome?**

Non-gonococcal urethritis, polyarthritis and conjunctivitis.
The conjunctivitis is the least common and is seen in only 30 percent of patients. Acute attacks respond well to NSAIDs.

❏❏ **What is the most common cause of immediate postpartum hemorrhage?**

Uterine atony followed by vaginal/cervical lacerations, and retained placenta or placental fragments.

❏❏ **What complications of rheumatoid arthritis require emergency treatment?**

Vasculitis. This should be promptly treated with systemic steroids, otherwise irreversible neuropathy may occur.

❏❏ **What is Felty's syndrome?**

Rheumatoid arthritis with splenomegaly and neutropenia. It is a late complication of rheumatoid arthritis.

❏❏ **What drugs are commonly known to induce a lupus reaction?**

Procainamide, hydralazine, isoniazid and phenytoin.

❏❏ **What is the most serious complication of dental infections, aside from possible respiratory compromise in Ludwig's angina?**

Septic cavernous sinus thrombosis.

❏❏ **What joint is <u>most common</u>ly affected with pseudogout?**

The knee. The causative agent is calcium pyrophosphate crystals.

❏❏ **What joint is <u>most commonly</u> affected with gout?**

The great toe MCP joint.

❏❏ **What are the complications of impetigo?**

Streptococcal induced impetigo can result in post-streptococcal glomerulonephritis.
It has not been shown to be associated with rheumatic fever.
Tx: erythromycin, dicloxacillin, cephalexin to help eliminate the skin lesions.
There is not clear proof that treatment prevents glomerulonephritis.

❏❏ What are the clinical features of rubella (German measles)?

Malaise, fever, headache, generalized lymphadenopathy, particularly the suboccipital and the posterior auricular nodes, with a pinkish maculopapular rash that first appears on the face.

❏❏ How does measles (Rubeola) typically present?

Fever, coryza and conjunctivitis. Pathognomonic Koplik's spots appear 2-4 d later on the buccal mucosa followed by the spreading maculopapular rash starting on the forehead and upper neck radiating to truck and extremities.

❏❏ The most common early manifestation of a significant radiation exposure is:

Nausea and vomiting.

❏❏ How does roseola infantum appear?

Roseola is typified by a high fever for three to four days, followed by a macular or maculopapular rash that is profuse on the chest and abdomen and mild on face and extremities. Patient feels well with rash.

❏❏ Describe the key features of the rash of Rocky Mountain Spotted Fever.

Rocky Mountain Spotted Fever is caused by Rickettsia rickettsii and is transmitted by Ixodidae ticks. Patients get sick, with high fever, headache, chills and muscular pain. On about the 4th d of fever, the rash begins on the wrists and ankles. The spread of rash is centripetal.

❏❏ The most effective dermal decontaminate following radiation exposure:

Wash with soap and water after removal of all clothes.

❏❏ Describe the rash of scarlet fever.

Sandpaper type texture rash beginning on the face, neck, chest, abdomen and spreads to extremities. Patients may have strawberry tongue.

❏❏ What is the most likely cause of unilateral transient loss of vision in a patient's eye (amaurosis fugax)?

Carotid artery disease. This is usually the result of platelet emboli from plaques in the arterial system.

❏❏ Syncope is a characteristic symptom of what valvular disease?

Aortic stenosis.

❏❏ What valvular lesion is most likely to cause syncope?

Aortic stenosis.

❏❏ The most common cause of a transudative pleural effusion?

Congestive heart failure.

❏❏ How does Landry-Guillain-Barré present?

Presentation in the third to fourth decade of a rapidly progressive ascending transverse myelitis. Weakness begins in lower extremities. Bulbar musculature may eventually be involved.
Decrease or loss of DTRs is relatively specific for this disorder, though tick paralysis and Diphtheria neurotoxin can share this feature.

❑❑ **How does a patient present with Eaton-Lambert Syndrome?**

Proximal weakness with aching muscles especially in the lower extremities. Cranial nerve involvement is very rare. Patients often have a dry mouth.
Unlike myasthenia gravis, which gets worse with activity, with E-L grip strength improves. There is no response to edrophonium test.

❑❑ **How is an acute hemorrhagic overdose of Coumadin best treated?**

Fresh frozen plasma, Vit K IM will help prevent subsequent hemorrhage.

❑❑ **Where does botulism toxin exert its effects?**

At the myoneural junction. It prevents the release of acetylcholine.

❑❑ **How does botulism present?**

Neurologic systems begin 24 - 48 hours after ingestion of contaminated foods. May start with nausea, vomiting or diarrhea.
Most common early neurologic complaints are related to the eye and bulbar musculature. Symptoms involve all muscles of the trunk and extremities. Intestinal and bladder involvement may include ileus and acute urinary retention.

❑❑ **Describe a patient with tick paralysis.**

A rapid progressive ascending paralysis that develops over one to two days. First systems occur in the extremities and trunk and move to bulbar musculature. It is almost identical to Guillain-Barré Syndrome.

❑❑ **Patient's with sickle cell trait most commonly present with:**

Hematuria and decreased urine concentrating ability.

❑❑ **Differentiate diphtheria with neurologic sequelae from toxicity due to botulism.**

Diphtheria vs. botulism - Diphtheria is an acute <u>febrile</u> illness with pseudomembranous oropharyngitis and cardiac involvement.

❑❑ **Differentiate neurologic sequela of botulism toxicity from neurologic deficits of Guillain-Barré syndrome.**

G-B is an ascending transverse myelitis. It does not begin with bulbar musculature.

❑❑ **How does infant botulism present?**

The usual source is raw honey. (Honey abusers, huh! We know your type...)
Presentation with lethargy, failure to thrive, progresses to paralysis and death.

❑❑ **What is the pathophysiology of myasthenia gravis?**

Circulatory antibody against ACh receptor which binds at the motor end plate. In myasthenics, ACh receptors are in short supply resulting in fatigable weakness.

❑❑ **What is the most serious transfusion reaction?**

Hemolytic. Treat with aggressive fluid replacement and Lasix.

❏❏ **What is the most common transfusion reaction?**

Febrile.

❏❏ **What diseases are associated with myasthenia gravis?**

Rheumatoid arthritis, pernicious anemia, SLE, sarcoidosis and thyroiditis. 10 - 25% have associated thymoma.

❏❏ **How does myasthenia gravis present?**

Muscular weakness with fatigability. Strength improves after resting. First muscles involved are usually the extraocular muscles (other bulbar muscles *may* present earlier). The first symptom is either diplopia or eyelid ptosis. Bright light may increase ptosis and diplopia and heat may increase muscle weakness. Proximal muscles are typically weakest. Respiratory muscle involvement can be life-threatening.

❏❏ **A patient presents with ocular, bulbar and limb weakness which gets worse during the day and decreases with resting - diagnosis?**

Myasthenia gravis.

❏❏ **The best emergent treatment of an Ellis III dental fracture in an adult:**

Cover tooth with moist cotton then dry aluminum foil, and refer immediately to an orthodontist.

❏❏ **What are some factors commonly associated with meningitis?**

Age less than 5 years or greater than 60 years, low socioeconomic status, male sex, crowding, black race, sickle cell disease, splenectomy, alcoholism, diabetes and cirrhosis, immunologic defects, dural defect from congenital, surgical or traumatic source, contiguous infections such as sinusitis, household contacts, malignancy, bacterial endocarditis, intravenous drug abuse and thalassemia major.

❏❏ **A patient has xanthochromic CSF with a low protein count. What is the most likely cause?**

Subarachnoid hemorrhage.

❏❏ **A patient has xanthochromic CSF with a high protein count (greater than 150 mg/dl). What is the most likely cause?**

Traumatic tap.

❏❏ **What disease is associated with periaqueductal petechial hemorrhages?**

Wernicke's disease.

❏❏ **What disorders are associated with cerebrocortical neuronal degeneration?**

Anoxic, hypoglycemic and hepatic encephalopathies.

❏❏ **What is the most commonly abused volatile substance?**

Toluene.

❏❏ **A patient presents with hypokalemia of 2.0, hyperchloremia and acidosis. What is the most likely toxicologic cause?**

Chronic toluene abuse.

❏❏ **A patient has been abusing nitrous oxide for a long time. What symptoms might be expected?**

Paresthesias and motor weakness may be present in chronic abusers. Such symptoms are often mistaken for symptoms of multiple sclerosis.

❏❏ **Describe the features of each of the three stages of PCP intoxication.**

Stage I - agitated or violent, normal vital signs.
Stage II - tachycardia, hypertension and unresponsive to pain.
Stage III - unresponsive, depressed respirations, seizures and death.

❏❏ **Should the urine be acidified in the treatment of PCP intoxication?**

Although acidification of the urine is theoretically advantageous, clinical experience has <u>not</u> shown this to be efficacious. Let's call that a "no."

❏❏ **Explain how methylene blue functions as an antidote for methemoglobinemia.**

A normal level of 3% methemoglobin is usually maintained by a NADPH - dependent enzyme. This enzyme capacity can be exceeded with oxidant poisoning.
Methylene blue enhances NADPH - dependent hemoglobin reduction by acting as a cofactor.
Methylene blue is usually only needed for MetHb levels > 30%; its dose is 1-2 mg/kg IV over 5 min.

❏❏ **A patient presents with belladonna alkaloid poisoning resulting in anticholinergic effects. Explain the dangers of treating this patient with physostigmine.**

Physostigmine acts to increase the acetylcholine levels. Doing so, it can precipitate a cholinergic crisis resulting in heart block and asystole. As a result, it is recommended to reserve physostigmine for life threatening anticholinergic complications.

Heart block and asystole.

❏❏ **Does botulism produce fever?**

No. This can be important in differentiating neurologic symptoms in a sick patient who could have diphtheria.

❏❏ **Describe a patient with Chlamydial pneumonia.**

Chlamydial pneumonia is usually seen in children 2 to 6 wk of age. The patient is afebrile. Patients do not appear toxic.

❏❏ **A patient has had three days of diarrhea which was abrupt in onset. The patient reports slimy green, malodorous stools that contain blood. In addition, the patient is febrile. What is the most likely cause?**

Salmonella.

❏❏ **Drug treatment for Campylobacter?**

Erythromycin or tetracycline.

❏❏ **In a child, does coarctation of the aorta typically cause cyanosis?**

No.

❏❏ **How much elemental iron will 100 mg of deferoxamine bind?**

About 8.5 mg of elemental iron is bound by 100 mg of deferoxamine.

❑❑ **Drug treatment for persistent Escherichia coli?**

Trimethoprim with sulfamethoxazole (TMP/SMX).

❑❑ **Drug treatment for Giardia lamblia?**

Quinacrine or metronidazole or furazolidone.

❑❑ **Drug treatment for persistent Salmonella?**

Ampicillin.
TMP/SMX.
Chloramphenicol.

❑❑ **Drug treatment for Shigella?**

TMP/SMX or Ciprofloxacin (if resistant).

❑❑ **Drug treatment for Yersinia?**

TMP/SMX.
Tetracycline.
3rd generation cephalosporin.

❑❑ **What are the 8 common clinical presentations of pediatric heart disease?**

Cyanosis, pathologic murmur, abnormal pulses, CHF, HTN, cardiogenic shock, syncope and tachyarrhythmias.

❑❑ **Complications of the use of sodium bicarbonate in severe metabolic acidosis include:**

Hypernatremia, paradoxical CSF acidosis, decreased oxygen unloading at the tissue level, hyperosmolality, dysrhythmias and hypokalemia.

❑❑ **What is the function of aldosterone?**

Aldosterone causes sodium conservation and K^+ excretion.
As a result, it causes increased resorption of sodium and fluid.

❑❑ **What drug will most rapidly decrease K^+?**

Calcium chloride IV (1 - 3 minutes).

❑❑ **What is a potential side effect of the use of Kayexalate?**

Kayexalate exchanges sodium for K^+. As a result, sodium overload and CHF may occur.

❑❑ **What is Addison's disease?**

Deficiency or absence of mineralocorticoid (aldosterone). This results in increased sodium excretion. Potassium is retained. The urine cannot concentrate.

This can lead to severe dehydration, hypotension and circulatory collapse.

Deficiency of cortisol (also produced in the adrenal cortex) leads to metabolic disturbances, weakness, hypoglycemia and deceased resistance to infection.

❑❑ **What metabolic conditions will potentiate the toxic cardiac effects of digoxin?**

Hypokalemia and hypercalcemia.

❏❏ **What is the initial treatment for hypercalcemia?**

Saline and furosemide.
Then, if you've not yet sent the patient to the floor, calcitonin, mithramycin, hydrocortisone, and indomethacin.

❏❏ **What conditions lead to hypocalcemia?**

Shock, impaired production, pancreatitis, hypomagnesemia, alkalosis, decreased serum albumin, hypoparathyroidism, osteoblastic mets, and fat embolism syndrome.

❏❏ **What vital sign might be affected with hypermagnesemia?**

Hypermagnesemia causes hypotension because it relaxes vascular smooth muscle. Deep tendon reflexes may disappear.

❏❏ **What is the immediate treatment of thyroid storm?**

1st	-Draw blood for Free T4 index and free T3 and cortisol levels.
2nd	-Supportive care (avoid aspirin - it may increase free T3 and T4).
3rd	-IV glucocorticoids - 300 mg hydrocortisone per day.
4th	-Inhibit thyroid hormone synthesis - propylthiouracil 900-1200 mg or methimazole 90 - 120 mg.
5th	-Retard thyroid hormone release (iodine 1g q 8 hours IV).
6th	-Block peripheral thyroid hormone effects (propranolol 1 mg q 1 min to total of 10 mg).

❏❏ **How is myxedema coma treated?**

IV thyroxine 400 - 500 mg infused slowly, then 50 - 100 mg every day. Caution, lower dose of thyroxine if cardiac ischemia or arrhythmias are present.

❏❏ **Common causes of hypercalcemia:**

PAM P SCHMIDT.

P = Parathormone
A = Addison's
M = Multiple Myeloma

P = Paget's

S = Sarcoidosis
C = Cancer
H = Hyperthyroidism
M = Milk - alkali Syndrome
I = Immobilization
D = Vitamin D Excess
T = Thiazides

❏❏ **What is the treatment for adrenal crisis?**

100 mg hydrocortisone (Solu-cortef) IV bolus and 100 mg hydrocortisone added to IV solution. Then, 200 mg hydrocortisone q 6 h for 24 hours.

(Refer to your preferred text for discussion of simultaneous testing and treatment with dexamethasone and corticotropin instead).

❏❏ **What are the signs and symptoms of Wernicke's encephalopathy?**

Oculomotor disturbances are common, usually with nystagmus and ocular palsies. Abnormal mentation and ataxia may be present. Ophthalmoplegias and nystagmus usually respond to thiamine, however, mental changes are often irreversible.

❏❏ **When does alcoholic ketoacidosis commonly occur?**

It usually occurs in chronic alcoholics after an interval of binge drinking followed by one to three days of protracted vomiting, abstinence and decreased food intake.

❏❏ **ECG changes associated with tricyclic antidepressant overdose?**

Prolongation of the PR, QRS and QT interval, as well as conduction defects such as bundle branch block, typically on the right.

❏❏ **What are the basic treatments for TCA overdose?**

Seizures   (MUST be stopped quickly 2° to acidosis! Paralyze if you have to.)
    Alkalinization
    Diazepam
    Phenobarbital
    Phenytoin (Some evidence suggests decreased effect in setting of CA OD)

Tachycardia
    Alkalinization, saline

Blocks and Ventricular Arrhythmias
    Alkalinization
    Phenytoin (Unproved)
    Lidocaine (Unstudied)

Hypotension
    Alkalinization
    Saline
    Pressors: NE, Epi
    Cardiopulmonary bypass or balloon pump assist
    Charcoal hemoperfusion

❏❏ **What drugs should be avoided in treatment of TCA overdose?**

Absolute - Procainamide. Also quinidine, disopyramide, flumazenil.

Relative - Corticosteroids, dopamine, isoproterenol, negative inotropes such as Ca- channel and ß-blockers, amiodarone, encainide and flecainide.

❏❏ **What dose of ASA will cause mild to moderate toxicity?**

200 - 300 mg/kg. Greater than 500 mg/kg is potentially lethal.

❏❏ **What is the ferric chloride test and what toxic ingestion does it detect?**

Add a few drops of 10% ferric chloride solution to a few drops of urine. Violet purple color indicates presence of salicylic acid. Ketones or phenothiazines can lead to false positive results.

❏❏ **What is the treatment of lithium overdose?**

Saline diuresis and hemodialysis.

❏❏ **What is the treatment for chloral hydrate overdose?**

Hemodialysis and/or charcoal hemoperfusion will clear the active metabolite, trichloroethanol.

❏❏ **What are the common effects of barbiturate overdose?**

Hypothermia, hyperventilation, venodilation with hypotension and
negative inotropic effect on the myocardium. Clear vesicles and bullae may also be seen.

❏❏ **What is the pediatric dose of naloxone?**

0.01 mg/kg to a dose of 0.8 mg, may repeat.

❏❏ **What electrolyte abnormality is commonly seen in salicylate toxicity?**

Hypokalemia.

❏❏ **What is the treatment for acetaminophen overdose?**

Charcoal, cathartics and N-acetylcysteine.

❏❏ **What electrolyte abnormality may mimic the signs and symptoms of hypocalcemia?**

Hypomagnesemia.

❏❏ **What are some key signs and symptoms of Thrombotic Thrombocytopenic Purpura (TTP).**

Thrombocytopenia, purpura, microangiopathic hemolytic anemia.
Presents with fever, fluctuating neurologic signs and renal complications. Untreated, the disease is almost uniformly fatal. Therapy includes steroids, splenectomy, plasmapheresis and exchange, and antiplatelet agents such as dipyridamole and aspirin.

❏❏ **How does a patient present with Boerhaave's syndrome?**

Boerhaave's syndrome is spontaneous esophageal perforation. It usually occurs after forceful vomiting. The patient suffers an acute collapse, chest and abdominal pain. A left pleural effusion is seen in 90 percent of patients on chest x-ray and most have mediastinal emphysema.

❏❏ **In what type of a patient is Staphylococcal pneumonia likely?**

Hospitalized, debilitated and drug abusing patients.

❏❏ **How low does the platelet count drop before spontaneous bleeding occurs .**

Below 50,000 per cubic millimeter spontaneous bleeding may occur.
CNS bleeds usually do not occur until counts drop below 10,000 per cubic millimeter.

❏❏ **What factors affect the prothrombin time (PT)? Which pathway is this?**

I, II, V, VII, and X. 125710.
Extrinsic.
PT is normal in hemophilia.
A normal PTT and increased PT suggests warfarin therapy, vitamin K deficiency, or liver disease.

❏❏ **What factors affect the partial thromboplastin time (PTT)? Which pathway is affected?**

VIII, IX, or XI. 8911.
Intrinsic.
Heparin increases PTT.

❏❏ **What affect will heparin or warfarin overdose have on the PT and PTT?**

Both cause increases in PT and PTT in excessive doses.

❏❏ **What are the five key lab findings in DIC?**

Increased PT, PTT, and fibrin degradation products.
Decreased fibrinogen and platelet levels.

❏❏ **In the thrombocytopenic patient, one unit of platelets will raise the platelet count by about how much?**

One unit raises the platelet count by $\approx 10,000 / mm^3$.

❏❏ **What are the classic findings of shaken baby syndrome?**

Failure to thrive, lethargy.
Seizures.
Retinal hemorrhages.
CT may show subarachnoid hemorrhage or subdural hematoma from torn bridging veins.

❏❏ **Define spondylolysis.**

Spondylolysis is a defect in the pars interarticularis.

❏❏ **Define spondylolisthesis.**

Spondylolisthesis is forward movement of one vertebral body on the vertebra below it.

❏❏ **Define spondylosis.**

Spondylosis is degenerative change in the vertebrae which may also include osteophyte formation at the disk spaces.

❏❏ **T/F - High fever in neonates with bacterial pneumonia usually <u>follows</u> a period of general fussiness and decreased feeding.**

True.

❏❏ **Chlamydia pneumonia is more likely to occur in the neonate after how many weeks of age?**

Three weeks.

❏❏ **Conjunctivitis is an associated finding in about what percentage of neonates with Chlamydia pneumonia?**

About 50%.

❏❏ **Neonates with Chlamydia pneumonia are usually tachypneic with a bad cough; are they febrile?**

Usually not.

❏❏ **What is the immediate treatment for cord prolapse?**

Displace the head cephalad.

❏❏ **What is the most common bacterium causing septic arthritis of the hip?**

Staphylococcus aureus.

❏❏ **What nerve may be injured in a distal femoral fracture?**

Peroneal nerve.

❑❑ **Newborns should stop losing weight by how many days after birth?**

About 6 days.

❑❑ **T/F - Stool color of neonates can be an important sign.**

False; with the exception of presence of blood, stool color is insignificant.

❑❑ **What is the difference between vomiting and regurgitation?**

Very little once it's on you!
Vomiting follows from forceful diaphragmatic and abdominal muscle contraction. Regurgitation occurs without effort.

❑❑ **Is regurgitation dangerous in an otherwise thriving neonate?**

No.
It can be dangerous for newborns with failure to thrive or respiratory problems and it may be associated with chronic aspiration.

❑❑ **Projectile vomiting in the neonate is often associated with pyloric stenosis. When this is the case, such vomiting becomes a prominent sign after how many weeks of age?**

About two to three weeks.

❑❑ **What is the name for diarrhea associated with sepsis, otitis media, UTI or other systemic disease?**

Parenteral diarrhea.

❑❑ **Infectious diarrhea is most commonly viral. What are the two <u>most</u> <u>common</u> viruses?**

Rotavirus and Norwalk virus.

❑❑ **T/F - Bacterial and parasitic etiologies of diarrhea in the neonate are rare.**

True.

❑❑ **What are some entities in the differential diagnosis of bloody diarrhea in the neonate?**

Necrotizing enterocolitis, bacterial enteritis, iatrogenic causes secondary to antibiotics, milk allergy.

❑❑ **Neonates with necrotizing enterocolitis are sick; what are some of the signs of sepsis to look for?**

Poor feeding, lethargy, fever, jaundice, abdominal distention, and poor color.

❑❑ **What should be considered in the case of a neonate who has never passed stool?**

Meconium ileus or plug, Hirschsprung's disease, intestinal stenosis or atresia.

❑❑ **Anal stenosis, hypothyroidism and Hirschsprung's disease can all present with what clinical sign?**

Constipation that was not initially present but which had onset prior to one month of age.

❑❑ **Describe the signs and symptoms, and x-ray tests, for diagnosing a slipped capital femoral epiphysis.**

Gradual onset of hip pain and stiffness with restriction of internal rotation; patient may walk with a limp. X-ray analysis should include both the anterior-posterior and lateral views of both hips. The slip of the epiphyseal plate posteriorly is best seen on the lateral view.

❏❏ **Describe the signs and symptoms of a patient with chondromalacia patellae.**

Chondromalacia patellae typically occurs in young, active females.
The pain is localized to the knee. There is no effusion and no history of trauma. Patella compression test is usually positive.

❏❏ **Describe the signs and symptoms of tarsal tunnel syndrome.**

Insidious onset of paresthesia, burning pain and numbness on the plantar surface of the foot. Pain radiates superiorly along the medial side of the calf. Rest decreases pain.

❏❏ **What is the cause of swimmer's itch (Schistosome dermatitis)?**

An invading cercariae.

❏❏ **Vector of malaria?**

Anopheles mosquito.

❏❏ **Insect vector of trypanosomiasis?**

Tsetse fly.

❏❏ **Infectious agent of elephantiasis?**

Nematode microfilaria.

❏❏ **What is the vector that transmits Chagas' disease (Trypanosoma Cruzi)?**

Reduviid (Assassin or kissing bug).

❏❏ **Cysticercosis is associated with:**

New onset seizure.

❏❏ **Hookworm is associated with what sort of anemia?**

Iron deficiency anemia.

❏❏ **Fish tapeworm (Diphyllobothrium latum) is associated with:**

Pernicious anemia.

❏❏ **Onchocerciasis (from Onchocerca volvalas) is associated with what visual deficit?**

Blindness.

❏❏ **Chagas' disease is associated with:**

Acute myocarditis. Trypanosoma Cruzi invades the myocardium resulting in myocarditis. Conduction defects may occur.

❏❏ **Roundworm is associated with:**

Small bowel obstruction.

❑❑ **Describe the presentation of a patient with post-extraction alveolitis:**

Pain of "dry socket" occurs on the 2nd or 3rd day after extraction.

❑❑ **Ludwig's angina typically involves what spaces in the head?**

The submental, the sublingual and submandibular spaces.

❑❑ **What are the signs and symptoms of a peritonsillar abscess?**

Sore throat, dysarthria (hot potato voice), odynophagia, ipsilateral otalgia, low grade fever, trismus, and uvular displacement.

❑❑ **What is the presentation of a patient with diphtheria?**

Sore throat, dysphagia, fever and tachycardia. A dirty tough gray fibrinous membrane that may be so firmly adherent that removal causes bleeding may be present in the oropharynx.
Corynebacterium diphtheriae exotoxin acts directly on cardiac, renal and nervous systems. Sure, it can cause ocular bulbar paralysis that may suggest botulism or, perhaps, myasthenia gravis.
The exotoxin may also cause flaccid limb weakness. Of note, such weakness may also include decreased or absent DTRs, a finding usually suggestive of Guillain-Barré or of tick paralysis (Dermacentor andersoni neurotoxin).

❑❑ **How does a patient present with a retropharyngeal abscess?**

Patients typically prefer a supine position. Retropharyngeal abscesses are common under 3 years of age. On examination, the uvula and tonsil are displaced away from the abscess. Soft tissue swelling and forward displacement of the larynx are present. Soft tissue x-ray films of the neck may assist in the diagnosis.

❑❑ **How does an adult with epiglottitis present?**

Pharyngitis and dysphagia are prominent symptoms. Adenopathy is uncommon. The patient may have a muffled voice and speak softly; hoarseness is rare. Pharyngitis is present and pain is out of proportion to objective findings.

❑❑ **What are the two most common pathogens in adult acute sinusitis?**

Streptococcus pneumoniae and Hemophilus influenzae.

❑❑ **What is rhinocerebral phycomycosis?**

Rhinocerebral phycomycosis, also known as mucormycosis, is a fungal infection typically seen in diabetic patients while in ketoacidosis, and in immunocompromised patients. The disease is rapidly fatal if not recognized and treated quickly. Treatment includes antifungal drugs and surgical debridement.

❑❑ **Where is the typical location of a Mallory-Weiss tear?**

The laceration typically occurs in the cardioesophageal region in the stomach, below the gastroesophageal junction. The bleeding usually stops spontaneously and does not typically require surgery. It can be diagnosed by endoscopy. It is associated with hiatal hernia.

❑❑ **Magnesium containing antacids may cause:**

Diarrhea.

❑❑ **Aluminum containing antacids may cause:**

Constipation.

❏❏ **What is the treatment for hepatic encephalopathy?**

Lactulose and poor per rectum neomycin.

❏❏ **When does an elevation of HBsAg occur in relation to symptoms of Hepatitis B?**

HBsAg always rises before clinical symptoms of hepatitis B.

❏❏ **Is hepatitis A associated with jaundice?**

Typically not, as more than 50 percent of the population have serologic evidence for hepatitis and do not recall being symptomatic.

❏❏ **Describe a patient with intussusception.**

Patients with intussusception are most likely very young. 70 percent occur within the first year of life. In children, the cause is thought to be secondary to lymphoid tissue at the ileocecal valve, whereas in adults, it is thought to be caused by local lesions, Meckel's diverticulum, or tumor. On exam, bowel sounds are usually normal. Intussusception typically involves the terminal ileum.   Meckel's diverticulum is the single most common intrinsic bowel lesion involved.

❏❏ **Are adhesions a common cause of bowel obstruction in the large bowel?**

No. They are very common in the small bowel, but do not be fooled; they are extremely uncommon in large bowel obstructions.

❏❏ **Should salmonella be treated?**

Only if symptomatic infection persists. Treat with ampicillin, TMP/SMX, or chloramphenicol.

❏❏ **What is the most common cause of acute food-borne disease?**

Staph aureus and the enterotoxins it produces.

❏❏ **What are the common features of Vibrio parahaemolyticus?**

Organism associated with oysters, clams and crabs.
Symptoms include cramps, vomiting, dysentery and explosive diarrhea. Severe infections are treated with tetracycline and chloramphenicol.

❏❏ **What types of anorectal abscesses can be drained in the emergency department?**

Perianal, submucosal, and pilonidal abscesses can be drained in the emergency department.
Ischiorectal and supralevator abscesses need to be drained in the operating room.

❏❏ **Painful, bright red rectal bleeding is most often due to:**

Anal fissure.
External hemorrhoids present with acute painful thrombosis and are not typically associated with constant, bright red bleeding.
Internal hemorrhoids present with <u>painless</u> bright red bleeding, usually with defecation.

❏❏ **Where is the narrowest part of the ureter?**

The ureterovesicular junction.

❏❏ **What percentage of kidney stones are radiopaque?**

90 percent. Most are made of calcium oxalate.

❑❑ **In a patient with acute testicular pain, relief of pain with elevation of the scrotum (Prehn's sign) is classically associated with:**

Epididymitis.

❑❑ **Drug of choice for treating urinary tract infection due to Proteus mirabilis?**

Ampicillin. This is common in young boys.

❑❑ **Most common organism causing epididymitis in a 20 year old?**

Chlamydia trachomatis.

❑❑ **How should hydralazine be dosed for a preeclamptic patient?**

Hydralazine is given in 5 mg boluses every 20 minutes until adequate BP control is achieved or a total of 20 mg is reached.

❑❑ **What is the antidote of overdose of magnesium sulfate?**

Calcium gluconate infusion.

❑❑ **In an ectopic pregnancy, is an adnexal mass a common finding?**

No. An adnexal mass is actually found in less than 50 percent of cases. Abdominal pain is the most frequent sign. Amenorrhea is the second most common sign.

❑❑ **As pCO_2 increases, pH will decrease. By how much is the pH expected to decrease for every 10 mm Hg increase in pCO_2?**

pH decreases by 0.08 units for each increase of 10 mm of pCO_2.

❑❑ **How much protamine is required to neutralize 100 units of heparin?**

1 mg of protamine will neutralize $\approx$ 100 units of heparin. The maximum dose of protamine is 100 mg.

❑❑ **What is the <u>most common</u> symptom of a PE?**

Chest Pain (88%)
Dyspnea (84%)

❑❑ **What is the <u>most common</u> sign of a PE?**

Tachypnea (92%)
Rales (58%)

❑❑ **What is the <u>most common</u> radiographic finding of a PE?**

An elevated hemidiaphragm (41%).

❑❑ **What is the <u>most common</u> ECG finding of a PE?**

T-wave inversion (42%)

❑❑ **Of patients with a PE, what percentage have a normal ECG?**

Normal (13%).

❑❑ **Of patients with a PE, what percentage of ECG's show the classic $S_1 Q_3 T_3$ pattern?**

$S_1 Q_3 T_3$ (12%), incidence is 18% with massive PE

❑❑ **What test is most sensitive for evaluating a PE?**

Perfusion scan is the <u>most</u> <u>sensitive</u> test, even more so than a pulmonary angiogram. Unfortunately, it is not a specific test, as 5 percent of normal volunteers will have an abnormal scan, and virtually any pulmonary pathology will produce an abnormal scan.

❑❑ **What organisms are most commonly present in a pulmonary abscess?**

Mixed anaerobes.

❑❑ **What are some causes of thoracic outlet syndrome?**

Compression of the subclavian artery by an anomalous cervical rib, compression of the neurovascular bundle as it passes through the interscalene triangle, and compression of the neurovascular bundle in the retroclavicular space anterior to the first rib when the arms are hyperabducted. Symptoms are typically produced when the shoulders are moved backward and downward.

The <u>most</u> <u>common</u> cause is a cervical rib.

❑❑ **What is the <u>most</u> <u>common</u> cause of endocarditis in IV drug abusers?**

Staphylococcus aureus, most commonly involving the tricuspid valve.

❑❑ **What are the classic signs and symptoms of aortic stenosis?**

Left heart failure, angina and exertional syncope.

❑❑ **What patient position will enhance the murmur of mitral stenosis?**

Left lateral decubitus.

❑❑ **What is optimal patient position and maneuver for auscultation of aortic insufficiency?**

Have the patient sit up and lean forward with the hands tightly clasped. During exhalation, listen at the left sternal border.

❑❑ **What murmurs will the Valsalva maneuver increase?**

Only IHSS. All other murmurs are diminished.

❑❑ **What is the most common valvular disorder in the United States?**

Mitral valve prolapse.

❑❑ **What is the most common cause of endocarditis in late onset prosthetic valve endocarditis?**

Streptococcus viridans.

❑❑ **Symptoms of endocarditis?**

Fever, chills, malaise, anorexia, weight loss, back pain, myalgia, arthralgia, chest pain, dyspnea, edema, headache, stiff neck, mental status changes, focal neurologic complaints, extremity pain, paresthesia, hematuria and abdominal pain.

❑❑ **Key physical finding of "malignant" hypertension?**

Papilledema.

❑❑ **Key diagnostic features of coarctation of the aorta?**

Rib notching seen on x-ray. Significant differences in the blood pressure between the upper and lower extremities.

❑❑ **What is an interesting diagnostic feature of aortic regurgitation?**

Head bobbing.

❑❑ **What is the most common arrhythmia associated with digitalis?**

PVC (60%).
Ectopic SVT (25%).
AV Block (20%).

❑❑ **What effect does furosemide have on calcium excretion?**

Furosemide causes increased calcium excretion in the urine.

❑❑ **What is the <u>most</u> <u>common</u> arrhythmia in mitral stenosis?**

Atrial fibrillation.

❑❑ **The <u>most</u> <u>common</u> cause of CHF in an adult is:**

Hypertension.

❑❑ **What is the differential diagnosis of pulmonary edema with a normal size heart?**

Constrictive pericarditis, massive MI, non-cardiogenic pulmonary edema, and mitral stenosis (not mitral regurgitation).

❑❑ **How does dobutamine differ from dopamine?**

Dobutamine decreases afterload with less tendency to cause tachycardia.

❑❑ **Describe Kerley A and Kerley B lines.**

Kerley A lines are straight, non-branching lines in the upper lung fields.

Kerley B lines are horizontal, non-branching lines at the periphery of the lower lung fields.

❑❑ **Does nifedipine typically effect preload or afterload?**

Nifedipine is a vasodilator whose primary effects are on afterload reduction.

❑❑ **What effect does the Valsalva maneuver have on the heart?**

Valsalva decreases blood return to both the right and left ventricles. All murmurs decrease in intensity except IHSS.

❑❑ **Does prednisone cross the placenta?**

No. Prednisone is metabolized through prednisolone which does not cross the placenta.

❑❑ **You see a patient with a severe high concentration burn of hydrofluoric acid burn. How do you treat this patient?**

In addition to topical jelly and cutaneous injections of calcium gluconate, provide IV treatment with 10 cc. of 10% Calcium Gluconate (not calcium chloride) diluted in 50 cc. of D_5W. This is given via a pump over 4 h.

❑❑ **How should an ocular burn secondary to hydrofluoric acid be treated?**

Use calcium gluconate in a 1% solution mixed with saline and irrigate the eyes with this solution. The solution is made by diluting one part of standard 10% calcium gluconate solution with ten parts of saline which produces a 1% solution.

❑❑ **What electrolyte is depleted in a victim of a hydrofluoric acid burn?**

Hydrofluoric acid results in <u>hypocalcemia</u>. Patients may require calcium replacement. Keep in mind that normal signs and symptoms of hypocalcemia such as Chvostek's sign do not typically appear with hypocalcemia secondary to HF.

❑❑ **A 35 y old female presents with altered mental status and a temperature of 105 °F. The patient's muscles are rigid and she feels very hot in the trunk but her extremities are cool. What diagnosis is likely?**

Neuroleptic malignant syndrome. High fever and muscle rigidity should make you suspect a diagnosis of neuroleptic malignant syndrome. Check the CPK.

❑❑ **How should a patient with neuroleptic malignant syndrome be treated?**

1) Ice packs to the groin and axilla.
2) Cooling blankets.
3) Fan.
4) Water mist evaporation.
5) Dantrolene at an IV rate of 0.8 to 3 mg/kg IV q 6 hours to a total of 10 mg/kg.

❑❑ **How should a patient with a black widow spider bite be treated?**

1) Consider antivenin.
2) Consider IV calcium gluconate.
3) Consider IV opiates plus IV benzodiazepines.

❑❑ **T/F - Centruroides scorpion antivenin should be administered for all Centruroides envenomations.**

NOT. False, false.
Scorpion antivenin is rarely necessary and is only typically used in children who have a severe (Grade IV) envenomation with peripheral motor and cranial nerve involvement. It is most important to use Centruroides antivenin only in severe cases as serum sickness or rash after administration is very common. In fact, as many as 60% of patients develop a rash or serum sickness secondary to this antivenin.

❑❑ **What is a significant complication of scorpion envenomation?**

Rhabdomyolysis.

❑❑ **In what states could a scorpion bite be deadly?**

Centruroides, which is the most toxic of scorpion stings, is only found in <u>Arizona</u>, California, Texas and New Mexico.

❑❑ **An elderly patient presents with the complaint of seeing halos around lights. What diagnosis is suspected?**

Glaucoma. Another presenting complaint of glaucoma is blurred vision. Also, consider digitalis toxicity.

❑❑ **A patient presents with back pain and complaints of incontinence. On exam, loss of anal reflex, and decreased sphincter tone is noted. What is your diagnosis?**

Cauda equina syndrome. The most consistent finding with cauda equina syndrome is <u>urinary retention</u>. On physical exam, expect saddle anesthesia, that is, numbness over the posterior superior thighs as well as numbness of the buttocks and perineum.

❑❑ **What is the most common site of lumbar disc herniations?**

98% of clinically important lumbar disc herniations are at the L4-5 or L5-S1 intervertebral levels.

Evaluate by checking for weakness of ankle and great toe dorsiflexors (L5). Also check pinprick sensation over the medial aspect of the foot (L5) and the lateral portion of the feet (S1).

❑❑ **What WBC count is expected during pregnancy?**

WBC counts of 15,000 to 20,000 are considered normal in pregnancy.

❑❑ **A trauma patient has a closed head injury with suspected elevated intracranial pressure. What treatments should be considered?**

1) Paralyze the patient and hyperventilate.
2) Maintain hypovolemia (fluid restrict).
3) Elevate the head of the bed to 30 degrees after the C-spine has been cleared.
4) Consider mannitol 500 ml. of a 20% solution over 20 minutes for a 70 kilogram adult.

Use of diuretics like furosemide is controversial. Steroids are no longer recommended. Barbiturate use is also not recommended. Mannitol use is also losing favor.

❑❑ **When monitoring a pregnant female trauma victim, who's vital signs are most sensitive - the mother's or those of the fetus?**

The fetal heart rate is more sensitive to inadequate resuscitation. Remember that the mother may lose 10 to 20% of her blood volume without change in vital signs whereas the baby's heart rate may increase or decrease above 160 or below 120 indicating significant fetal distress. Most common pitfall is failure to adequately resuscitate the mother!

❑❑ **What two findings on physical exam are indicative of uterine rupture?**

Loss of uterine contour and palpable fetal part.

❑❑ **What physical exam findings may be discovered in abruptio placenta?**

Rapidly increasing fundal height secondary to bleeding into the uterus or a higher than expected fundal height.

❑❑ **What is the <u>number one</u> risk factor for uterine rupture?**

Previous cesarean section.

❑❑ **How should a diagnostic peritoneal lavage be performed for a pregnant patient?**

Use an open supraumbilical approach. Always make sure an NG tube and Foley are in place.

❑❑ **A gravid woman is sent to the OB floor for cardiotocographic monitoring after a motor vehicle accident. What findings will suggest problems with the fetus?**

On the OB floor, they will look for uterine contractions at a rate of greater than 8 per minute. They will also watch for late decelerations. Late deceleration are a slowing of the fetal heart rate near the end of a contraction.

❏❏ **An unconscious, 60 y old patient presents to the ED with a head injury. An ECG shows significant ST segment elevation. What is your concern?**

Although MI should be considered, don't forget the possibility of an intracerebral hemorrhage. This may also cause significant ST segment elevation.

❏❏ **Why should the use of atropine be considered in a pediatric patient prior to intubation?**

Many pediatric patients develop bradycardia associated with intubation. This can be prevented by pre-treatment with atropine (dose is 0.01 mg/kg).

❏❏ **What size tracheotomy tube is appropriate for an adult female and for an adult male?**

An adult female generally requires #4 tracheostomy tube and an adult male requires a #5.

❏❏ **After use of ketamine in a pediatric patient, what effects are expected?**

The child will have eyes wide open with a glassy stare, nystagmus, hyperemic flush and hypersalivation. There will also be a slight rise in the heart rate. A very rare complication of ketamine use is laryngospasm. Hallucinations are a common side-effect in children over the age of 10; as a consequence, ketamine should be restricted to use only in patients under the age of 10.

Ketamine may also cause sympathetic stimulation which increases intracranial pressure, and may cause random movements of the head and extremities. It is thus not a good sedative for children going to CT scan.

❏❏ **Contraindications to TAC?**

Mucus membranes, burns, and large abrasions. TAC used on the tongue and mucus membranes has led to status epilepticus and patient death.

❏❏ **Why are quinolones contraindicated in children?**

Quinolones impair cartilage growth.

❏❏ **A patient presents with a symmetric weakness which has been progressive over several days to weeks and has associated paresthesia. Diminished reflexes are noted. Diagnosis?**

Guillain-Barré syndrome. Other signs and symptoms are diminished reflexes, minimal loss of sensation, paresthesias, and leg weakness.

❏❏ **How is Guillain-Barré syndrome diagnosed in the ED?**

Suspect the diagnosis based on signs and symptoms, but confirmation requires nerve conduction studies performed as an inpatient.

❏❏ **What is the dose of acyclovir (Zovirax) used to treat herpes zoster infections in an immunocompetent adult?**

800 mg. po. five times per day for 7 to 10 days.
For herpes simplex genitalis, the dose is much lower, 200 mg. po. five times a day for ten days!

❏❏ **A patient is brought to the ED after exposure to ammonia gas. What are your chief concerns?**

Ammonia gas affects the upper respiratory tract and may cause significant laryngeal and tracheal edema. Administer warm humidified O_2 to soothe the bronchial tract. Bronchodilators may also be given by nebulization for bronchospasm. Be ready to intubate if severe upper airway edema occurs.

❏❏ What signs and symptoms would lead to consideration of hyperbaric oxygen treatment for a patient with CO poisoning?

History of, or current, unconsciousness, arrhythmia or ischemia, neurologic impairment greater than a mild headache, and/or a carboxyhemoglobin level over 40%. Some now recommend tx for levels greater than 25% and greater than 15% for a gravid woman.

❏❏ What are the indications for giving digitalis specific Fab?

Ventricular arrhythmias.

$K^+ > 5.5$ mEq/L.
Unresponsive bradyarrhythmias.

Some authors refer to an ingestion of more than 0.3 mg/kg as requiring Fab (Digibind).
The dose of Fab is:

   # vials required = 1.33 x mg ingested,

or   use formula to determine dose based on serum digoxin level,
or   give 10 vials (40 mg Fab each) if amount ingested is not known.

Adolescents and children have an even higher sensitivity to the serious complications of digoxin overdose and may need Fab therapy with ingestion of less than the recommended level of 0.3 mg. per kilogram.

Remember - in an acute overdose situation, the serum level of digitalis is unreliable in evaluating toxicity. Digitalis levels typically only become accurate after 4 to 6 hours; this is too long to wait for treatment.

❏❏ You give digoxin specific antibody (Fab) to a digoxin-toxic patient with an elevated digoxin level. A repeat digoxin level is obtained after this treatment and it is much <u>higher</u> than the previous level! What gives? Didn't the Fab work?

Digoxin assay measures free <u>and</u> bound digoxin, the latter increases ≈ 15 x via binding to Fab.

❏❏ What electrolyte change is expected with a serious digoxin ingestion?

Expect hyperkalemia. After Fab, potassium level may drop quickly and the patient may become hypokalemic. Monitor carefully.

❏❏ A near drowning victim is comatose and intubated with a diagnosis of severe pulmonary edema. What specific pulmonary treatment should be provided in the Emergency Department?

It is important to give these patients PEEP early. PEEP will decrease intrapulmonary shunting and prevent terminal airway closure.

Great quotes series:

   "Victory at all costs, victory in spite of all terror, victory however long and hard the road may be; for without victory there is no survival."

                    Sir Winston Leonard Churchill, Speech, House of Commons, 13 May, 1940.

❏❏ There are four types of hypersensitivity reactions. Name them in order:

Hypersensitivity Reaction	Mediator	Example
Type 1 - Immediate	IgE binds allergen, includes mast cells and basophils	Food allergy. **Asthma in children.**
Type 2 - Cytotoxic	IgG & IgM antibody reactions to antigen on cell surface activates complement and killers	Blood transfusion rxn. ITP, hemolytic anemia. The least common rxn.
Type 3 - Immune complex, Arthrus	Complexes activate complement	Tetanus toxoid in sensitized persons. **Poststreptococcal glomerulonephritis.**
Type 4 - Cell mediated, delayed hypersensitivity	Activated T-lymphocytes	Skin tests

❏❏ **What distinguishes heat stroke from heat exhaustion?**

Heat exhaustion is progressive loss of electrolytes and body fluid depletion. Therapy is rehydration.

Heat stroke occurs when body temperature exceeds 42 °C and enzyme systems cease to function normally. As a result, there is necrosis, denaturing, and organ failure. Heat stroke requires much more aggressive treatment than simple fluid rehydration.

Remember - in patients with an altered sensorium and a core temperature above 42 °C, always suspect heat stroke. Half of patients will be diaphoretic.

❏❏ **What lab abnormalities may be found with heat stroke?**

High elevations in SGOT, SGPT and LDH.

❏❏ **How should a patient with heat stroke be treated?**

1) Cool the patient with lukewarm water and fans.
2) Pack the axillae, neck and groin with ice.
3) Give fluids cautiously as large boluses of fluids may precipitate pulmonary edema.
4) Treat shivering with chlorpromazine (Thorazine) 25 to 50 mg IV.

❏❏ **What complications can result from heat stroke?**

Renal failure, rhabdomyolysis, DIC, and seizures. Remember antipyretics will not help.

❏❏ **You are currently working locum tenens in <u>Arizona</u>, California, Texas and Mexico. As these states will have the deadly Centruroides scorpion, you are particularly concerned with scorpion sting treatment. How should a scorpion sting be treated?**

A scorpion sting should be treated with local ice compresses, analgesics, and perhaps antidote. Patients who have extremity jerking, blurred vision, slurred speech, or hypersalivation probably will require antivenin as this represents a Grade IV envenomation with peripheral motor and cranial nerve involvement.

❏❏ **Describe the appearance of a black widow spider bite?**

Two tiny red marks with surrounding erythematous patch. The initial bite may be painless. If a "pinprick" type bite is followed by abdominal cramps, think of a black widow spider. Exam reveals abdominal rigidity without true tenderness. Patients are restless and move about the gurney. Antivenin should probably be given to patients who are pregnant, younger than 16 and older than 65, and symptomatic. It also should be given to patients with underlying cardiac disease.

Other treatments include calcium, diazepam (Valium), or methocarbamol (Robaxin). Traditional treatment also includes calcium gluconate.

❏❏ **What conditions may make the end tidal CO_2 monitor inaccurate?**

Monitor may be falsely yellow due to contamination from acid dilutants and drugs such as lidocaine-HCl and epinephrine-HCl. Contamination with vomitus or acid dilutants may produce false readings.

❏❏ **You are having a hard time remembering which anesthetics are amides and which anesthetics are esters. What is a fairly easy way of telling these two classifications of anesthetics apart?**

The word amide has an "i" in it and so do the am"i"des (the "I" in "caine" doesn't count).

> Lidocaine (Xylocaine).
> Bupivacaine (Marcaine).
> Mepivacaine (Carbocaine).
>
> Esters on the other hand have no "i",
> Procaine (Novocain)
> Cocaine
> Tetracaine (Pontocaine)
> Benzocaine.

So remember - those with i's are amides. (In the first syllables only, the caines don't count! Thanks Pat!)

❏❏ **An elderly patient presents with sudden onset of severe abdominal pain followed by a forceful bowel movement. Diagnosis?**

Acute mesenteric ischemia. Keep in mind that abdominal series may be normal early in acute mesenteric ischemia. Possible late x-ray findings include:

Absent bowel gas, ileus, gas in the intestinal wall and thumb-printing of the intestinal mucosa.
In most cases, films are normal or not specifically suggestive. Expect heme-positive stools. Patients especially prone to mesenteric ischemia include those with CHF and chronic heart disease.

❏❏ **Under what conditions does neurogenic pulmonary edema occur?**

Neurogenic pulmonary edema is commonly associated with increased intracranial pressure. It is commonly seen with head trauma, subarachnoid hemorrhage, and even with seizures.

❏❏ **A patient had a very severe headache two days ago. The headache is now subsiding and physical exam is normal. Should the possibility of a subarachnoid hemorrhage be evaluated, and if so, how?**

Yes. CT.
However, a significant percentage of scans will be negative 48 hours after intracranial hemorrhage.
LP done 2 to 3 days after a bleed should still be positive and xanthochromia typically persists for 7 to 10 days.

❏❏ **What are the classic signs and symptoms of adrenal insufficiency?**

Fatigue, weakness, GI symptoms, anorexia, hypotension, and dehydration. May also have the classic clue - history of chronic steroid use. Order plasma cortisol level. Remember - cortisol level should be drawn prior to giving steroid therapy.

❏❏ **What is the initial treatment for adrenal insufficiency (don't worry about Rx while Dx)?**

Fluids and hydrocortisone IV in a typical dose of 100 to 200 mg.

❏❏ **An elderly patient presents with altered mental status, a history of IDDM and is hypoglycemic. Core temperature is 32 °C. What endocrinologic condition is likely?**

Myxedema coma.
Other clues to look for are history of thyroid surgery, hypothyroidism, and use of anti-thyroid medications.

❏❏ **What three conditions may cause a falsely low sodium concentration?**

Pseudohyponatremia may be caused by:

Hyperglycemia.
Hyperlipidemia.
Hyperproteinemia.

❏❏ **A patient presents with very low sodium and you suspect SIADH. What lab findings would confirm the diagnosis?**

Serum osmolality should be low and urine sodium and osmolality should both be high.
Remember - treatment of severe symptomatic hyponatremia includes a loop diuretic such as furosemide and simultaneous infusion of small boluses of 3% saline over 4 hours or 0.9 normal saline. Too rapid a correction of hyponatremia may result in neurologic sequelae.

❏❏ **A young competitive figure skater presents with a complaint of generalized weakness following practice. What might be the cause of this profound weakness?**

Hypokalemic "paralysis" is a cause of acute weakness.

❏❏ **How may hyperglycemic, hyperosmolar, non-ketotic coma be differentiated from DKA?**

Serum osmolality is higher in NKHC.
$NaHCO_3$ is normal in NKHC and depleted in DKA.
pH is usually maintained at >7.2 in NKHC.

❏❏ **How should non-ketotic hyperosmolar coma be treated?**

Fluids, fluids and more fluids. Such patients can be as much as 12 liters deficient. Give normal saline until adequate blood pressure and urinary output are established. Follow with half normal saline. When blood glucose falls to 250 to 300 mg, the solution should be changed to saline and glucose to avoid cerebral edema.
It is important to note that these patient's require very little insulin. Give as little as 5 to 10 units of insulin IV.
These patients are commonly deficient in potassium and will need 10 to 15 mEq per hour once urine flow has been established.
This disorder has a grave prognosis with up to a 50% mortality for severe cases.

❏❏ **T/F - Phenytoin is the drug of choice for a patient with non-ketotic hyperosmolar coma who experiences a seizure.**

False. Phenytoin is contraindicated in patients with hyperglycemic, hyperosmolar, non-ketotic coma. Drugs of choice for treating this seizure disorder are lorazepam (Ativan) or diazepam (Valium). Phenobarbital use is also appropriate.

❏❏ **For what types of overdoses is activated charcoal <u>not</u> indicated?**

Alcohol ingestion, electrolytes, heavy metals, lithium, hydrocarbons and caustic ingestions.

❏❏ **A young patient has a threatened abortion in the first trimester. Laboratory studies reveal she is Rh negative and her husband is Rh positive. Treatment?**

The patient will need 50 μg of Rh immunoglobulin (RhoGAM) IM. After the first trimester, the dose is increased to 300 μg IM.

❑❑ **What type of blood test is used to determine if a patient needs RhoGAM therapy?**

A Kleihauer-Betke checks for fetomaternal bleeding.

❑❑ **What are the signs and symptoms of preeclampsia?**

Upper abdominal pain, headache, visual complaints, cardiac decompensation, creatinine greater than 2, proteinuria greater than 100 mg per deciliter, and a blood pressure of greater than 160 mm Hg systolic or 110 mm Hg diastolic.

Preeclampsia is most common in nulliparous women late in pregnancy, typically after 20 weeks gestation. Look for edema, hypertension, and proteinuria to diagnose these patients.

The ED treatment for preeclampsia is IV hydralazine titrated to a blood pressure of 90 to 110 diastolic using 5 mg boluses q 20 to 30 minutes. Blood pressure must be lowered slowly to avoid compromising the uteroplacental blood flow. Patients with moderate to severe preeclampsia need IV magnesium (though its true utility is not well demonstrated).

❑❑ **What is the most commonly missed hip fracture?**

Femoral neck fracture.

❑❑ **Which is more common - a medial or a lateral tibial plateau fracture?**

The lateral tibial plateau is most commonly fractured. If AP and lateral films are negative, follow-up with oblique views if suspicious of a tibial plateau fracture.

❑❑ **What is the most commonly missed fracture in the elbow region?**

A radial head fracture. Like the navicular fracture, radiographic signs of a radial head fracture may not show up for days after the injury. A positive fat pad sign may be the only finding suggestive of this injury.

❑❑ **What are the two most common errors made in the intubation of a neonate?**

1) Placing the neck in hyperextension - this moves the cords even more anteriorly.
2) Inserting the laryngoscope too far.

❑❑ **What is the most common cause of food-borne <u>viral</u> gastroenteritis?**

Norwalk virus commonly found in shell fish.

❑❑ **What are the symptoms of "Chinese Restaurant" syndrome?**

Headache, dizziness, abdominal discomfort, facial flushing, and chest or facial burning. Symptoms typically start within an h of eating Chinese food.

❑❑ **A patient is in anaphylactic shock. She happens to be taking ß-blockers. She is not responding to epinephrine. What alternative agents might you consider?**

Norepinephrine, diphenhydramine, and glucagon.

❑❑ **A young boy is presented for evaluation after suffering a coral snake bite. He appears to be fine. What is appropriate management?**

Admit to the Intensive Care Unit and be ready for respiratory arrest. Coral snake bites appear minor at first. When symptoms begin, the patient may quickly progress to respiratory arrest. Coral snake venom is neurotoxic.

❑❑ **Describe the appearance of a coral snake.**

The snake is red, yellow and black. There is a black spot on the head. It is a round snake.

Coral snake bites typically do not cause immediate local pain whereas viper bites do.
(Red on yellow, kill a fellow!)

❏❏ **What type of rattlesnake bite leads to most deaths?**

Diamond back rattlesnake is the cause of nearly all lethal snake bites in the United States. The Diamond Back accounts for only 3% of snake bites seen. Treat with 10 to 20 vials of antivenin.

❏❏ **How does a stupid idiot recognize a pit viper?**

If he gets close enough, he will observe an elliptical pupil that looks like a football stood on end and the heat sensing pits.

❏❏ **What are some more common entities in the differential diagnosis of a limp or gait abnormality in a child?**

Legg-Calvé-Perthes disease (avascular necrosis of the femoral head), Osgood-Schlatter disease, avulsion of the tibial tubercle, infection, toxic transient tenosynovitis, patellofemoral subluxation, chondromalacia patella, slipped capital femoral epiphysis, septic arthritis, metatarsal fracture, proximal stress fracture, and toddler fracture (spiral tibia fracture).

❏❏ **What are the treatment recommendations for a patient with cluster headache?**

Treat similarly to migraine except skip ß-blockers, add O_2, try lidocaine 4% in the ipsilateral nostril.

❏❏ **What is the treatment for trigeminal neuralgia?**

Carbamazepine (Tegretol) 100 to 200 mg. tid. Obtain baseline CBC and platelet count before starting carbamazepine.

❏❏ **What is the only absolute contraindication to IVP?**

Profound hypotension - the kidneys won't be perfused. Two relative contraindications are renal insufficiency with a creatinine greater than 1.6 and a history of allergic reactions.

❏❏ **What markers indicate that an HIV positive patient is at increased risk for opportunistic infections like PCP?**

An absolute CD-4 count of less than 200.

CD-4 lymphocytic percentage less than 20%.

❏❏ **What are the National Institutes of Health treatment recommendations for spinal cord injury?**

Give high dose methylprednisolone (Solu-medrol) 30 mg/kg bolus over 15 minutes followed by 45 minutes normal saline drip. Over the subsequent 23 hours the patient should receive an infusion of 5.4 mg/kg/h of methylprednisolone.

❏❏ **What is the <u>most</u> <u>common</u> cause of small bowel obstruction in the surgically virgin abdomen?**

Incarcerated hernia.

❏❏ **A patient with a temperature of 29 °C develops V-fib. Is defibrillation likely to be successful?**

Defibrillation should be attempted but is unlikely to be successful at temperatures less than 29 °C.

❑❑ **T/F - The presentation of infectious endocarditis in an IV drug abusing patient does <u>not</u> usually include a murmur.**

TRUE. Less than 1/2 present with a murmur.

❑❑ **How is a retropharyngeal abscess diagnosed on plain films of a one year old child?**

Look for prevertebral thickening of the soft tissues. More than 3 mm suggests the possibility of a retropharyngeal abscess. Air/fluid level may be present.

If still unsure, order a CT of the neck. On CT scan retropharyngeal abscesses are just anterior to the vertebral column, will appear in only a few cuts, and appear as a gray area of about the same density as the spinal canal on CT.

❑❑ **In what age child is use of an <u>un</u>cuffed tube most appropriate?**

Children under 6 should receive an uncuffed tube.

❑❑ **A straight (Miller) blade is preferred for intubating children of less than what age?**

4 y.

❑❑ **What is the Parkland formula for treating a pediatric burn victim?**

Ringer's lactate 4 ml/ %BSA/ kg over 24 h with 1/2 given in first 8 h.

❑❑ **Large burns in children less than 5 years of age may require:**

Colloid (5% Albumin or FFP) at 1 ml/ %BSA/ kg/ d

❑❑ **A burned pediatric patient is receiving fluids per the Parkland formula. How much *additional* fluid should be given for maintenance requirements?**

    100 ml/kg/d for each kg up to 10 kg
+   50 ml/kg/d for each kg from 10-20 kg
+   20 ml/kg/d for each kg thereafter.

❑❑ **When examining a lateral adult C-spine film, the predental space, that is the area between the dens and the anterior arch of C1, looks particularly wide. What width space is normal for an adult?**

Normal is 2.5 to 3 mm.

If this width is greater than 3 mm, consider that the transverse ligament has ruptured or is at least lax.

❑❑ **What is the upper limit of normal of prevertebral soft tissue at C3?**

Anything greater than 5 mm suggests hematoma or fracture.

❑❑ **What disease is commonly associated with central retinal vein occlusion?**

Hypertension.

❑❑ **What are common eye findings in patients with AIDS?**

Cotton wool spots and CMV retinitis.

❑❑ **What is Purtscher's retinopathy?**

Purtscher's retinopathy is associated with thoracic injuries and broken bones. Findings include retinal hemorrhage and cotton wool spots.

❑❑ **What are the common features of central vertigo?**

   1) Symptoms are gradual and continuous.
   2) Focal signs may be present.
   3) Hearing loss is rare.
   4) Nausea and vomiting.

❑❑ **What are the signs and symptoms of peripheral vertigo?**

   1) Symptoms are usually <u>acute</u> and <u>intermittent</u>.
   2) Hearing loss is <u>common</u>, nausea and vomiting are severe.

❑❑ **In the evaluation of retropharyngeal abscess, what is the most common age of the patient, how do they present, what diagnostic tests are used in the evaluation, and what treatment modalities are recommended?**

   Retropharyngeal abscess is most commonly seen in children less than 4 years of age.

   Usual presentation is with dysphagia, muffled voice, stridor, sensation of a lump in the throat. Patients usually prefer to lie supine.

   Diagnosis is made with a soft tissue lateral neck film which may demonstrate edema and air/fluid levels. CT may be useful.

   Treatment includes airway, IV antibiotics and admission to the ICU. Intubation may rupture the abscess.

❑❑ **The causes of epiglottitis include:**

   Hemophilus influenzae is by far <u>most</u> <u>common.</u>
   Pneumococcus, staphylococcus, and Branhamella may also be causes.
   Presentation is most common among children within a few years of age 5.
   Dogma to <u>never</u> attempt direct visualization of epiglottis is being questioned.

❑❑ **What is the most common cause of Ludwig's angina?**

   Ludwig's angina is often associated with dental infections. Hemolytic streptococcus or mixed anaerobic infections are most common.

   It is commonly seen in elderly and debilitated patients. It often presents with sublingual pain, protruding tongue, dysphonia, brawny induration, and stridor.

❑❑ **A set of perennial favorites from our friend, René Le Fort! What is a Le Fort I fracture?**

   A maxilla fracture extending to the nasal aperture often missed on x-ray.

❑❑ **What is a Le Fort II fracture?**

   A "pyramidal" fracture extends vertically through the maxilla, through maxillary sinuses and infraorbital rims and across nasal bridge. Usually confirmed with Waters' view.

❑❑ **What is a Le Fort III fracture?**

   Craniofacial dysfunction includes fracture through the frontozygomatic suture lines, across the orbits and through the base of the nose. Le Fort I or II may also be present.

❑❑ **What is the usual cause of facial cellulitis in children less than 3 years of age?**

   H. influenzae.
   In adults- Staph or Strep.

❑❑ **A trauma patient presents with a complaint of severe burning pain in the upper extremities and associated neck pain. On physical exam, the patient has good strength in his upper extremities and no obvious neurologic deficits in the lower extremities. Although the C-spine series is negative, what problem is still suspected?**

Central cord syndrome. This injury is due to hyperextension of the spinal cord.

Diagnostic findings include upper extremity neurologic symptoms and minimal or no lower extremity symptoms.
Tingling, paresthesias, burning pain, and severe weakness or paralysis in the upper extremities with little or no symptoms in the lower extremities.

❑❑ **An asthmatic patient suddenly develops a supraventricular tachycardia. Blood pressure is normal and the QRS complex is also narrow. What therapy is most appropriate?**

Verapamil.

Avoid the use of adenosine as it is relatively contraindicated and may exacerbate bronchospasm in asthmatic patients. Also avoid ß-blockers.

❑❑ **How is a laryngeal fracture diagnosed on plain films?**

On a lateral soft tissue x-ray of the C-spine, check for retropharyngeal air, and elevation of the hyoid bone. The hyoid bone is usually at the level of C3 if there is no evidence of a laryngeal fracture.

Elevation of the hyoid bone above C3 suggests a laryngeal fracture.

❑❑ **Differentiate between a hypertensive emergency and a hypertensive urgency.**

Elevated BP + end organ damage = hypertensive emergency.
Elevated BP + no symptoms or signs of end organ damage = hypertensive urgency; usually DBP > 115 mm Hg. Requires acute treatment.

❑❑ **A patient presents with a history of forehead contusion. She cannot move her arms; lower extremity strength is intact. X-rays of the neck are normal. What is the suspected diagnosis?**

Central cord syndrome. We just did this!
Management includes maintaining C-spine precautions, CT or MRI of the C-spine and neurosurgical consultation.

❑❑ **What are the antibiotics of choice in a wound resulting from a skin diving incident?**

Ciprofloxacin or TMP/SMX.

❑❑ **How should a jelly fish sting be treated?**

Rinse with saline.
Apply 5% acetic acid (vinegar) locally to the wound for approximately 30 minutes. In addition, corticosteroid agents may be applied topically. No antibiotics are necessary.
Tetanus prophylaxis.
Chironex flexeri antivenin only for this coelenterate.

❑❑ **A young man was found on the street by police and is brought to the ED. He has a temperature of 105 °F, altered mental status and muscle rigidity. You find a bottle of thioridazine (Mellaril) in his pocket. What conditions should be considered?**

Meningitis, encephalitis, hyperthyroidism, anticholinergic or strychnine poisoning and heat stroke come to mind. Another disease that should be considered is neuroleptic malignant syndrome.

Patients may also have hypotension, hypertension, and tachycardia.

❑❑ **When does dysbaric air embolism typically occur?**

DAE always develops within minutes of surfacing after a dive. Symptoms are sudden and dramatic and include loss of consciousness, focal neurologic symptoms such as monoplegia, convulsions, blindness, confusion, and sensory disturbances.

Sudden loss of consciousness or other acute neurologic deficits immediately after surfacing is due to DAE unless proven otherwise. Treatment includes high flow oxygen and rapid transport for hyperbaric oxygen treatment.

❑❑ **A patient's blood gases reflect a mixed metabolic acidosis and respiratory alkalosis; what cause immediately comes to mind?**

Salicylate intoxication.

❑❑ **A two y old has jammed a pencil into her lateral soft palate. What complication might develop?**

Ischemic stroke is a complication of soft palate pencil injuries that results in contralateral hemiparesis.

❑❑ **What is the appropriate paralyzing agent to use when intubation is required in a seizing patient?**

Use pancuronium (Pavulon) as succinylcholine has greater tendency to increase serum potassium and to increase ICP.

❑❑ **Distinguish the key differences between strychnine and tetanus poisoning:**

Tetanus poisoning produces constant muscle tension whereas strychnine produces tetany and convulsions with episodes of relaxation between muscle contractions.

❑❑ **What is the common name for Dermacentor andersoni?**

Wood tick.

❑❑ **What neurologic disorder presents similarly to symptoms caused by Dermacentor andersoni (Wood Tick) bite?**

Guillain-Barré. Recall that tick paralysis may have decreased or absent DTRs as a clinical finding. Such DTRs may also be found associated with diphtheria exotoxin.

❑❑ **What nerve supplies taste to the anterior two thirds of the tongue, the lacrimal and salivary glands?**

Cranial nerve VII.

❑❑ **What disease is associated with anti-acetylcholine receptor antibodies that affect the post-synaptic neuromuscular site and is seen more commonly in females with a peak incidence in the third decade of life?**

Myasthenia gravis. 50% of myasthenia gravis patients have thymomas and 75% have lymphoid hyperplasia.

❑❑ **What antibiotics should be avoided in myasthenia gravis patients?**

Polymyxin and aminoglycosides have curare-like properties and may cause paralysis in these patients.

❑❑ **A baby presents to your emergency department with no facial movement, the lids sag and the child has a poor suck. She does not seem to move much and seems very weak. What causes do you consider?**

Myasthenia gravis or baby botulism.

❏❏ **A patient complains of pronounced weakness when attempting to climb stairs and even becomes tired when they do such simple tasks as brushing their teeth. Diagnosis?**

Myasthenia gravis.

❏❏ **What is the treatment for myasthenia gravis?**

Steroids, thymectomy, immunosuppressive drugs, plasmapheresis, and cholinergic agents such as pyridostigmine.

❏❏ **What disease is tick paralysis very similar to?**

It is very Guillain-Barré like.

❏❏ **Eaton-Lambert syndrome is associated with what class of diseases?**

Malignancies, particularly oat-cell carcinoma.
Symptoms include aching muscle pain and weakness (the latter usually less than associated with MG); cranial nerves are not usually involved.
Muscle strength may increase with repeated action in contradistinction to greater weakness with use encountered in MG.

❏❏ **What is a chalazion?**

This is a Meibomian gland granuloma.

❏❏ **How should a chalazion be treated?**

Surgical curettage.

❏❏ **Patient presents with eye pain. She has a constricted pupil, ciliary flush, and red injected sclera at the limbus. Diagnosis?**

Acute iritis.

❏❏ **A patient presents with loss of central vision. Likely diagnosis?**

A retrobulbar neuritis is likely. MS is associated with about 25% of cases of retrobulbar neuritis.

Macular degeneration and central retinal vein occlusion can also lead to loss of central vision.

❏❏ **I am used to treat acute angle closure glaucoma (and occasionally in vain attempts to treat retinal artery occlusion). I also play a role in treatment and prevention of acute mountain sickness. I decrease aqueous humor production via my mechanism of being a carbonic anhydrase inhibitor. What is my name?**

Acetazolamide (Diamox).

❏❏ **A patient presents with fever, neck pain or neck stiffness and trismus. Exam reveals pharyngeal edema with tonsil displacement and edema of the parotid area. Diagnosis?**

PARAPHARYNGEAL Abscess.

❏❏ **A patient presents with hearing loss, nystagmus, complaint of facial weakness, and diplopia. Vertigo is provoked with sudden movement. A lumbar puncture reveals elevated CNS protein. What diagnosis is suspected?**

An acoustic neuroma.

❏❏ **Can a parapharyngeal abscess present with an associated finding of edema in the area of the parotid gland?**

Yes.

❏❏ **In a trauma patient, facial dimpling of the cheek is associated with:**

Zygomatic arch fracture.

❏❏ **What x-rays should be ordered to diagnose a fracture of the zygoma?**

A jug handle, Water's view or submental view.

❏❏ **What are the key features of Stevens-Johnson Syndrome?**

It is a bullous form of erythema multiforme with involvement of mucous membranes. It may cause corneal ulcerations, anterior uveitis and blindness.

❏❏ **Blood is originating from a tooth after trauma. What Ellis classification?**

3.

❏❏ **What are the most common drugs causing TEN?**

Phenylbutazone, barbiturates, sulfa drugs, anti-epileptics and antibiotics.

❏❏ **Rhomboid shaped crystals from a joint aspiration are associated with:**

Pseudogout.

❏❏ **Needle shaped crystals are associated with:**

Gout.

❏❏ **What is the most common site of aseptic necrosis?**

The hip.

❏❏ **Acute treatment for gout?**

Colchicine, indomethacin and other NSAIDs.

❏❏ **Most common presentation of a Charcot's joint?**

A swollen ankle and a" bag of bones" appearance on x-ray.

❏❏ **On x-ray you see Charcot's joints.   Diagnosis?**

Diabetes.

❏❏ **What is the most common cause of Charcot's joint?**

Diabetic peripheral neuropathy.

❏❏ **What is the most common tendon affected in calcified tendonitis?**

The supraspinatus.

❏❏ **Which epicondyle is involved in tennis elbow?**

The lateral epicondyle.

❑❑ **What is the <u>most</u> <u>common</u> and second most common site of infectious arthritis?**

The knee is the most common and the hip is the second most common.
Staphylococcus is the <u>most</u> <u>common</u> cause.

❑❑ **At what cervical level is the hyoid bone normally found?**

The third cervical vertebra.
If the hyoid is above this level a laryngeal fracture should be suspected.

❑❑ **At what cervical level is the thyroid located?**

Level of the fourth cervical vertebra.

❑❑ **What is the most common site of cervical disc herniation?**

C5-C6. Patient will complain of bilateral shoulder pain.

❑❑ **What nerve is located in the tarsal tunnel?**

The tibial nerve.

❑❑ **A patient has difficulty squatting and arising. Likely spinal pathology?**

L4 root compression with involvement of quadriceps.
(Don't even *think about* X-linked Duchenne's muscular dystrophy!)

❑❑ **What STD pathogens cause *painful* ulcers?**

Type II Genital Herpes and chancroid.

STD	Ulcer	Node
Genital Herpes	**Painful**	Painful
Chancroid	**Painful**	Painful
Syphilis	Painless	Less Painful
Lymphogranuloma Venereum	Painless	Moderately

❑❑ **A patient presents with a complaint of pain at the site of the deltoid insertion with radiation into the back of the arm (C5 distribution). On exam, there is increased pain with active abduction from 70° - 120°. X-rays reveal calcification at the tendinous insertion of the greater tuberosity. Diagnosis?**

Supraspinatus tendonitis.

❑❑ **Absent knee jerk. What level?**

L4.

❑❑ **Absent Achilles reflex. What level?**

S1.

❑❑ **Paresthesia of the great toe. Level?**

L5.

❏❏ **Paresthesia of the little toe. Level?**

S1.

❏❏ **What is the most common site of compartment syndrome?**

Anterior compartment of the leg.

❏❏ **Describe the leg position associated with an anterosuperior hip dislocation.**

Anterosuperior - External rotation and slight abduction. In the pubic type, the hip is extended and in the iliac type, it is slightly flexed.

❏❏ **Describe the leg position associated with an obturator hip dislocation.**

In an obturator dislocation there is external rotation, flexion and abduction.

❏❏ **Posterior hip dislocation - leg position?**

Internal rotation, flexion and adducted. Most common type.

❏❏ **A patient in the ED cannot recall ever having a tetanus shot. The nurse gives him a tetanus shot. Later, he develops a hypersensitivity reaction and recalls that he recently had a tetanus shot. What type of reaction does he have?**

Type 3 - arthrus reaction.
Type 3 reactions are caused by immune complexes or antigen-antibody complexes that activate complement and platelets forming aggregates and complexes with IgE.

❏❏ **A positive TB test is what type of reaction?**

Type 4 - cell mediated, delayed hypersensitivity.
Type 4 reactions do not involve complement or antibodies.

❏❏ **What drugs commonly cause erythema multiforme?**

Carbamazepine, penicillin, sulfa, pyrazolone, phenytoin, barbiturates.

❏❏ **What <u>aerobe</u> is <u>most commonl</u>y found in cutaneous abscesses?**

Staphylococcus aureus.

❏❏ **What is the most common gram negative aerobe found in cutaneous abscesses?**

Proteus mirabilis.

❏❏ **Describe the Gram stain appearance of Staphylococcus aureus.**

Gram positive cocci in grape-like clusters.

❏❏ **What is the <u>most common</u> cause of cellulitis in children less than 3 years of age?**

Hemophilus influenzae.

❏❏ **What is the <u>most common</u> cause of cellulitis in the adult?**

Staphylococcus aureus.

❑❑ **What is the cause of erysipelas?**

Group A , ß-hemolytic streptococci.

❑❑ **How is erysipelas treated?**

Penicillin.

Erythromycin for penicillin allergic patients.

❑❑ **What is the most common cause of toxic shock syndrome?**

Staphylococci. Toxins C and F are the proteins that mediate toxic shock syndrome.

❑❑ **A child presents to the ED with a history of fever, conjunctival hyperemia, and erythema of the mucus membranes with desquamation. Diagnosis?**

Kawasaki's Disease. Remember - Kawasaki's Disease may have lesions resembling erythema multiforme.

❑❑ **Clostridium tetanus, a Gram and anaerobe, produces a neurotoxin. Is it an endotoxin or an exotoxin?**

Tetanospasmin is an exotoxin. Its major effect is prevention of transmission of inhibitory neurons in anterior horn cells resulting in motor system disinhibition.

❑❑ **What are some of the common causes of prerenal acute renal failure?**

Volume depletion and decreased effective volume (CHF, sepsis, cirrhosis).

❑❑ **What are the causes of acute renal failure which are renal in nature?**

Acute Tubular Necrosis, acute interstitial nephritis, acute glomerulonephritis and vascular disease.

❑❑ **What are the causes of post-renal failure?**

Ureteral and urethral obstruction.

❑❑ **What findings mark the presentation of a patient with rapidly progressive glomerulonephritis?**

Most common - hematuria.
Also edema (periorbital), HTN, ascites, pleural effusion, rales, and anuria.

❑❑ **What arrhythmia is frequently encountered during renal dialysis.**

Hypokalemia induced ventricular fibrillation.

❑❑ **In which trimester of pregnancy is UTI and pyelonephritis most common?**

Third.

❑❑ **What is inflammation of the foreskin called?**

Balanitis or balanoposthitis.

❑❑ **What is phimosis?**

A condition in which the foreskin cannot be retracted posterior to the glans. The preliminary treatment is a dorsal slit.

❑❑ **What is paraphimosis?**

A condition in which the foreskin is retracted posterior to the glands and cannot be advanced over the glans.

❑❑ **What are causes of priapism?**

Prolonged sex, leukemia, sickle cell trait and disease, blood dyscrasias, pelvic hematoma or neoplasm, syphilis, and urethritis.
Drugs - Phenothiazines, prazosin, tolbutamide, anticoagulants, corticosteroids.

❑❑ **What causes a green to gray frothy vaginal discharge with mild itching.**

Trichomonas vaginitis. On physical exam, the cervix may have a strawberry appearance (20%).

❑❑ **Describe the presentation of a patient with Gardnerella vaginitis?**

On physical exam, note a frothy, gray-white, fishy smelling vaginal discharge. Wet mount may show clue cells (clusters of bacilli on the surface of epithelial cells).

Sherlock Holmes always uses his magnifying lens to look for *Clues* in the *Garden*.

❑❑ **Do you know why I *hate* it when my foot falls asleep during the day?**

It'll be up all night!

❑❑ **Sulfamethoxazole may lead to hemolysis in a patient with:**

G6PD deficiency.

❑❑ **What disease is associated with <u>painless</u> bright red bleeding per vagina in the third trimester?**

Placenta previa.

❑❑ **<u>Painful</u> third trimester vaginal bleeding likely represents?**

Abruptio placenta.

❑❑ **What affect does pregnancy have on BUN and creatinine?**

Both the creatinine and BUN are decreased. This is as the result of increased renal blood flow and increased glomerular filtration rate.

❑❑ **When can one auscultate the fetal heart?**

Ultrasound-   6 weeks.

Doppler-   10 - 12 weeks.

Stethoscope-   18 - 20 weeks.

❑❑ **Describe a Brudzinski sign:**

Flexion of the neck produces flexion of the knees.

❑❑ **Describe Kernig's sign:**

Extension of the knees from the flexed thigh position results in strong passive resistance.

❑❑ **What is the normal opening pressure in a spinal tap?**

15 cm H_2O.

❑❑ **What is the normal CSF protein level?**

40 mg/dl

❑❑ **What opening pressure and protein level are expected in bacterial meningitis?**

Opening pressure of near 30 cm H_2O and protein level of greater than 150 mg/dl. Glucose level will drop with bacterial meningitis, with TB and with fungal infections.

❑❑ **What does the India ink test show?**

Cryptococcus neoformans.

❑❑ **What is the most significant pathophysiologic mechanism of death from cyclic antidepressants?**

Myocardial depression, including hypotension and conduction blocks.

❑❑ **Of patients who die from CA overdose, what percentage are awake and alert at the time of first prehospital contact?**

25%.

❑❑ **What are some common side effects of phenothiazine use?**

Malaise, hyperthermia, tachycardia, anticholinergic effects, and quinidine-like membrane stabilization. The most dangerous side effect is neuroleptic malignant syndrome.

❑❑ **How should stable ventricular tachyarrhythmias associated with phenothiazine overdose be treated?**

Lidocaine and phenytoin.

❑❑ **Which antibiotic may either increase or decrease lithium secretion?**

Tetracycline.

❑❑ **How is lithium overdose treated?**

Lavage, saline diuresis, furosemide, and hemodialysis.
Alkalinization *may* be appropriate.

❑❑ **Is phenobarbital more quickly metabolized by children or by adults?**

Adults. Neonates are especially slow at metabolizing phenobarbital.

❑❑ **How should barbiturate poisoning be treated?**

Supportive, charcoal, alkalinization of the urine, charcoal hemoperfusion or hemodialysis.

❑❑ **What drugs increase the half-life of phenytoin?**

Sulfonamides, isoniazid, dicumarol, and chloramphenicol.

❑❑ **What hypersensitivity skin rashes are noted with phenytoin use?**

Lupus-like and Stevens-Johnson syndrome.

❑❑ **What are the cardiac effects of phenytoin?**

Inhibits sodium channels, decreases the effective refractory period and automaticity in the Purkinje fibers. Little effect on QRS width or action potential duration.

❏❏ **What is the lethal dose of phenytoin?**

20 mg/kg.

❏❏ **What symptoms are expected with a phenytoin level of > 20, of > 30, and of > 40 μg/ml?**

> 20 - lateral gaze nystagmus.
> 30 - lateral gaze nystagmus plus increased vertical nystagmus with upward gaze.
> 40 - lethargy, confusion, dysarthrias, and psychosis.

❏❏ **In endocarditis (all comers), what is the most commonly involved cardiac valve?**

Mitral > Aortic > Tricuspid > Pulmonic.

❏❏ **Infectious endocarditis in an IV drug abuser most commonly affects which valve?**

#1 - Tricuspid.
#2 - Pulmonary.

❏❏ **What is the most common causative bacterium associated with right-sided endocarditis in IV drug abusers?**

S. aureus.
Left- sided endocarditis in IV drug abusers is likely due to E. coli, streptococcus, Klebsiella, Pseudomonas and Candida.

❏❏ **A heroin addict presents with pulmonary edema. What is the best treatment?**

Naloxone, O_2 and ventilatory support.
Don't bother using diuretics. This seems like a good test question.

❏❏ **What is the most common neurologic complication of IV drug abuse?**

Nontraumatic mononeuritis - painless weakness 2 -3 h after injection.

❏❏ **Name two frequently observed organisms causing septic arthritis in drug addicts.**

Serratiae and Pseudomonas.
These are rare causes in non-addicts.

❏❏ **An alcoholic patient presents with complaints of abdominal pain and blurred vision. The patient is very photophobic and blood gases reveal a metabolic acidosis. Diagnosis?**

Methanol poisoning. These patients may describe seeing something resembling a snowstorm.

❏❏ **What is the mechanism of action of clonidine?**

Clonidine is a central acting α-agonist. It leads to decreased sympathetic outflow and lowers catecholamine levels.

❏❏ **What is the lethal dose of methanol?**

30 ml.
Formate levels in methanol poisoning are greatest in vitreous humor.

❏❏ **What alcohol poisoning is suggested by a plasma bicarbonate level of zero (cipher, null, empty set, zip, Ø)?**

Methanol.

It also produces a large osmolar gap and large anion gap. Methanol poisoning is treated with IV ethanol and hemodialysis.

❏❏ **Positive birefringent calcium oxalate crystals are pathognomonic for poisoning with what substance?**

Ethylene glycol.
The lethal dose of ethylene glycol is 100 ml.

❏❏ **What are the signs and symptoms of ethylene glycol poisoning?**

Hallucinations, nystagmus, ataxia, papilledema, and a large anion gap.

❏❏ **How should ethylene glycol poisoning be treated?**

Gastric lavage, sodium bicarbonate, thiamine and pyridoxine, IV ethanol and hemodialysis.

❏❏ **What are the major lab findings in a patient with isopropanol poisoning?**

Elevated osmolal gap.
Acetonemia and acetonuria. Acetone.
Ø acidosis.

❏❏ **A patient presents to the ER with ataxia, altered mental status, and sixth nerve palsy. What is your diagnosis?**

Wernicke's encephalopathy.

❏❏ **What are the signs and symptoms of isopropanol poisoning?**

Sweet odor of breath (acetone), hypotension and hemorrhagic gastritis, CNS depression from isopropanol and from its metabolite, acetone.

❏❏ **What is the treatment of cocaine toxicity?**

Sedate with benzodiazepine.
Treat unresponsive hypertension with nitroprusside or phentolamine.
Return to text book to re-read discussion of <u>worsening</u> symptoms with ß-adrenergic antagonists.

❏❏ **Vertical nystagmus?**

<u>PCP</u>.
(O.K., there *are* some other causes...brainstem disease, vestibular disease.)

❏❏ **X-ray finding in a patient with salicylate toxicity:**

Noncardiogenic pulmonary edema.

❏❏ **Describe central nervous system affects of salicylate poisoning:**

Lethargy, confusion, seizures, and respiratory arrest.

❏❏ **Salicylate levels should ideally be checked how long after an ingestion?**

6 h.

❑❑ **What is the minimum likely toxic dose of salicylates?**

150 mg/kg.

❑❑ **Salicylate <u>level</u>, measured at 6 h after ingestion, greater than _____ is associated with toxicity.**

45 mg/dl.

❑❑ **ACEtaminophen <u>level</u>, measured 4 ACEs after ingestion, greater than _____ is associated with toxicity.**

150 µg/ml.

❑❑ **For what drugs will alkalinization of the urine increase excretion?**

CA's, salicylates, and long-acting barbiturates.
May be of some use to enhance lithium excretion.

❑❑ **What are the signs of salicylate poisoning?**

Hyperventilation, hyperthermia, mental status changes, nausea, vomiting, abdominal pain, dehydration, diaphoresis, ketonuria, metabolic acidosis, and respiratory alkalosis.

❑❑ **A child presents with lethargy, seizures, and hypoglycemia. A history of several days of preceding viral syndrome symptoms is elicited. Name two disorders that should be considered.**

Reye's syndrome and salicylate intoxication.

❑❑ **What laboratory test can aid in evaluation of a possible toxic iron ingestion?**

Total iron binding capacity measured 3 to 5 hours after ingestion.
If serum iron level is significantly less than the total iron binding capacity, a toxic iron ingestion is less likely.

❑❑ **What is the antidote for a toxic ingestion of iron?**

Deferoxamine chelates only free iron.

❑❑ **Deferoxamine should be given for a serum iron level greater than:**

350 µg/dl.

❑❑ **Deferoxamine should be given for what ratio of serum iron to total iron binding capacity?**

Give deferoxamine if serum iron is > total iron binding capacity.

❑❑ **How many hours after an iron ingestion should total iron binding capacity be measured. Feel the Force, Luke; we just did this.**

3-5 h.

❑❑ **What type of hydrocarbons are most toxic?**

"Oh no...not that reverse viscosity stuff!"

Kinematic viscosity (u), shear rates unrelated to apparent viscosity (∂) neglecting Fähraeus-Lindqvist effect.

O.K. - Thus, substances with <u>low</u> viscosities (measured in Saybolt Seconds Universal (SSU)) are <u>more</u> toxic than higher viscosity compounds. Your gasoline, kerosene and paint thinner (all aliphatic hydrocarbons with SSU's of < 60), are all more toxic than your motor oil, your tar and your petroleum jelly, which all have SSUs > 100.

Of the compounds with SSUs < 60, the most toxic are those that are not aliphatic, including your benzene, toluene, xylene and tetrachloroethylene.

❏❏ **What is the most reliable site for detecting central cyanosis?**

The tongue.

❏❏ **You are taking boards and are presented with a patient with a history of placement of an aortic graft or of abdominal aortic aneurysm. The patient has been vomiting up some coffee ground emesis. What infrequent entity needs to be considered?**

The dreaded aortoenteric fistula. These patients may present with a limited herald bleed before massive bleeding develops.
A CT showing air in the periaortic area is indicative of need for immediate surgery.

❏❏ **What is a common complication of pancuronium?**

Tachycardia from its vagolytic action.
Pancuronium tachycardia can give you an ulcer; that is Pantac can give you an ulcer!

❏❏ **What is the most common cause of hypermagnesemia in a patient with renal failure?**

Patient use of compounds high in magnesium, such as antacids.
This can result in neuromuscular paralysis.
Consider IV calcium.
Saline and furosemide assisted diuresis may not help this patient with renal failure, so consider dialysis.

❏❏ **How much energy should be used in cardioversion of an unstable infant with a wide complex tachycardia?**

0.5 to 1.0 J/kg.

❏❏ **How much energy should be used to cardiovert unstable VF in an infant?**

2 J/kg.

❏❏ **What is the most common malposition of the nasotracheal tube?**

Into the piriform sinus. The second most common malposition is the esophagus.

❏❏ **What is the <u>most</u> <u>common</u> physical sign of a PE?**

Tachypnea.

❏❏ **What are the three most common presenting signs of aortic stenosis?**

Syncope, angina, and heart failure.

❏❏ **When do CK levels first begin to rise and when do they peak in an MI?**

CK - MB earliest rise 6-8 h.
Peak 24-30 h.
Normalizes 48 h.

❏❏ **When does LDH first begin to rise and when does it peak in an MI?**

LDH-I (from heart) earliest rise 12 to 24 h.
Peak 48 to 96 h.

❑❑ **What is the effect of nitrates on preload and afterload?**

Nitrates mostly dilate veins and venules to decrease preload.

❑❑ **Inferior wall MIs commonly lead to what two types of heart block (via mechanism of damage to autonomic fibers in the atrial septum giving increased vagal tone impairing AV node conduction)?**

First degree AV block.
Mobitz Type I (Wenckebach) second-degree AV block.
Sinus bradycardia can also occur.

Progression to complete AV block is not common.

❑❑ **Anterior wall MIs may directly damage intracardiac conduction. This may lead to what type of arrhythmias?**

The dangerous type! Mobitz II second-degree AV block that can suddenly progress to complete AV block.

❑❑ **What are some of the potential, sometimes rare, complications of Mycoplasma pneumonia?**

Non-pulmonary: Hemolytic anemia, aseptic meningitis, encephalitis, Guillain-Barré syndrome, pericarditis, and myocarditis.

Pulmonary: ARDS, atelectasis, mediastinal adenopathy, pneumothorax, pleural effusion and abscess.

❑❑ **Under what conditions should Staphylococcal pneumonia be considered as a possible diagnosis?**

Although it only accounts for 1% of bacterial pneumonias, it should be considered in patients with sudden chills, hectic fever, pleurisy and cough, especially following a viral illness such as measles or influenza.

❑❑ **Of the following anesthetics, which has the shortest duration of action - lidocaine, procaine, bupivacaine or mepivacaine?**

Procaine.

❑❑ **Differential diagnosis of a ring lesion on CT scan:**

Toxoplasmosis, lymphoma, fungal infection, TB, CMV, Kaposi's, and hemorrhage.

❑❑ **Does erythema multiforme itch?**

Not typically. It may be tender.

❑❑ **A patient presents with granuloma inguinale. What does it look like?**

Papular, nodular or vesicular painless lesions. These can progress to extensive destruction of local tissues. Cause is Calymmatobacterium granulomatis.

❑❑ **What causes chancroid?**

Hemophilus ducreyi.
Painful necrotic ulcerative lesions and painful nodes.

❑❑ **Describe lesions associated with Chlamydia.**

Painless shallow ulcerations, papular or nodular lesions or herpetiform vesicles wax and wane.

❏❏ **What type of diarrhea causing disease may be transmitted by pets?**

Yersinia.

❏❏ **What state is associated with akinetic mutism?**

N. Dakota is a bucolic state.
Akinetic mutism is an abulic state (which is like a coma vigil). Patients seem awake and may have eyes open. They respond to questions very slowly.
The cause is typically due to depressed frontal lobe function.

❏❏ **What is normal blood pressure in a newborn?**

60 mmHg.

❏❏ **What is the initial drug of choice to treat SVT in a pediatric patient.**

Adenosine 0.1 mg/kg is drug of choice.
Digoxin 0.02 mg/kg may take ≈ 4 h for conversion.
Verapamil may be used in children > 2 years of age. It is contraindicated in younger children due to several deaths.
Synchronized cardioversion at 0.5-1.0 J/kg.

❏❏ <u>**After**</u> **the first mo of life, what is the number one cause of meningitis and of pneumonia in children?**

Most common cause of meningitis after the first mo of life is H. influenza.

Most common cause of pneumonia after the first mo of life is S. pneumoniae; H. influenza is the second most common cause.

For bacteremia in children greater than one mo, the <u>most</u> <u>common</u> causes are S. pneumoniae (70%) and H. influenza (20%) of the time.

❏❏ **Discuss infantile spasms.**

Onset is by 3 to 9 months of age, typically lasts seconds, and may occur in single episodes or bursts. The EEG is most often abnormal.
85% of these patients go on to be mentally handicapped.

❏❏ **Erythema multiforme can be associated with which anticonvulsants?**

Phenobarbital, phenytoin and carbamazepine.

❏❏ **Hepatic failure is commonly associated with what anticonvulsant?**

Valproic acid.

❏❏ **A patient presents with fever, neck pain and trismus. Exam reveals pharyngeal edema with tonsil displacement and edema of the *parotid* area. Diagnosis?**

PARAPHARYNGEAL abscess.

❏❏ **Does H. influenza typically cause abscesses?**

No.

❏❏ **What drugs, activities and cooking habits are associated with increasing clearance of theophylline (decreasing the theophylline level)?**

Phenytoin, phenobarbital, cigarette smoking and charcoal Bar-B-Queing.

❏❏ **Anaphylaxis is a common cause of what type of renal failure?**

Prerenal.

❏❏ **What are the end products of methanol, of ethylene glycol and of isopropyl alcohol metabolism?**

Methanol   - formate.
Ethylene glycol   - oxalate and formate.
Isopropyl alcohol   - acetone.

❏❏ **What type of alcohol ingestion is associated with hypocalcemia?**

Ethylene glycol.

❏❏ **What type of alcohol ingestion is associated with hemorrhagic pancreatitis?**

Methanol.

❏❏ **Arsenic produces an odor on the breath similar to what?**

Garlic.

❏❏ **When does ECM show up in Lyme disease?**

Stage I - 3 to 32 days after the bite.

❏❏ **For what disorder is vigorous digital massage of the orbit indicated?**

Central retinal artery occlusion.
DO NOT do this in central vein occlusion!

❏❏ **What pathogen is suggested by a pneumonia with a single rigor?**

Pneumococcus.

❏❏ **What pathogen does a strawberry cervix suggest?**

Trichomonas.

❏❏ **What are the key features of Ellis Type I, II, and III?**

Enamel, dentin, pulp.
Enamel, dentin, pulp. Pulp bleeds.

❏❏ **What is the vector and causative organism of Lyme disease?**

The vector is Ixodes dammini and the organism is Borrelia burgdorferi. It is the most frequently transmitted tick-borne disease.

❏❏ **Q fever cause:**

Coxiella burnetii, aka Rickettsia burnetii.
First found in Dermacentor andersonii tick.
Fever, headache, malaise, chest pain.

❏❏ **A hordeolum is:**

A Meibomian gland infection, usually of upper lid.

❏❏ **Ludwig's angina pathology:**

Hemolytic streptococci, staphylococcus, mixed aerobes and anaerobes.

❏❏ **The three most common locations of malignant melanoma:**

1) Skin.
2) Eye.
3) Anal canal.

❏❏ **What is the initial dose of blood to be given in children?**

10 ml/kg of packed RBCs.

❏❏ **What is achalasia?**

Disorder of esophageal motility and incomplete relaxation of the lower esophagus.

❏❏ **Suspected mesenteric ischemia may be virtually confirmed by what invasive exam other than laparotomy?**

Angiography.

❏❏ **Enterotoxin producing organisms that can cause food poisoning:**

Clostridium.
Staph aureus.
Vibrio cholerae.
E. coli.

❏❏ **Antibiotics should be avoided in what infectious diarrhea?**

Salmonella. Clear exceptions are in severe cases of diarrhea in immunocompromised patients and in children less than 6 months of age.

❏❏ **Anal fissures:**

Crohn's.

❏❏ **Diphtheria - growth medium:**

Loffler's medium or tellurite.
O.K.

❏❏ **Three disorders that are associated with decreased DTRs:**

Guillain-Barré.
Tic paralysis due to Dermacentor andersoni (Wood Tick) bite.
Diphtheria exotoxin.

❏❏ **What is the <u>most common</u> cause of bacterial pneumonia in children greater than 4 weeks of age?**

S. pneumoniae is the <u>most common</u>.
H. influenza is the second most common.

❏❏ **Likely cause of CHF in a premature infant?**

Premature infants = PDA.

❏❏ **Likely cause of CHF presenting in the first 3 d of life?**

First 3 d = transposition of the great vessels which will cause cyanosis and failure.

❏❏ **Likely cause of CHF presenting in the first week of life?**

First week = hypoplastic left ventricle.

❏❏ **Likely cause of CHF presenting in the second week of life?**

Second week = coarctation.

❏❏ **Do you treat Shigella with antibiotics?**

In general, yes.

❏❏ **What is a pinguecula?**

It is a yellowish nodule, particularly on the nasal aspect of the eye, but it may be lateral. Often caused by wind and dust.

❏❏ **What is a pterygium?**

It is a chronic growth over the medial or lateral aspect of the cornea approaching the pupil. It is much thicker than pingueculae.

❏❏ **What is the most common cause of painless upper GI bleeding in an infant or child?**

Varices from portal hypertension.

❏❏ **What is the most common cause of major painless lower GI bleeding in an infant or child?**

Meckel's diverticulum.

❏❏ **Common cause of orbital cellulitis:**

Staph aureus.

❏❏ **Who should receive prophylaxis after exposure to Neisseria meningitidis?**

People living with the patient or having close intimate contact.

❏❏ **Name some common hydrocarbons that are considered to be most toxic and have SSU's of less than 60.**

Aromatic hydrocarbons, halogenated hydrocarbons, mineral seal oil, kerosene, naphtha, turpentine, gasoline and lighter fluid.

Others considered less toxic have SSU's greater than 100, such as grease, diesel oil, mineral oil, petroleum jelly, paraffin wax, and tar.

❏❏ **What drug is absolutely contraindicated in the treatment of hydrocarbon poisoning?**

Epinephrine as it sensitizes the myocardium, potentially leading to arrest.

❏❏ **What drug is contraindicated in a glue sniffing patient?**

Epinephrine. Like solvent abusers, these patients may be scared to death.

❏❏ **What is a delayed complication of acid ingestion?**

Pyloric stricture.

❏❏ **What is the difference between carbamates and organophosphates?**

Carbamates produce similar symptoms as organophosphates, however, the bonds in carbamate toxicity are reversible.

❏❏ **What are key signs and symptoms of organophosphate poisoning?**

Ataxia, abdominal pain and cramping, blurred vision, seizures, ataxia and miosis.

❏❏ **A patient presents with miotic pupils, muscle fasciculations, diaphoresis and diffuse oral and bronchial secretions. The patient has an odor of garlic on his breath. What is your diagnosis?**

Organophosphate poisoning.

❏❏ **What ECG changes may be associated with organophosphate poisoning?**

Prolongation of the QT interval, and ST and T wave abnormalities.

❏❏ **What is the key laboratory finding in the diagnosis of organophosphate poisoning?**

Decreased red blood cell cholinesterase activity.
The serum cholinesterase level (pseudocholinesterase) is more sensitive but less specific. RBC cholinesterase is regenerated slowly and can take months to approach normal levels.

❏❏ **Treatment of organophosphate poisoning?**

Decontaminate, charcoal, atropine and pralidoxime prn.

❏❏ **What are the key features in the diagnosis of Trench foot?**

Exposure must be for one to two days of wet, cold temperatures above freezing.
Trench foot represents a superficial partial burn with no deep tissue damage.

❏❏ **What is chilblain?**

Chilblain is prolonged exposure to dry cold.

❏❏ **At about what core body temperature does shivering cease?**

30 to 32 °C.

❏❏ **What is the sequence of arrhythmia development in a patient with hypothermia?**

Bradycardia ' Atrial fibrillation ' Ventricular fibrillation ' Asystole.

❏❏ **What is the common pathogen in a cat bite?**

Pasteurella multocida.

❏❏ **What would you expect to find in the hippocampus of a patient with rabies?**

Negri bodies. Incubation for rabies is 30 to 60 days. Treatment includes cleaning of the wound, rabies immune globulin, and Human Diploid Cell Vaccine. Remember, 1/2 the rabies immune globulin goes around the wound and the other half goes IM.

❏❏ **How do you treat the bite of a megalopyge opercularis caterpillar?**

Calcium gluconate, 10 ml of a 10% solution IV.
Stings cause immediate rhythmic pain.

❏❏ What kind of tick transmits Rocky Mountain Spotted Fever?

The female andersoni tick. It transmits rickettsia rickettsii.

❏❏ What is the most common symptom in Rocky Mountain Spotted Fever?

Headache occurs in 90% of patients.

❏❏ Describe the rash of Rocky Mountain Spotted Fever.

It is a macular rash, 2 to 6 mm in diameter, and located on the wrists and palms, spreading to the soles and trunk.

❏❏ What tick transmits Lyme disease?

The Ixodes dammini tick.
Spirochete Borrelia burgdorferi is diagnosed by culture on Kelly's medium.

❏❏ Describe skin lesion seen in Lyme disease.

A large distinct circular skin lesion called erythema chronicum migrans. It is an annular erythematous lesion with central clearing.

❏❏ Describe a patient with tick paralysis.

Bulbar paralysis, ascending flaccid paralysis, paresthesias of hands and feet, symmetric loss of deep tendon reflexes and respiratory paralysis.

❏❏ What drug is contraindicated in a Gila monster bite?

Meperidine (Demerol).
(May be synergistic with venom!)

What is the causative organism of otitis externa?

Pseudomonas.

❏❏ Signs and symptoms of Lyme Disease, stages I-III:

I   Erythema Chronicum Migrans.
     Malaise, fatigue, headache, arthralgias, fever, chills.

II   Neurologic, cardiac.
     Headache, meningoencephalitis, facial nerve palsy, radiculoneuropathy, ophthalmitis and 1°, 2° and 3° AV blocks.

III Arthritis.
     Knee > shoulder > elbow > TMJ > ankle > wrist > hip >hands > feet.

❏❏ A diver levels off at 33 feet. How many atmospheres of pressure is he experiencing?

Two. Sea level is one, 33 feet is two, 66 feet is three, etc.

❏❏ After a diver surfaces, she immediately experiences aphasia, paralysis and blindness. Diagnosis?

Dysbaric air embolism.

❑❑ **After a blast injury, the most life threatening injury is likely to have occurred where?**

In the lungs.

❑❑ **Describe the wound resulting from AC .**

AC produces an entrance and exit wound of similar size.
The damage from AC is usually worse than that from DC.

❑❑ **Describe a DC wound.**

Small entrance wound, large exit wound.

❑❑ **What type of arrhythmia does lightning produce?**

It is a DC and produces asystole.

❑❑ **What type of arrhythmia does AC tend to produce?**

Ventricular fibrillation.

❑❑ **A patient, who works in a plant that makes chemical deodorizers presents after exposure to phenol. Possible field treatment?**

Clean the patient with olive oil and water.

❑❑ **What are the most common complaints in a patient with carbon monoxide poisoning?**

The most common is headache. Also dizziness, weakness, and nausea.

❑❑ **What signs and symptoms are expected after radiation exposures of 100 REM, 300 REM, 400 REM and 2000 REM, less than two hours post exposure?**

100 REM produces nausea and vomiting.
300 REM produces erythema.
400 REM produces diarrhea.
2000 REM produces seizures.

❑❑ **What drug blocks the uptake of radioactive iodine?**

Potassium iodine.

❑❑ **Psilocybin mushroom is associated with:**

Hallucinations.

❑❑ **With brain stem herniation, is decorticate or decerebrate posturing expected?**

Decerebrate posturing (hyperextension)
Decorticate posturing is flexion of the upper extremities and extension of the lower extremities.

❑❑ **A patient presents after experiencing trauma to the head. The patient has an elevated systolic blood pressure and bradycardia. Diagnosis?**

Cushing reflex.

❑❑ **What are the three components to the Glasgow coma scale, and how many points is each worth?**

Eye opening (4).

Verbal response (5).
Motor response (6).

❑❑ **What is the name for a flexion mechanism fracture through the anterior aspect of a vertebral body that is associated with ligamentous damage and an anterior cord syndrome?**

A teardrop fracture.

❑❑ **Describe the corneal reflex.**

Conducted by the ophthalmic branch of the 5th nerve and the afferent branch of the facial (7th) nerve.

❑❑ **What is the most unstable cervical spine injury?**

Rupture of transverse atlantal ligament > dens fracture > burst fracture (flexion teardrop) > bilateral facet dislocation.

❑❑ **What is the eponym for a C1 burst fracture from vertical compression?**

Jefferson fracture.

❑❑ **A patient in a motor vehicle accident sustains a hyperextension injury of the neck. Plain films reveal a C2 bilateral facet fracture through the pedicles. You describe this fracture in consultation with the neurosurgeon. What type of fracture have you described?**

A Hangman's fracture.

❑❑ **A patient has an avulsion fracture of the spinous process of C7 with a history of a hyperflexion mechanism. Diagnosis?**

Clay shoveller's fracture - fracture involving the spinous process of C6, C7, or T1. The mechanism is usually flexion or a direct blow.

❑❑ **A patient suffers a bilateral interfacetal dislocation. What is your concern?**

Injury occurs as a result of flexion and is very unstable with ligament disruption.

❑❑ **What is the most unstable <u>fracture</u> of the cervical spine?**

A dens fracture with rupture of the atlantal ligament.

❑❑ **Stable or unstable: a Clay shoveller's fracture?**

Stable.

❑❑ **Stable or unstable: fracture of the posterior arch of C1?**

Stable.

❑❑ **Name the four stable cervical spine fractures.**

Simple wedge.
Clay shovelers.
Pillar.
C1 posterior neural arch.
The rest are unstable or potentially unstable!

❑❑ **A patient presents with a history of a blow to the forehead. Her neck was hyperextended. Patient complains of weakness in the arms with minimal weakness in the lower extremities. Diagnosis?**

Central cord syndrome.

❑❑ **You see a patient with an obvious traumatic spinal cord lesion. On physical exam, he has motor paralysis, loss of gross proprioception and loss of vibratory sensation on one side, and loss of pain and temperature sensation on the opposite side. Diagnosis?**

Brown-Séquard's syndrome.

❑❑ **What is the most common cause of shock in patients with blunt chest trauma?**

Pelvic (or extremity) fracture.

❑❑ **What is a frequent complication of ethmoid sinusitis?**

Orbital cellulitis.

❑❑ **What is the most common site of aspiration pneumonitis?**

Right lower lobe.

❑❑ **What is the most common ECG finding associated with a myocardial contusion?**

ST-T wave abnormalities.

❑❑ **What is the <u>most</u> <u>common</u> valvular injury associated with blunt cardiac injury?**

A ruptured aortic valve.

❑❑ **What is the most common site of a traumatic aortic laceration?**

The vast majority occur just distal to the left subclavian artery.

❑❑ **What is the most common x-ray finding in traumatic rupture of the aorta?**

Widening of the superior mediastinum.

❑❑ **What is the most accurate x-ray finding in traumatic rupture of the aorta?**

Rightward deviation of the esophagus more than 1 - 2 cm.

❑❑ **A patient presents with a history of high speed traumatic injury to the chest. On physical exam, a systolic murmur over the precordium is auscultated The patient has a slightly hoarse voice. The nurse tells you the pulse is also stronger in the upper extremities. Diagnosis?**

Traumatic rupture of the aorta.

❑❑ **A patient presents with a history of chest trauma, a systolic murmur and an infarct pattern on ECG. Diagnosis?**

Traumatic ventricular septal defect.

❑❑ **A person with a history of a motor vehicle accident has x-ray findings of retroperitoneal air seen on a flat plate of the abdomen. What is a likely diagnosis?**

Duodenal injury. Tentative test is a contrast study. Extravasation confirms a duodenal injury.

❑❑ **On an x-ray of the hand, the AP view shows a triangular shaped lunate. Diagnosis?**

Lunate dislocation.
Lateral films will show a cup spilling out water.

❏❏ **What x-ray view is required to diagnose a perilunate dislocation?**

Lateral view.

❏❏ **A patient presents describing a snapping sensation in the wrist and a click. Diagnosis:**

Scaphoid dislocation.

❏❏ **X-ray of the hand reveals a 3 mm space between the scaphoid and the lunate. Diagnosis?**

Scaphoid dislocation.

❏❏ **In a boxer's fracture, how much angulation of the 5th metacarpal neck is acceptable.**

50 degrees.

❏❏ **What ligament in the hand is commonly injured in a fall while skiing?**

Thumb MCP joint ulnar collateral ligament rupture (Gamekeeper's thumb).

❏❏ **Posterior dislocation of the shoulder is often missed with a standard radiographic shoulder series. What x-ray view aids in diagnosis?**

The scapular "Y" view.

❏❏ **Name the four muscles of the rotator cuff.**

Supraspinatus, infraspinatus, teres minor and the subscapularis. Patients with a rotator cuff tear will not be able to fully abduct or to internally or externally rotate the arm normally.

❏❏ **What is the usual mechanism of injury in a supracondylar fracture?**

A fall on the outstretched arm.

❏❏ **What artery is commonly injured with a supracondylar fracture?**

Brachial artery.

❏❏ **What nerve is commonly injured with a supracondylar fracture?**

Injury to the anterior interosseous nerve, which is a branch of the median nerve.

❏❏ **Elbow X-ray. Posterior fat pad sign! Diagnosis?**

Occult fracture such as a supracondylar fracture of the humerus. Posterior fat pad seen on a lateral radiograph of the flexed elbow is usually due to hemarthrosis caused by a fracture.

❏❏ **What nerve injury is associated with a medial epicondyle fracture?**

Ulnar nerve.

❏❏ **About how many liters of blood can a patient lose in the retroperitoneal space?**

About 6 liters.

❏❏ **Which type of pelvic fracture has the greatest amount of bleeding?**

Vertical sheer.

❑❑ **A patient presents to the emergency department with a history of a limp. Physical exam reveals pain with extension and abduction of the hip. Diagnosis?**

Greater trochanteric fracture, the result of an avulsion at the insertion site of the gluteus medius.

❑❑ **A patient presents with a history of hearing an audible pop in the knee and ankle as he fell. Diagnosis?**

Tear of the anterior cruciate and Achilles tendon rupture.

❑❑ **What nerve may be injured with a knee dislocation?**

The peroneal nerve.

❑❑ **What is the most common site of a stress fracture in the foot?**

Second and third metatarsal.

❑❑ **What is the most frequent cause of superior vena cava obstruction?**

Bronchogenic carcinoma.

❑❑ **What is the most common level of malignant spinal cord compression?**

Thoracic.

❑❑ **What is the most common site of bursitis?**

Olecranon.

❑❑ **What is the most common cause of subarachnoid hemorrhage in teenagers?**

AV malformations.

❑❑ **A patient presents with a painful, red eye and a decrease in visual acuity. What is the differential?**

Central corneal lesions, glaucoma, and iritis.

❑❑ **What is the most common symptom of acute mesenteric ischemia?**

Abdominal pain.

❑❑ **Where does pulmonary embolism rank in terms of lethality in the United States?**

It is the third most common cause of death in the United States.
About 650,000 cases occur annually with overall mortality of 8%.

❑❑ **What are the most common findings of osteomyelitis on x-ray?**

Periosteal elevation and demineralization.

❑❑ **For what conditions is hydralazine commonly used?**

Treatment of preeclampsia and eclampsia.

❑❑ **What is the most common cause of acute aortic regurgitation?**

Infectious endocarditis.

❑❑ **What is the most common congenital valvular disease?**

Bicuspid aortic valve.

❑❑ **What infarct is most commonly associated with acute mitral regurgitation?**

Inferior wall.

❑❑ **What metabolic abnormality is commonly associated with hypercalcemia?**

Up to 1/3 will have hypokalemia.

❑❑ **What form of hepatitis is most commonly transmitted through blood transfusions?**

Hepatitis C.

❑❑ **On funduscopic exam, microaneurysms and soft exudates are typical of:**

Hypertension.

❑❑ **On funduscopic exam, macular microaneurysms and hard exudates are typical of:**

Diabetes.

❑❑ **In a patient with retrobulbar optic neuritis, what is the most likely cause?**

Multiple sclerosis.

❑❑ **How is pancuronium reversed?**

Atropine and neostigmine.

❑❑ **What are the initial symptoms of a patient with hypocalcemia?**

Paresthesias around the mouth and fingertips, irritability, hyperactive deep tendon reflexes and seizures.

❑❑ **What ECG change is associated with hypocalcemia?**

Prolonged T waves.

❑❑ **A patient is digitalis toxic. What electrolytes will need to be replaced?**

It is important to replace potassium and magnesium.

❑❑ **What is the most common complication of verapamil and how should it be treated?**

Hypotension, treated with calcium gluconate IV over several minutes, glucagon can follow.

❑❑ **Third degree heart block is often seen in what type of myocardial infarction?**

Acute anterior wall myocardial infarction.

❑❑ **What is the most common arrhythmia associated with Wolff-Parkinson-White syndrome?**

PAT. The patient presents with angina, syncope, and shortness of breath.

❑❑ **How may mydriasis caused by mydriatics and anticholinergic drugs be distinguished from those caused third cranial nerve compression?**

Pilocarpine. Pilocarpine will reverse cranial nerve compression but will have no effect on anticholinergic drugs or mydriatics.

❏❏ **During CPR, the mean cardiac index is what percentage of normal?**

25%.

❏❏ **Outline treatment of atrial flutter.**

Cardioversion 25 to 50 joules, verapamil, digoxin, propranolol, procainamide, and quinidine.

❏❏ **How should atrial fibrillation be treated?**

Procainamide, digoxin, verapamil, and propranolol.
Cardioversion with 100 to 200 joules.

❏❏ **Why is verapamil a bad choice to treat ventricular tachycardia?**

Verapamil could increase heart rate and decrease blood pressure, without converting the rhythm.

❏❏ **What drugs should never be used in atrial fibrillation with Wolff-Parkinson-White?**

Digitalis, verapamil, and phenytoin.
Atrial fibrillation with Wolff-Parkinson-White should be treated with cardioversion or procainamide.

SVT with Wolff-Parkinson-White should be treated with verapamil or adenosine.

❏❏ **What does VVI mean?**

Ventricular pace, ventricular sense, and inhibited.

❏❏ **What complications can result from excessive lidocaine administration?**

Seizures and methemoglobinemia.

❏❏ **Name the drug of choice for Wolff-Parkinson-White with atrial flutter or fibrillation?**

Procainamide.

❏❏ **What makes the first heart sound?**

Closure of the mitral valve and left ventricular contraction.

❏❏ **What makes the second heart sound?**

Closure of the pulmonary and aortic valves.

❏❏ **What is the cause of the third heart sound.**

This is caused by the deceleration of blood flowing into the ventricle when the ventricle reaches its final stages of filling.

❏❏ **What is the cause of the fourth heart sound?**

It is caused by vibrations of the left ventricular muscle, the mitral valve and the left ventricular flow tract.

❏❏ **What is a common pathologic cause of an S_3?**

Congestive heart failure.

❑❑ **What is the pathologic cause of an S$_4$?**

Often decreased left ventricular compliance due to acute ischemia.
Other causes include: aortic stenosis, subaortic stenosis, HTN, coronary artery disease, myocardiopathy, anemia and hyperthyroidism.

❑❑ **What is the chief effect of dopamine and what is the chief complication of dopamine?**

The chief effect is prompt elevation of blood pressure with ß-adrenergic effects at low doses and α-adrenergic effects at high doses.
The primary complication is tachycardia which unfortunately, increases myocardial oxygen demand.

❑❑ **What is the chief effect of dobutamine?**

Dobutamine increases the cardiac contractility. It has only minor effects on peripheral α-receptors.
It can increase cardiac output without increasing blood pressure.

❑❑ **What effect does morphine have on preload and afterload?**

Morphine decreases both preload and afterload.

❑❑ **Does furosemide affect preload or afterload?**

Furosemide decreases preload.

❑❑ **What is the most common cause of post splenectomy sepsis?**

Streptococcus pneumonia.

❑❑ **What laboratory findings are expected in a child with pyloric stenosis?**

Hypokalemia, hypochloremia, and metabolic alkalosis.

❑❑ **What is the most common cause of tricuspid regurgitation?**

Right heart failure secondary to left heart failure, typically caused by mitral stenosis.

❑❑ **What drug is preferred to treat hypertension in a patient with renal failure?**

Labetalol (metabolized in the liver).

❑❑ **Treatment for a propranolol overdose?**

Glucagon.

❑❑ **Preferred treatment for a patient with hypertensive encephalopathy?**

Nitroprusside and labetalol.

❑❑ **What are the x-ray findings in ischemic bowel disease?**

"Thumb" printing on the plain film and a ground glass appearance with absence of bowel gas.

❑❑ **A patient with currant jelly sputum is likely to have what type of pneumonia?**

Klebsiella or type 3 Pneumococcus.

❑❑ **What two diseases does the deer tick, Ixodes dammini, transmit?**

Lyme disease and Babesia.

❏❏ **How do patients present with Babesia infection?**

Intermittent fever, splenomegaly, jaundice, and hemolysis. The disease may be fatal in patients without spleens. The disease can simulate rickettsial diseases like Rocky Mountain spotted fever. Treatment is with clindamycin and quinine.

❏❏ **Time for a food question! There are 9 questions in this book that deal with either strawberry tongue, strawberry cervix, currant jelly sputum or currant jelly stool. Describe the pathology associated with each of these.**

Strawberry tongue - Scarlet fever, Kawasaki's disease.
Strawberry cervix - Trichomonas.
Currant jelly sputum - Klebsiella, less commonly type 3 Pneumococcus.
Currant jelly stool - Intussusception.

❏❏ **What is the most frequently transmitted tick-borne disease?**

Lyme disease.
Causative agent - spirochete Borrelia burgdorferi.
Vector - Ixodes dammini (deer tick) also I. pacificus, Amblyomma americanum, and Dermacentor variabilis.

❏❏ **What is the <u>second</u> <u>most</u> <u>common</u> tick borne disease?**

Rocky Mountain spotted fever.
Causative agent - Rickettsia rickettsii.
Vector - Female Ixodid ticks Dermacentor andersoni (wood tick) and D. variabilis (American dog tick).

❏❏ **If you melt enough dry ice, can you swim without getting wet?**

Probably not!

BIBLIOGRAPHY

BOOKS/ARTICLES:

Adler, J.N. & Plantz, S.H. Emergency Medicine Pearls of Wisdom (3rd. Ed.). Watertown: Mt. Auburn Press, 1994.

Adler, J.N. & Plantz, S.H. Emergency Medicine Pearls of Wisdom (1st Ed.). 1993.

Advanced Cardiac Life Support. Dallas: American Heart Association, 1992.

Advanced Trauma Life Support. Chicago: American College of Surgeons, 1990.

Anderson, J.E. Grant's Atlas of Anatomy (8th Ed.). Baltimore: Williams & Wilkins, 1983.

Auerbach, P.S. Management of Wilderness and Environmental Emergencies (2nd Ed.). St. Louis: C.V. Mosby Company, 1989.

Bakerman, S. A B C'S of Interpretive Laboratory Data (2nd Ed.). Greenville: Interpretive Laboratory Data, Inc., 1984.

Barkin, R.M. Emergency Pediatrics (3rd Ed.). St. Louis: C.V. Mosby Company, 1990.

Berkow, R. The Merck Manual (15th Ed.). Rahway: Merck Sharp & Dohme Research Laboratories, 1987.

Bork, K. Diagnosis and Treatment of Common Skin Diseases. Philadelphia: W.B. Saunders Company, 1988.

Bryson, P.D. Comprehensive Review in Toxicology (2nd Ed.) Aspen Publishers, Inc., 1989

Dambro, M.R. Griffith's 5 Minute Clinical Consult. Williams and Wilkins, 1996.

DeGowin, E.L. Bedside Diagnostic Examination (4th Ed.). New York: Macmillan Publishing Co. Inc., 1981.

Diagnostic and Treatment Guidelines on Domestic Violence, AMA Publication.

Diagnostic and Treatment Guidelines on Sexual Assault, AMA Publication.

Firearm Violence: Community Diagnosis and Treatment, Publication and slide show of Physicians for Social Responsibility

Fitzpatrick, T.B. Color Atlas and Synopsis of Clinical Dermatology. New York: McGraw-Hill Publishing Company, 1990.

Harris, J.H. The Radiology of Emergency Medicine (2nd Ed.). Baltimore: Williams and Wilkins, 1981.

Harrison, T.R. Principles of Internal Medicine (11th Ed.). New York: McGraw-Hill Book Company, 1987.

Harwood-Nuss, A. The Clinical Practice of Emergency Medicine. Philadelphia: J.B. Lippincott Company, 2nd. Ed, 1996.

Harwood-Nuss, A. The Clinical Practice of Emergency Medicine. Philadelphia: J.B. Lippincott Company, 1991.

Hoppenfeld, S. Physical Examination of the Spine and Extremities. Norwalk: Appleton-Century-Crofts, 1976.

Leaverton, P.E. A Review of Biostatistics (3rd Ed.). Boston: Little Brown and Company, 1986.

Marriott, H.J.L. Practical Electrocardiography (7th Ed.). Baltimore: Williams and Wilkins, 1983.

Moore, K.L. Clinically Oriented Anatomy. Baltimore: Williams & Wilkins, 1982.

Perkins, E.S. An Atlas of Diseases of the Eye (3rd Ed.). London: Churchill Livingstone, 1986.

Physicians' Desk Reference (50th Ed.). Oradell: Medical Economics Company Inc., 1996.

Plantz, SH. Emergency Medicine PreTest, Self-Assessment and Review, McGraw- Hill, 1990.

Plantz, S.H. & Adler, J.N. Emergency Medicine Pearls of Wisdom, Second Edition. Watertown: Mount Auburn Press, 1993.

Rivers, C.S. Preparing for the Written Board Exam in Emergency Medicine. Milford: Emergency Medicine Educational Enterprises, Inc. 1992.

Robbins, S.L. Pathologic Basis of Disease (3rd Ed.). Philadelphia: W.B. Saunders Company, 1984.

Rosen, P. Emergency Medicine Concepts and Clinical Practice (3rd Ed.). St. Louis: Mosby Year Book, 1992.

Rowe, R.C. The Harriet Lane Handbook (11th Ed.). Chicago: Year Book Medical Publishers, Inc., 1987.

Simon, R.R. Emergency Orthopedics The Extremities (2nd Ed.). Norwalk: Appleton & Lange, 1987.

Simon, R.R. Emergency Procedures and Techniques (2nd Ed.). Baltimore: Williams and Wilkins, 1987.

Slaby, F. Radiographic Anatomy. New York: John Wiley & Sons, 1990.

Squire, L.F. Fundamentals of Radiology (3rd Ed.). Cambridge: Harvard University Press, 1982.

Stedman, T.L. Illustrated Stedman's Medical Dictionary (24th Ed.). Baltimore: Williams & Wilkins, 1982.

Stewart, C.E. Environmental Emergencies. Baltimore: Williams and Wilkins, 1990.

Textbook of Pediatric Advanced Life Support. Dallas: American Heart Association, 1988.

The Hand Examination and Diagnosis (2nd Ed.). London: Churchill Livingstone, 1983.

The Hand Primary Care of Common Problems (2nd Ed.). London: Churchill Livingstone, 1990.

The Physician's Guide to Domestic Violence, Salber and Taliaferro, Volcano Press, 1995

Tintinalli, J.E. Emergency Medicine A Comprehensive Study Guide (4th Ed.). New York: McGraw-Hill, Inc., 1996.

Tintinalli, J.E. Emergency Medicine A Comprehensive Study Guide (3rd Ed.). New York: McGraw-Hill, Inc., 1992.

Tsang T, Demby AM. Penile fracture with urethral injury. The Journal of Urology, 1992;147:466-468.

Weinberg, S. Color Atlas of Pediatric Dermatology (2nd Ed.). New York: McGraw-Hill, 1990.

Weiner, H.L. Neurology for the House Officer (4th Ed.). Baltimore: Williams & Wilkins, 1989.

Wilkins, E. W. Emergency Medicine (3rd Ed.). Baltimore: Williams & Wilkins, 1989.

COURSES/CONFERENCES:

Eye Emergencies, Chicago, IL 1991.

ENT Emergencies, Chicago, IL 1991.

CRIT Course, Springfield, MA 1992.

Emergency Medicine Board Review, Chicago, IL 1991.

Emergency Medicine Specialty Review, Chicago, IL 1991.

Emergency Medicine Interactive Review, Boca Raton, FL 1992.

Emergency Medicine Board Review, Columbus, OH 1992.

EMS: A Trauma Update. Sponsored by Boston Medflight, Plymouth, MA 1994.

Selected Topics in Emergency Medicine. Sponsored by MGH and Brigham and Women's Hospitals and Harvard Medical School, Boston, MA 1995 and 1996.

Emergency Medicine: Update and Current Practice. Sponsored by MGH ED and Harvard Medical School, Boston, MA 1994, 1995, 1996.

Update on New Techniques and Review of Established Principles of Management of Cerebrovascular Emergencies. Sponsored by MGH Brain Aneurysm/AVM Center, Neurointensive Care Unit and ED, Boston, MA 1996.

SAEM Annual Scientific Assembly, Denver, CO 1996; Washington, D.C. 1995.

American Academy of Emergency Medicine, Scientific Assembly 1995 (Philadelphia, PA), 1996 (Las Vegas, NV).

American Academy of Emergency Medicine, Emergency Medicine Written Board Review Course, Las Vegas, NV 1996.